Jørgen Nordling • Jean-Jacques Wyndaele
Joop P. van de Merwe • Pierre Bouchelouche
Mauro Cervigni • Magnus Fall
Editors

Bladder Pain Syndrome

A Guide for Clinicians

Springer

Editors
Jørgen Nordling
Department of Urology
Herlev Hospital
University of Copenhagen
Herlev, Denmark

Joop P. van de Merwe
Departments of Immunology and Internal Medicine
Erasmus MC, University Medical Center Rotterdam
Rotterdam, The Netherlands

Mauro Cervigni
Department of Urogynecology S. Carlo-IDI
Department Obstetrics and Gynecology
Catholic University
Rome, Italy

Jean-Jacques Wyndaele
Department of Urology
University Hospital Antwerp and Antwerp University
Edegem, Belgium

Pierre Bouchelouche
Department of Clinical Biochemistry
Koege Hospital
University of Copenhagen
Copenhagen, Denmark

Magnus Fall
Department of Urology
Institute of Clinical Sciences
Sahlgrens Academy at University of Gothenburg
Göteborg, Sweden

ISBN 978-1-4899-9617-6 ISBN 978-1-4419-6929-3 (eBook)
DOI 10.1007/978-1-4419-6929-3
Springer New York Heidelberg Dordrecht London

Printed on acid-free paper

Springer is part of Springer Science+Business Media (www.springer.com)

Preface

In 2007 ESSIC (International society for the study of Bladder Pain Syndrome) proposed not more to use the name Interstitial Cystitis (IC) and replace the name with Bladder Pain Syndrome (BPS) [1]. The reason was that no uniform definition existed of IC and the problems arising from the lack of generally approved diagnostic criteria caused enormous problems both clinically and in research. To change a name of a disease is not something you do without careful consideration. It may have severe implications for patients, and their organizations with their aim at IC, and also for insurance and reimbursement practices in different health systems around the world.

When A.J.C. Skene in 1887 introduced the name Interstitial Cystitis (IC) he referred to an inflammatory disease: "When the disease has destroyed the mucus membrane partly or wholly and extended to the muscular parietes, we have what is known as interstitial cystitis…". [2]. After the introduction of cystoscopes around the beginning of the last century, it was found that the disease had some specific cystoscopic features. These were first described by G.L. Hunner in female patients with severe frequency and pain, appearing as focal red bleeding areas, and he named them elusive ulcers [3, 4]. However, these inflammatory infiltrates are not ulcers, but rather focal inflammatory lesions with a central fragility resulting in a provoked crack or deep wound when the bladder is distended [5]. So in the beginning of the nineteenth century IC was a well-defined disease with microscopic and cystoscopic findings of characteristic inflammatory lesions in the bladder wall, mostly in female patients with severe frequency and bladder pain.

But in 1949 J.R. Hand described "small discrete submucosal hemorrhages, showing variations in form … dot-like bleeding points … little or no restriction to bladder capacity" and he claimed these "glomerulations" as a typical cystoscopic finding in IC [6]. Subsequently, IC became a real elusive disease with a total lack of a proper definition and proper diagnostic tools. E. Messing and T. Stamey underlined this in their paper from 1978 where they described IC as a diagnosis of exclusion in patients with the characteristic symptoms and glomerulations under anesthesia [7]. Unintentionally, the confusion became even greater after the introduction of the initial NIDDK criteria in 1988 [8] and the final NIDDK criteria in 1990 [9].

The NIDDK criteria were not meant as diagnostic, but rather as a means to select comparable patient populations for clinical trials. Nevertheless, these criteria became a worldwide standard for the diagnosis of IC. But the NIDDK criteria included two symptoms: Pain *or* urgency, and two cystoscopic findings: Hunner lesion *or* glomerulations. Urgency has later become the cardinal symptom of Overactive Bladder Syndrome (OAB) and the dispute concerning what exact nature or kind of urgency is characteristic for OAB and what kind for IC [10] is still running.

The problem of definitions was first considered in a terminology report of the International Continence Society in 2002 [11]. The following year, during the first International Conference on IC in Japan in 2003, the worldwide confusion concerning IC became evident [12]. Major differences in the concept of IC were brought to light. Some regarded IC as a frequency-urgency syndrome with or without pelvic pain. Some regarded IC as a cystoscopically defined disease and many did not really know what they should mean. As a consequence of this confusion ESSIC was founded in 2004. Annual meetings and busy Internet discussions in the following years resulted in the 2008 proposal to use the term bladder pain syndrome as the overall denomination, to include all patients with bladder pain within the definition, since interstitial cystitis rather describes a special phenotype with deep inflammation of the bladder wall.

The editors of this book have therefore tried to replace the name interstitial cystitis (IC) with bladder pain syndrome (BPS) throughout the book. The name IC is, however, maintained if the text refers to obvious historical data based on the concept of IC at that time, e.g., in the chapter on epidemiology.

The process of going from IC to BPS has brought major changes in our concepts and knowledge of this disease and we are therefore very happy getting the opportunity to gather all these new data and ideas in the present book.

Herlev, Denmark — Jørgen Nordling
Edegem, Belgium — Jean-Jacques Wyndaele
Rotterdam, The Netherlands — Joop van de Merwe
Copenhagen, Denmark — Pierre Bouchelouche
Rome, Italy — Mauro Cervigni
Göteborg, Sweden — Magnus Fall

References

1. van de Merwe JP, Nordling J, Bouchelouche P, Bouchelouche K, Cervigni M, Daha LK, et al. Diagnostic criteria, classification, and nomenclature for painful bladder syndrome/interstitial cystitis: an ESSIC proposal. Eur Urol. 2008;53(1):60–7.
2. Skene AJC. Diseases of the bladder and urethra in women. New York: William Wood; 1887.
3. Hunner GL. A rare type of bladder ulcer in women; report of cases. Boston Med Surg J. 1915;172:660–4.
4. Hunner GL. A rare type of bladder ulcer. Further notes, with a report of eighteen cases. JAMA 70(4), 203–12.

5. Nordling J, Fall M, Hanno P. Global concepts of bladder pain syndrome (interstitial cystitis). World J Urol. 2012;30(4):457–64.
6. Hand JR. Interstitial cystitis: report of 223 cases (204 women and 19 men). J Urol. 1949;61:291–310.
7. Messing EM, Stamey TA. Interstitial cystitis: early diagnosis, pathology, and treatment. Urology. 1978;12(4):381–92.
8. Gillenwater JY, Wein AJ. Summary of the National Institute of Arthritis, Diabetes, Digestive and Kidney Diseases Workshop on Interstitial Cystitis, National Institutes of Health, Bethesda, Maryland, August 28–29, 1987. J Urol 1988;140(1):203–6.
9. Interstitial Cystitis. London: Springer Verlag; 1990.
10. Abrams P, Hanno P, Wein A. Overactive bladder and painful bladder syndrome: there need not be confusion. Neurourol Urodyn 2005;24(2):149–50.
11. Abrams P., Cardozo L., Fall M., Griffiths, D., Rosier, P., Ulmsten, U., van Kerrebroeck, P., Victor, A., Wein, A. The standardisation of terminology in lower urinary tract function. Report from the Standardisation sub-committee of the International Continence Society. Neurourol Urodyn. 2002;21:167–78.
12. Ueda T. The legendary beginning of the International Consultation on Interstitial Cystitis. Int J Urol. 2003;10 Suppl:S1–S2.

Contents

Contributors

Maria Avolio Institute of Public Health and Preventive Medicine, National Observatory in Health in the Italian Regions, Catholic University "Sacro Cuore", Rome, Italy

Z. Chad Baxter, MD Urology, Center for Pelvic Health and Reconstructive Surgery, Smith Institute for Urology, North Shore—LIJ School of Medicine, New Hyde Park, NY, USA

Kirsten Bouchelouche, MD, DMSc Smooth Muscle Research Center, Department of Clinical Biochemistry, Koege Hospital, University of Copenhagen, Copenhagen, Denmark

Pierre Bouchelouche, MD Smooth Muscle Research Center, Department of Clinical Biochemistry, Koege Hospital, University of Copenhagen, Copenhagen, Denmark

Mauro Cervigni, MD Department of Urogynecology, S. Carlo-IDI, Rome, Italy

Department Obstetrics and Gynecology, Catholic University, Rome, Italy

Mahindra Chincholkar, MD, FRCA, FFPMRCA Department of Pain Management, Salford Royal Hospital, Salford, UK

Dominique El-Khawand, MD Division of Female Pelvic Medicine and Reconstructive Surgery, Department of Obstetrics and Gynecology, Drexel University College of Medicine, Philadelphia, PA, USA

Magnus Fall, MD, PhD Department of Urology, Institute of Clinical Sciences, Sahlgrens Academy at University of Gothenburg, Göteborg, Sweden

Jennifer Yonaitis Fariello, MSN, CRNP Urology Division, Department of Obstetrics and Gynecology, FPMRS, The Pelvic and Sexual Health Institute, Drexel University College of Medicine, Philadelphia, PA, USA

Justin I. Friedlander, MD The Arthur Smith Institute for Urology, North Shore-Long Island Jewish Health System, New Hyde Park, NY, USA

Philip M. Hanno, MD, MPH Division of Urology, Department of Surgery, Hospital of the University of Pennsylvania, Philadelphia, PA, USA

Amy Rejba Hoffmann, MSN The Pelvic and Sexual Health Institute, Philadelphia, PA, USA

John Hughes, MBBS, FRCA, FFPMRCA Pain Management Unit, The James Cook University Hospital, Middlesbrough, UK

Paul P. Irwin, MCh, FRCSI(Urol) Michael Heal Department of Urology, Mid Cheshire Hospitals NHS Trust, Leighton Hospital, Crewe, Cheshire, UK

Christina Kåbjörn-Gustafsson Department of Pathology, Sahlgrenska University Hospital, Gothenburg, Sweden

Mikael Leppilahti, MD, PhD Seinäjoki Central Hospital, Seinäjoki, Finland

Helen R. Levey, DO, MPH The Arthur Smith Institute for Urology, North Shore–Long Island Jewish Health System, New Hyde Park, NY, USA

Silvia Malaguti, MD Clinical Neurophysiology, Clinical Neurophysiology and Biomechanics of Pelvic Floor Dysfunctions, Milan, Italy

Jane M. Meijlink, BA Hons International Painful Bladder Foundation (IPBF), Rotterdam, The Netherlands

Salma Mohammed, MBBS, FRCA Pain Management Unit, Anaesthesia, Intensive Care & Pain Medicine, The James Cook University Hospital, Middlesbrough, UK

Robert M. Moldwin, MD Urology Division, The Arthur Smith Institute for Urology, North Shore-Long Island Jewish Health System, New Hyde Park, NY, USA

Urology Department, The Hofstra University School of Medicine, New Hyde Park, NY, USA

Simone Montagnoli Social Health Division, Dynamic and Clinical Psychology, Research Department, Institute of Social Affairs, Rome, Italy

Loredana Nasta Italian Interstitial Cystitis Association, Rome, Italy

Franca Natale, MD Department of Urogynecology, S. Carlo-IDI Hospital, Rome, Italy

J. Curtis Nickel, MD, FRCSC Urology Department, Kingston General Hospital, Queen's University, Kingston, ON, Canada

Jørgen Nordling, MD, Dr.med.Sci., FEBU Department of Urology, Herlev Hospital, University of Copenhagen, Herlev, Denmark

Paulo Dinis Oliveria, MD, PhD Department of Urology, Hospital de São João, Porto, Portugal

Ralph Peeker Department of Urology, Sahlgrenska University Hospital, Gothenburg, Sweden

Claus Riedl, MD Urology Department, Landesklinikum Thermenregion Baden, Baden, Austria

Mirja Ruutu, MD, PhD, FEBU Department of Urology, Helsinki University Central Hospital, Helsinki, Finland

Jukka Sairanen, MD, PhD Department of Urology, Helsinki University Central Hospital, Helsinki, Finland

Hina M. Sheth, MS, PT, OCS, MTC Rebalance Physical Therapy, Philadelphia, PA, USA

Barbara Shorter, RD, CDN Didactic Program in Dietetics, Department of Nutrition, Long Island University, Brookville, NY, USA

Gianfranco Tajana, MD Department of Pharmaceutical and Biomedical Sciences (FARMABIOMED), University of Salerno, Salerno, Italy

Dean A. Tripp, PhD Departments of Psychology, Anesthesia & Urology, Queen's University, Kingston, ON, Canada

Arndt van Ophoven, MD, PhD Division of Neuro-Urology, Marienhospital Herne, University Hospital of Bochum, Herne, Germany

Joop P. van de Merwe, MD, PhD Departments of Immunology and Internal Medicine, Erasmus MC, University Medical Center Rotterdam, Rotterdam, The Netherlands

John W. Warren, MD Medicine and Epidemiology and Public Health, University of Maryland School of Medicine, Baltimore, MD, USA

Kristene E. Whitmore, MD Urology Division, Department of Obstetrics and Gynecology, FPMRS, The Pelvic and Sexual Health Institute, Drexel University College of Medicine, Philadelphia, PA, USA

Jean-Jacques Wyndaele, MD, DSci, PhD Department of Urology, University Hospital Antwerp and Antwerp University, Edegem, Belgium

Andrey Zaytsev Department of Urology, Moscow State Medical Stomatological University, Moscow City Hospital, Moscow, Russia

Chapter 1
Historical Perspective

Philip M. Hanno

As with most disorders, how we arrived at our current concept of bladder pain syndrome (BPS) depends upon knowledge of the historical perspective underlying the syndrome. It was a true change in the paradigm that resulted in what had been considered a rare, pure bladder disease with specific endoscopic and common pathologic findings into a much more prevalent chronic pain syndrome diagnosed almost exclusively by symptomatic criteria. Changes in nomenclature parallel the history [1].

Historical reviews confirm that interstitial cystitis (IC) was recognized as a pathologic entity during the nineteenth century [2, 3]. Joseph Parrish, a Philadelphia surgeon, described three cases of severe lower urinary tract symptoms in the absence of a bladder stone in an 1836 text [4], and termed the disorder "tic doloureux of the bladder." Teichman argues that this may represent the first description of interstitial cystitis [5]. Fifty years later Skene used the term interstitial cystitis to describe an inflammation that has "destroyed the mucous membrane partly or wholly and extended to the muscular parietes" [6].

Early in the twentieth century, at a New England Section meeting of the American Urological Association, Guy Hunner reported on eight women with a history of suprapubic pain, frequency, nocturia, and urgency lasting for an average of 17 years [7, 8]. He drew attention to the disease, and the red, bleeding areas he described on the bladder wall came to have the pseudonym "Hunner's ulcer." As Anthony Walsh [9] observed, this has proven to be unfortunate. In the early part of the twentieth century, the very best cystoscopes available gave a poorly defined and ill-lit view of the fundus of the bladder. It is not surprising that when Hunner saw red and bleeding areas high on the bladder wall, he believed they were ulcers. For the next 60 years, urologists would look for ulcers and fail to make the diagnosis in their absence. The disease was thought to be focal, rather than a pancystitis. As has been pointed out

P.M. Hanno, M.D., M.P.H. (✉)
Division of Urology, Department of Surgery, Hospital of the University of Pennsylvania, Philadelphia, PA, USA
e-mail: hannop@uphs.upenn.edu

J. Nordling et al. (eds.), *Bladder Pain Syndrome: A Guide for Clinicians*,
DOI 10.1007/978-1-4419-6929-3_1, © Springer Science+Business Media New York 2013

by Dr. Magnus Fall, the so-called ulcer was really a vulnus (*a solution of continuity, or separation by external violence, of parts naturally united*) [10] or wound seen in the bladder only upon distention.

In 1949 Hand [11] authored the first comprehensive review about the disease, reporting 223 cases. The majority of his findings have relevance even today. His clinical description bears repeating. "I have frequently observed that what appeared to be a normal mucosa before and during the first bladder distention showed typical interstitial cystitis on subsequent distention." He notes, "small, discrete, submucosal hemorrhages, showing variations in form … dot-like bleeding points … little or no restriction to bladder capacity." He portrays three grades of disease, with grade three matching the small-capacity, scared bladder described by Hunner. Sixty-nine percent of patients were grade one and only 13% were grade three.

Walsh [9] later coined the term "glomerulations" to describe the petechial hemorrhages that Hand had described. But it was not until Messing and Stamey [12] discussed the "early diagnosis" of IC that attention turned from looking for an ulcer to make the diagnosis to the concepts that (1) symptoms and glomerulations at the time of bladder distention under anesthesia were the disease hallmarks and (2) the diagnosis was primarily one of exclusion.

IC was like your Aunt Minnie: (*"She is hard to define, but you know her when you see her"*). Bourque's description is almost 60 years old and is worth recalling. "We have all met, at one time or another, patients who suffer chronically from their bladder; and we mean the ones who are distressed, not only periodically but constantly, having to urinate often, at all moments of the day and of the night, and suffering pains every time they void. We all know how these miserable patients are unhappy, and how those distressing bladder symptoms get finally to influence their general state of health physically at first, and mentally after a while" [13].

This description and others like it were not suitable for defining this disease in the late twentieth century. What was needed was a definition that would help physicians make the diagnosis and design research studies to learn more about the problem in a uniform manner in nations around the world. Physician interest and government participation in research were sparked through the efforts of a group of frustrated patients led by Dr. Vicki Ratner, an orthopedic surgeon residing in New York City, who founded the first patient advocacy group, the Interstitial Cystitis Association in the living room of her small New York City apartment in 1984 [14, 15]. The first step was to develop a working definition of the disease. The modern history of BPS is best viewed through the development of the modern definition.

Evolution of Definition

While it would seem that defining this syndrome should not be difficult, the pillars of the symptom complex—frequency, pain, and an urgent desire to void—all have intrinsic problems for a clinically useful definition. Large variation in the degree of bother with varying rates of frequency [16] makes a symptomatic diagnosis of IC based on an absolute number of voids subject to question, and frequency per volume of intake or even the concept of "perception of frequency" as a problem may be more accurate than an absolute number. Pain can be difficult for the physician or patient to localize. Urgency can mean something different to patients and to clinicians [17].

In an effort to define IC so that patients in different geographic areas, under the care of different physicians, could be compared, the National Institute of Diabetes and Digestive and Kidney Diseases (NIDDK) held a workshop in August 1987 at which consensus criteria were established for the diagnosis of IC [18]. These criteria were not meant to define the disease for the clinician, but rather to ensure that groups of patients included in basic and clinical research studies would be relatively comparable. After pilot studies testing the criteria were carried out, the criteria were revised at another NIDDK workshop a year later [19]. These criteria are presented in Table 1.1.

Although meant initially to serve only as a research tool, the NIDDK "research definition" became a de facto definition of this disease, diagnosed by exclusion and colorfully termed a "hole in the air" by Hald [20]. Certain of the exclusion criteria served to make one wary of a diagnosis of IC, but could not be used for categorical exclusion of such a diagnosis. However, because of the ambiguity involved, it was determined that these patients should be eliminated from research studies or categorized separately. In particular, exclusion criteria 4, 5, 6, 8, 9, 11, 12, 17, and 18 are only relative. What percentage of patients with idiopathic sensory urgency has IC is unclear [21]. The specificity of the finding of bladder glomerulations has come into question [22–24]. Similarly, the sensitivity of glomerulations is also unknown, but clearly patients with IC symptoms can demonstrate an absence of glomerulations under anesthesia [25, 26]. Hunner's lesions have been historically considered rare and exist in less than 15% of patients in this author's experience and in the experience of others [27]. A California series found 20% of patients to have ulceration [28]. Specific pathologic findings represent a glaring omission from the criteria, because there is a lack of consensus as to which pathologic findings, if any, are required for, or even suggestive of, a tissue diagnosis [24, 29–31], while some maintain that histopathologic criteria in classic Hunner disease are well defined [32, 33].

The unexpected use of the NIDDK research criteria by the medical community as a definition of IC led to concerns that many patients suffering from this syndrome might be misdiagnosed. The multicenter Interstitial Cystitis Database (ICDB) study through NIDDK accumulated data on 424 patients with IC, enrolling patients from May 1993 through December 1995. Entry criteria were much more symptom driven than those promulgated for research studies [34] and are noted in Table 1.2. In an analysis of the defining criteria [35, 36], it appeared that the NIDDK research criteria fulfilled their mission. Fully 90% of expert clinicians agreed that patients diagnosed with IC by those criteria in the ICDB indeed had the disorder. However, 60% of patients deemed to have IC by these experienced clinicians would not have met NIDDK research criteria. Thus, IC remained a clinical syndrome defined by some combination of chronic symptoms of urgency, frequency, and/or pain in the absence of other reasonable causation. Whereas IC symptom and problem indices have been developed and validated [37, 38], these are not intended to diagnose or define IC but rather to measure the severity of symptomatology and monitor disease progression or regression [39].

Table 1.1 National institute of diabetes and digestive and kidney diseases (NIDDK) diagnostic criteria for interstitial cystitis

To be diagnosed with interstitial cystitis, patients must have either glomerulations on cystoscopic examination or a classic Hunner ulcer, and they must have either pain associated with the bladder or urinary urgency. An examination for glomerulations should be undertaken after distention of the bladder under anesthesia to 80–100 cm H_2O for 1–2 min. The bladder may be distended up to two times before evaluation. The glomerulations must be diffuse—present in at least three quadrants of the bladder—and there must be at least ten glomerulations per quadrant. The glomerulations must not be along the path of the cystoscope (to eliminate artifact from contact instrumentation). The presence of any one of the following excludes a diagnosis of interstitial cystitis:

1. Bladder capacity of greater than 350 mL on awake cystometry using either a gas or a liquid filling medium
2. Absence of an intense urge to void with the bladder filled to 100 mL of gas or 150 mL of liquid filling medium
3. The demonstration of phasic involuntary bladder contractions on cystometry using the fill rate just described
4. Duration of symptoms less than 9 months
5. Absence of nocturia
6. Symptoms relieved by antimicrobial agents, urinary antiseptic agents, anticholinergic agents, or antispasmodic agents
7. A frequency of urination while awake of less than 8 times per day
8. A diagnosis of bacterial cystitis or prostatitis within a 3-month period
9. Bladder or ureteral calculi
10. Active genital herpes
11. Uterine, cervical, vaginal, or urethral cancer
12. Urethral diverticulum
13. Cyclophosphamide or any type of chemical cystitis
14. Tuberculous cystitis
15. Radiation cystitis
16. Benign or malignant bladder tumors
17. Vaginitis
18. Age younger than 18 years

From Wein AJ, Hanno PM, Gillenwater JY: Interstitial cystitis: An introduction to the problem. In: Hanno PM, Staskin DR, Krane RJ, Wein AJ editors. Interstitial Cystitis. London: Springer-Verlag, 1990, p 13–15

Nomenclature and Taxonomy

The literature over the last 170 years has seen numerous changes in description and nomenclature of the disease. The syndrome has variously been referred to as tic doloureux of the bladder, interstitial cystitis, cystitis parenchymatosa, Hunner's ulcer, panmural ulcerative cystitis, urethral syndrome, and painful bladder syndrome [3, 5–7, 13, 40, 41]. The term "interstitial cystitis," which Skene is credited with coining and Hunner brought into common usage, is a misnomer; in many cases not only is there no interstitial inflammation, but also, histopathologically, there may be no inflammation at all [24, 42–44]. By literally focussing exclusively on the urinary

Table 1.2 Interstitial cystitis database (ICDB)

Study eligibility criteria
1. Providing informed consent to participate in the study
2. Willing to undergo a cystoscopy under general or regional anesthesia when indicated, during the course of the study
3. At least 18 years of age
4. Having symptoms of urinary urgency, frequency, or pain for more than 6 months
5. Urinating at least 7 times per day, or having some urgency or pain (measured on linear analog scales)
6. No history of current genitorurinary tuberculosis
7. No history of urethral cancer
8. No history of bladder malignancy, high-grade dysplasia, or carcinoma in situ
9. Males: No history of prostate cancer
10. Females: No occurrence of ovarian, vaginal, or cervical cancer in the previous 3 years
11. Females: No current vaginitis, clue cell, trichomonas, or yeast infections
12. No bacterial cystitis in the previous 3 months
13. No active herpes in the previous 3 months
14. No antimicrobials for urinary tract infections in previous 3 months
15. Never having been treated with cyclophosphamide
16. No radiation cystitis
17. No neurogenic bladder dysfunction (e.g., due to a spinal cord injury, stroke, Parkinson's disease, multiple sclerosis, spina bifida, or diabetic cystopathy)
18. No bladder outlet obstruction (determined by urodynamic investigation)
19. Males: No bacterial prostatitis for previous 6 months
20. Absence of bladder, ureteral, or urethral calculi for previous 3 months
21. No urethritis for previous 3 months
22. Not having had a urethral dilation, cystometrogram, bladder cystoscopy under full anesthesia, or a bladder biopsy in previous 3 months
23. Never having had an augmentation cystoplasty, cystectomy, cystolysis, or neuroectomy
24. Not having a urethral stricture of less than 12 French

From Simon LJ, Landis JR, Erickson DR, Nyberg LM. The interstitial cystitis data base study: concepts and preliminary baseline descriptive statistics. Urology 1997;49:64–75

bladder, the term interstitial cystitis furthermore does not do justice to the condition from both the physician's and the patient's perspective. The textual exclusiveness ignores the high comorbidity with various pelvic, extra-pelvic, and non-urological symptoms and associated disorders [45] that frequently precede or develop after the onset of the bladder condition [46].

With the formal definition of the term "painful bladder syndrome" by the ICS in 2002, the terminology discussion became an intense international focal point [47].

- In Kyoto at the ICICJ in March 2003, it was agreed that the term "interstitial cystitis" should be expanded to "interstitial cystitis/chronic pelvic pain syndrome" when pelvic pain is at least of 3 months duration and associated with no obvious treatable condition/pathology [48].
- The European Society for the Study of Interstitial Cystitis (ESSIC) held its first meeting in Copenhagen soon after Kyoto. Nomenclature was discussed, but no

decision was reached, as the meeting concentrated on how to evaluate patients for diagnosis [49].

- At the 2003 meeting of the NIDDK titled, "Research Insights into Interstitial Cystitis," it was concluded that "interstitial cystitis" will ultimately be replaced as a sole name for this syndrome. It will be a gradual process over several years. At the meeting it was referred to as "interstitial cystitis/painful bladder syndrome" in keeping with International Continence Society nomenclature [50].
- At the 2004 inaugural meeting of the Multinational Interstitial Cystitis Association in Rome, it was concluded that the syndrome should be referred to as "painful bladder syndrome/interstitial cystitis" or "PBS/IC" to indicate an intellectual and taxonomical hierarchy within the acronym [50].
- The International Consultation on Incontinence in 2004, cosponsored by the ICS and Societe Internationale d'Urologie in association with the World Health Organization, included the syndrome as a part of its consultation. The chapter in the report was titled, "painful bladder syndrome (including interstitial cystitis)," suggesting that the IC formed an identifiable subset within the broader syndrome. Because such a distinction is difficult to define, within the body of the chapter, coauthored by nine committee members and five consultants from four continents, it was referred to as PBS/IC (one inclusive entity) [30]. Interstitial cystitis may be a subgroup that encompasses those patients with typical histological and cystoscopic features [51], but what these features are is still controversial and somewhat vague.
- In June 2006 Abrams and colleagues published an editorial focussing on the nomenclature problem [52]. They noted: "It is an advantage if the medical term has clear diagnostic features that translate to a known pathophysiologic process so that effective treatment may be given. Unfortunately, the latter is not the case for many of the pain syndromes suffered by patients seen at most pain, gynecological, and urological clinics. For the most part these 'diagnoses' describe syndromes that do not have recognized standard definitions, yet imply knowledge of a pathophysiologic cause for the symptoms. Unfortunately the terminology used to describe the condition may promote erroneous thinking about treatment on the part of physicians, surgeons and patients. These organ based diagnoses are mysterious, misleading and unhelpful, and can lead to therapies that are misguided or even dangerous." The editorial went on to note that a single pathologic descriptive term (interstitial cystitis) for a spectrum of symptom combinations ill serves patients. The umbrella term "painful bladder syndrome" was proposed, with a goal to define and investigate subsets of patients who could be clearly identified within the spectrum of PBS. It would fall within the rubric of chronic pelvic pain syndrome. Sufferers would be identified according to the primary organ that appears to be affected on clinical grounds. Pain not associated with an individual organ would be described in terms of the symptoms.One can see in this the beginnings of a new paradigm that might be expected to change the emphasis of both clinical and basic science research, and that removes the automatic presumption that the end-organ in the name of the disease should necessarily be the sole or primary target of such research.

- At the major biannual IC research conference in the fall of 2006, held by the National Institute of Diabetes, Digestive, and Kidney Disorders (Frontiers in Painful Bladder Syndrome/Interstitial Cystitis), the ESSIC group was given a block of time with which to present their thoughts and conclusions. Because (1) the term PBS did not fit into the taxonomy of other pelvic pain syndromes such as urethral or vulvar pain syndromes, (2) as defined by the International Continence Society missed over a third of afflicted patients [53], and (3) is a term open to different interpretations, ESSIC suggested that Painful Bladder Syndrome be redesignated as BPS, followed by a type designation based on findings at hydrodistention and pathology (see Chap. 4). Although neither cystoscopy with hydrodistention nor bladder biopsy was prescribed as an essential part of the evaluation, by categorizing patients as to whether either procedure was done, and if so, the results, it is possible to follow patients with similar findings and study each identified cohort to compare natural history, prognosis, and response to therapy [54].
- As Baranowski et al. conceived it in early 2008, BPS is thus defined as a pain syndrome with a collection of symptoms, the most important of which is pain perceived to be in the bladder [55]. IC is distinguished as an end-organ, visceral-neural pain syndrome, whereas BPS can be considered a pain syndrome that involves the end-organ (bladder) and neuro-visceral (myopathic) mechanisms. In IC, one expects end-organ primary pathology. This is not necessarily the case in the broader BPS.

Recent international consultations have essentially agreed that the nomenclature of "interstitial cystitis" should be revised. The International Consultation on Incontinence used the term "BPS" [56]. The ESSIC group has also adopted this name for the syndrome (http://www.essic.org/). This change implies that it is the symptoms that drive treatment, and the question as to whether "interstitial cystitis" should refer to a distinct subgroup of the bladder pain syndrome is, as yet, unclear. East Asian urologists representing institutions in Taiwan, Japan, and Korea have settled on the terms "interstitial cystitis" and "hypersensitive bladder syndrome," the former paralleling the NIDDK research definition and the latter including patients with hypersensitivity and urinary frequency with or without bladder pain [57]. The issue has been finessed by the American Urological Association in its 2011 guidelines by referring to the disorder as "Interstitial Cystitis/Bladder Pain Syndrome" [58].

References

1. Hanno PM. Re-imagining interstitial cystitis. Urol Clin North Am. 2008;35(1):91–9.
2. Parsons JK, Parsons CL. The historical origins of interstitial cystitis. J Urol. 2004;171(1):20–2.
3. Christmas TJ. Historical aspects of interstitial cystitis. In: Sant GR, editor. Interstitial Cystitis. Philadelphia: Lippincott-Raven; 1997. p. 1–8.

4. Parrish J. Tic doloureux of the urinary bladder. Practical observations on strangulated hernia and some of the diseases of the urinary organs. Philadelphia: Key and Biddle; 1836. p. 309–13.
5. Teichman JM, Thompson IM, Taichman NS. Joseph Parrish, tic doloureux of the bladder and interstitial cystitis. J Urol. 2000;164(5):1473–5.
6. Skene AJC. Diseases of the bladder and urethra in women. New York: William Wood; 1887.
7. Hunner GL. A rare type of bladder ulcer. Further notes, with a report of eighteen cases. JAMA. 1918;70(4):203–12.
8. Hunner GL. A rare type of bladder ulcer in women; report of cases. J Boston Med Surg. 1915;172:660–4.
9. Walsh A. Interstitial cystitis. In: Harrison JH, Gittes RF, Perlmutter AD, et al., editors. Campbell's Urology. 4th ed. Philadelphia: W B Saunders; 1978. p. 693–707.
10. Ruddock EH. Modern medicine and surgery on homeopathic principles. London: Homeopathic Publishing Company; 1874.
11. Hand JR. Interstitial cystitis: report of 223 cases (204 women and 19 men). J Urol. 1949;61:291–310.
12. Messing EM, Stamey TA. Interstitial cystitis: early diagnosis, pathology, and treatment. Urology. 1978;12(4):381–92.
13. Bourque JP. Surgical management of the painful bladder. J Urol. 1951;65:25–34.
14. Ratner V, Slade D, Whitmore KE. Interstitial cystitis: a bladder disease finds legitimacy. J Womens Health. 1992;1:63–8.
15. Ratner V, Slade D. Interstitial cystitis: a women's health perspective. In: Sant GR, editor. Interstitial cystitis. Philadelphia: Lippincott-Raven; 1997. p. 257–60.
16. Fitzgerald M, Butler N, Shott S, Brubaker L. Bother arising from urinary frequency in women. Neurourol Urodyn. 2002;21:36–41.
17. Hanno PM, Chapple CR, Cardozo LD. Bladder pain syndrome/interstitial cystitis: a sense of urgency. World J Urol. 2009;27:717–21.
18. Gillenwater JY, Wein AJ. Summary of the National Institute of Arthritis, Diabetes, Digestive and Kidney Diseases Workshop on Interstitial Cystitis, National Institutes of Health, Bethesda, Maryland, August 28–29, 1987. J Urol. 1988;140(1):203–6.
19. Wein A, Hanno PM, Gillenwater JY. Interstitial cystitis: an introduction to the problem. In: Hanno PM, Staskin DR, Krane RJ, Wein AJ, editors. Interstitial cystitis. London: Springer; 1990. p. 13–5.
20. George NJR. Preface. In: George NJR, Gosling JA, editors. Sensory disorders of the bladder and urethra. Berlin: Springer; 1986. p. vii.
21. Frazer MI, Haylen BT, Sissons M. Do women with idiopathic sensory urgency have early interstitial cystitis? Br J Urol. 1990;66(3):274–8.
22. Waxman JA, Sulak PJ, Kuehl TJ. Cystoscopic findings consistent with interstitial cystitis in normal women undergoing tubal ligation. J Urol. 1998;160(5):1663–7.
23. Erickson DR. Glomerulations in women with urethral sphincter deficiency: report of 2 cases (corrected). J Urol. 1995;153(3 Pt 1):728–9.
24. Tomaszewski JE, Landis JR, Russack V, Williams TM, Wang LP, Hardy C, et al. Biopsy features are associated with primary symptoms in interstitial cystitis: results from the interstitial cystitis database study. Urology. 2001;57(6 Suppl 1):67–81.
25. Awad SA, MacDiarmid S, Gajewski JB, Gupta R. Idiopathic reduced bladder storage versus interstitial cystitis. J Urol. 1992;148(5):1409–12.
26. Al Hadithi H, Tincello DG, Vince GS, Richmond DH. Leukocyte populations in interstitial cystitis and idiopathic reduced bladder storage. Urology. 2002;59(6):851–5.
27. Sant GR. Interstitial cystitis. Monogr Urol. 1991;12:37–63.
28. Koziol JA. Epidemiology of interstitial cystitis. Urol Clin North Am. 1994;21(1):7–20.
29. Hanno P, Levin RM, Monson FC, Teuscher C, Zhou ZZ, Ruggieri M, et al. Diagnosis of interstitial cystitis. J Urol. 1990;143(2):278–81.
30. Hanno P, Baranowski A, Fall M, Gajewski JB, Nordling J, Nyberg L, et al. Painful bladder syndrome (including interstitial cystitis). In: Abrams PH, Wein AJ, Cardozo L, editors. Incontinence, chap. 23, vol. 2. 3rd ed. Paris: Health Publications Limited; 2005. p. 1456–520.

31. Tomaszewski JE, Landis JR, Brensinger C, Hardy C, et al. Baseline associations among pathologic features and patient symptoms in the national interstitial cystitis data base. J Urol. 1999;161S:28.
32. Fall M, Johansson SL, Aldenborg F. Chronic interstitial cystitis: a heterogeneous syndrome. J Urol. 1987;137:35–8.
33. Johanson SL, Fall M. Clinicla features and spectrum of light microscopic changes in interstitial cystitis. J Urol. 1990;143:1118–24.
34. Simon LJ, Landis JR, Erickson DR, Nyberg LM. The interstitial cystitis data base study: concepts and preliminary baseline descriptive statistics. Urology. 1997;49(5A Suppl):64–75.
35. Hanno PM, Landis JR, Matthews-Cook Y, Kusek J, et al. Interstitial cystitis: issues of definition. Urol Integr Invest. 1999;4(4):291–5.
36. Hanno PM, Landis JR, Matthews-Cook Y, Kusek J, Nyberg Jr L. The diagnosis of interstitial cystitis revisited: lessons learned from the National Institutes of Health Interstitial Cystitis Database study. J Urol. 1999;161(2):553–7.
37. Goin JE, Olaleye D, Peters KM, Steinert B, Habicht K, Wynant G. Psychometric analysis of the University of Wisconsin interstitial cystitis scale: implications for use in randomized clinical trials. J Urol. 1998;159(3):1085–90.
38. O'leary MP, Sant GR, Fowler Jr FJ, Whitmore KE, Spolarich-Kroll J. The interstitial cystitis symptom index and problem index. Urology. 1997;49(5A Suppl):58–63.
39. Moldwin R, Kushner L. The diagnostic value of interstitial cystitis questionnaires. J Urol. 2004;171(4 Suppl):96.
40. Dell JR, Parsons CL. Multimodal therapy for interstitial cystitis. J Reprod Med. 2004;49(3 Suppl):243–52.
41. Powell NB, Powell EB. The female urethra: a clinico-pathological study. J Urol. 1949;61:557–70.
42. Rosamilia A, Igawa Y, Higashi S. Pathology of interstitial cystitis. Int J Urol. 2003;10(Suppl):S11–5.
43. Lynes WL, Flynn SD, Shortliffe LD, Stamey TA. The histology of interstitial cystitis. Am J Surg Pathol. 1990;14(10):969–76.
44. Denson MA, Griebling TL, Cohen MB, Kreder KJ. Comparison of cystoscopic and histological findings in patients with suspected interstitial cystitis. J Urol. 2000;164(6):1908–11.
45. Clauw DJ, Schmidt M, Radulovic D, Singer A, Katz P, Bresette J. The relationship between fibromyalgia and interstitial cystitis. J Psychiatr Res. 1997;31(1):125–31.
46. Wu EQ, Birnbaum H, Kang YJ, Parece A, Mallett D, Taitel H, et al. A retrospective claims database analysis to assess patterns of interstitial cystitis diagnosis. Curr Med Res Opin. 2006;22(3):495–500.
47. Abrams PH, Cardozo L, Fall M, Griffiths D, Rosier P, Ulmsten U, et al. The standardisation of terminology of lower urinary tract function: report from the standardisation sub-committee of the international continence society. Neurourol Urodyn. 2002;21:167–78.
48. Ueda T, Sant GR, Hanno PM, Yoshimura N. Interstitial cystitis and frequency-urgency syndrome (OAB syndrome). Int J Urol. 2003;10(Suppl):S39–48.
49. Nordling J, Anjum FH, Bade JJ, Bouchelouche K, Bouchelouche P, Cervigni M, et al. Primary evaluation of patients suspected of having interstitial cystitis (IC). Eur Urol. 2004;45(5):662–9.
50. Hanno P, Keay S, Moldwin R, Vanophoven A. International consultation on IC - Rome, September 2004/forging an international consensus: progress in painful bladder syndrome/interstitial cystitis report and abstracts. Int Urogynecol J Pelvic Floor Dysfunct. 2005;16 Suppl 1:S2–34.
51. Peeker R, Fall M. Toward a precise definition of interstitial cystitis: further evidence of differences in classic and nonulcer disease. J Urol. 2002;167(6):2470–2.
52. Abrams P, Baranowski A, Berger R, Fall M, Hanno P, Wesselmann U. A new classification is needed for pelvic pain syndromes – are existing terminologies of spurious diagnostic authority bad for patients? J Urol. 2006;175:1989–90.
53. Warren JW, Meyer WA, Greenberg P, Horne L, Diggs C, Tracy JK. Using the International Continence Society's definition of painful bladder syndrome. Urology. 2006;67(6):1138–42.

54. van de Merwe JP, Nordling J, Bouchelouche P, Bouchelouche K, Cervigni M, Daha LK, et al. Diagnostic criteria, classification, and nomenclature for painful bladder syndrome/interstitial cystitis: an ESSIC proposal. Eur Urol. 2008;53(1):60–7.
55. Baranowski A, Abrams P, Berger R, Buffington CA, Williams CD, Hanno P, et al. Urogenital pain- time to accept a new approach to phenotyping and, as a consequence, management. Eur Urol. 2008;53:33–6.
56. Hanno P, Lin AT, Nordling J, Nyberg L, van Ophoven A, Ueda T. Bladder pain syndrome. In: Abrams P, Cardozo L, Khoury S, Wein A, editors. Incontinence. Paris: Health Publication Ltd; 2009. p. 1459–518.
57. Homma Y, Ueda T, Tomoe H, Lin AT, Kuo HC, Lee MH, et al. Clinical guidelines for interstitial cystitis and hypersensitive bladder syndrome. Int J Urol. 2009;16(7):597–615.
58. Hanno PM, Burks D, Clemens JQ, Dmochowski R, Erickson D, Fitzgerald MP, et al. AUA guideline for the diagnosis and treatment of interstitial cystitis/bladder pain syndrome. J Urol. 2011;185(6):2162–70.

Chapter 2
Epidemiology

Mirja Ruutu, Mikael Leppilahti, and Jukka Sairanen

Reliable epidemiological studies on PBS/IC are difficult to perform due to inconsistency of diagnostic criteria and rarity of the disease. The situation is very different from cancer epidemiology, where incidence and prevalence figures are based on solid histopathological criteria and mortality data from population registries. Most data on PBS/IC epidemiology come from the United States and some from the Western European countries. Lately, some important studies have emerged from Asia.

Most epidemiological studies seem to concentrate on an estimation of the disease prevalence. Because IC is a nonfatal disease with unclear starting events, it is very difficult to evaluate its incidence, which could only be theoretically calculated from longitudinal prevalence figures.

Methodological Problems in PBS/IC Epidemiology

The majority of epidemiological studies are reports from single institutions or local areas, and the diagnosis is determined by respective urologists, gynaecologists or other health care physicians. Such patient cohorts are not representative for the whole population. If NIDDK criteria for the disease diagnosis [1] are followed, the prevalence

Editorial Comment Epidemiological studies have not yet been performed based on the definition of Bladder Pain Syndrome (BPS). Previous epidemiological studies have therefore been based on the different, elusive, non-specific criteria existing for Interstitial Cystitis (IC) and Painful Bladder Syndrome (PBS). To avoid misunderstandings the name of the condition is therefore kept as IC, PBS or PBS/IC in this chapter.

M. Ruutu, M.D., Ph.D., F.E.B.U. (✉) • J. Sairanen, MD, PhD
Department of Urology, Helsinki University Central Hospital, Helsinki University, Helsinki, Finland
e-mail: Mirja.Ruutu@hus.fi

M. Leppilahti, MD, PhD
Seinäjoki Central Hospital, Seinäjoki, Finland

J. Nordling et al. (eds.), *Bladder Pain Syndrome: A Guide for Clinicians*,
DOI 10.1007/978-1-4419-6929-3_2, © Springer Science+Business Media New York 2013

figures remain low because early or mild cases are then not recognised. It has been estimated that strict application of those criteria would miss more than 60% of patients regarded as definitively or probably having IC [2]. Population-based studies are more representative from the epidemiological point of view. Only few such studies have been carried out. The reported prevalence figures seem to be higher compared with institutional studies. The already classic Interstitial Cystitis Symptom Index (ICSI) and Interstitial Cystitis Problem Index questionnaire has been validated only in patients meeting the NIDDK criteria compared with a control group without symptoms [3], and later monitoring changes in patients diagnosed with IC [4]. Despite these validations the formula does not define whether urgency is painless or associated with pain and relieved after voiding, differential diagnosis with overactive bladder is therefore problematic. Pelvic Pain and Urgency/Frequency (PUF) symptom scale has been developed to recognise IC patients amongst heterogenic patient groups who also seek medical advice for suspected gynaecological conditions and validated by comparison of the results with potassium sensitivity test in these patients [5]. It has not been tested in genuine population-based studies and most likely overestimates the number of women having IC. Neither of the above-mentioned questionnaires seem to have sufficient specificity to perform as the only diagnostic tool [6].

The recent epidemiological studies include PBS in the nomenclature, alone or in combination PBS/IC, but not BPS as is advised by ESSIC [7]. In further studies the different categories of PBS should be defined more clearly.

Institutional and Health Care-Based Epidemiological Studies

The first report on epidemiology of IC was published from Finland in 1975 [8]. This investigation was based on the number of patients treated in the intake area of Helsinki University Hospital and led to a prevalence estimation of 18.1 females per 100,000 and 10.6 per 100,000 for both genders. In this study an estimated figure for IC incidence was also given, that being 1.2 new cases per 100,000 females yearly.

An early epidemiological study from the United States was based on three different sources: urologists, IC patients and a sample from the general population [9]. This survey yielded an IC case prevalence estimation of 30 per 100,000.

In the National Household Interview Survey (NHIS), 20,561 participants were asked if they ever had symptoms of a urinary tract infection that lasted 3 months or longer, and if they were told at the time of those persistent symptoms that they had PBS or IC [10]. In this survey, 110 women and 8 men were regarded as having IC, leading to a prevalence estimation of 500 per 100,000.

In another large study, the Nurses Health Study I and II, the prevalence of IC was estimated to be 52 per 100,000 in females with diagnosis by cystoscopy and 67 per 100,000 in those with a prior IC diagnosis [11].

A study by Bade from the Netherlands showed an estimated prevalence of 8–16 females per 100,000 based on physician-assigned diagnosis [12]. An inquiry among

Table 2.1 Institutional and respective epidemiological studies on IC

Author (ref)	Year	Estimated prevalence per 100,000
Oravisto [8]	1975	18.1 women, 10.6 both genders
Held [9]	1990	30 both genders
Bade [12]	1995	8–16 women
Jones [10]	1997	870 women
Curhan [11]	1999	52–67 women
Miki [13]	2000	4.5 women

300 urologists in Japan yielded a much lower prevalence of 4.5 per 100,000 females [13]. The above-mentioned institutional studies are depicted in Table 2.1.

The patient material seen by urologists and other physicians in different institutions may vary greatly. The Canadian PIE-study (Prostatitis, Interstitial Cystitis and Epididymitis Study) revealed that the percentage of patients seen by urologists in a 2-week audit period was lower for academic urologists (1.3%) compared with community urologists (3.4%). The same study [14] showed that 2.5% of patients seen by male urologists had IC whereas the respective figure was as high as 7.7% for female urologists. Thus the inconsistencies in target populations and diagnostic methods used make the comparison of the institutional epidemiological studies difficult.

Population-Based Epidemiological Studies

There are only a few truly population-based studies on PBS/IC (Table 2.2).

The first study using ICSI-questionnaire was published as late as 2002 [15]. The questionnaire was mailed to randomly selected 2,000 Finnish women 18–71 years old from the national population register. After a new mail at 6 weeks of an identical questionnaire to those who had not responded, altogether 1,343 women replied (67.2%). After exclusions for incompletely filled questionnaires, institutionalisation or refusal to participate the final analysable study group consisted of 1,331 women (66.6%). Overall 73% of them had few or no symptoms (score 0–3), while 15% had mild (score 4–6), 9% had moderate (score 7–11) and 3% had severe (score 12 or greater) symptoms. Respectively, 78% experienced no problem (score 0–3), 13% had mild problems (4–6), 7% had moderate problems (7–11) and 2% had severe problems (12 or greater). After exclusion of women with urinary infection during the last month, 86 of 1,331 (6.5%) reported a moderate or severe symptom score combined with a moderate or severe problem score (7 or greater). Eleven women (0.8%) reported severe symptoms and problems (12 or greater), and 6 (0.45%) of them fulfilled the criteria for probable IC.

Later the same author reported the results of clinical examination of the responders who had moderate or severe symptoms at the original survey [16]. This investigation showed that the estimated prevalence of clinically confirmed probable IC in women was 230 per 100,000 and that of possible/probable IC was 530 per 100,000.

Table 2.2 Population-based epidemiological studies on PBS/IC (Q = questionnaire)

Author (ref no.)	Year	No. of subjects	Gender	Prevalence	Method
Leppilahti [15]	2002	2,000	Female	450	Mailed Q (ICSI)
Leppilahti [16]	2005	2,000	Female	230–300	Clinical confirmation of the study above
Rosenberg [17]	2004	1,218	Female	570 12,600	Q (ICSI) in primary care Q (PUF)
Temml [18]	2007	1,143	Female	306	Q (ICSI) + clinical
Clemens [19]	2007	5,506	Both	830–2,710 women 250–1,220 men	Interview with Q's
Litford [20]	2009	67,095	Female	2,300	Mailed Q
Inoue [21]	2009	80,367	Female	265	Internet-based Q
Choe [22]	2010	2,323	Female	261	Telephone survey (Q)

The corrected estimates taking into account those women who did not undergo clinical examination for various reasons but had high symptom scores were 300 per 100,000 for probable IC and 680 per 100,000 for possible/probable IC.

Rosenberg and Hazzard conducted a survey among all female patients 18–71 years old who presented for a routine visit in primary care during 9 months [17]. These women were administered both ICSI and PUF questionnaires. Of the 1,218 eligible subjects, 74.5% scored 0–3 in ICSI, 16.5% had mild symptoms (score 4–6), 7% had moderate symptoms (7–11) and 2.0% had severe symptoms (12 or greater). The problem index was distributed as follows: 89.6% had no problems, 5.7% had mild problems, 3.3% had moderate problems and 1.4% had severe problems (12 or greater). Altogether 14 women reported severe symptoms and problems including 7 who filled the criteria of probable IC according to Leppilahti [15]. The estimated prevalence was thus 0.57% (570 per 100,000). Of the 965 patients with PUF score, the total percentage of women predicted to have IC was as high as 12.6% (12,600 per 100,000).

Another European study from Austria [18] appeared 5 years after the Finnish study. Women attending a voluntary health survey project in Vienna underwent a detailed health investigation and completed ICSI questionnaire as well as other questionnaires including items on pain, quality of life and sexual aspects. The study comprised 1,143 women of whom 162 were excluded due to urinary tract infection, missing urinalysis or incompletely answered questionnaires. Of the remaining 981 women, 57.9% had no IC symptoms, 25.9% had mild, 13.9% moderate and 2.3% severe symptoms (score 12 or greater). Using the same definitions as Leppilahti [15], the overall prevalence of IC in the Vienna female population was 306 per 100,000. The strength of this study is that the patients underwent a health examination having also urinalysis taken to exclude infection.

The BACH Survey (Boston area population based, random sample, cross-sectional epidemiological study of a broad range of urological symptoms, funded by NIDDK) accomplished a 2-h person interview on 5,506 individuals [19]. Of them, 252 were excluded due to history of various urogenital cancers or neurological diseases affecting bladder function. The survey questionnaire included questions about bladder pain, urinary frequency, urinary urgency and nocturia. Many questions were extracted from ICSI. PBS was defined with eight various symptom complexes. The prevalence of PBS symptoms was 0.83–2.71% in women and 0.25–1.22% in men depending on the definitions used. The symptoms were equally common in white, black and Hispanic individuals and more common in lower socioeconomic group compared with middle and upper status.

All participants in the Nurses' Health Study ($n=67,095$) were mailed a simple question asking whether in the last 10 years they had experienced pain, discomfort or burning in the pelvis or bladder for more than 3 months in row and accompanied by urinary frequency or urgency [20]. Those who answered yes ($n=4,005$) received a supplementary larger questionnaire with PBS symptom and bother scores. Of the 3,042 supplementary questionnaire respondents, 1,548 (51%) confirmed symptoms consistent with a diagnosis of PBS. The overall prevalence was calculated as 2,395 per 100,000 women. Using an alternate question to exclude cases with urge incontinence, the respective figure was 1,946 per 100,000. Another alternate question to include pain with bladder filling and relief with voiding led to a prevalence figure of 2,133 per 100,000 [20]. The final estimated figure on PBS in this large survey was 2.3%.

Recently, two large important studies have emerged from Asia. Japanese investigators conducted an Internet-based survey among randomly selected women in different age groups [21]. Questionnaires with socioeconomic data and the ICSI questionnaire were sent to little over 80,000 women, of whom 32,074 (39.9%) responded. The response rate was as expected, based on other earlier Internet experiences. Responders with severe symptoms (12 or greater in ICSI), nocturia twice or more and pain (two points or more) were defined as possible cases of PBS. The total number of these women in different age groups was 85 leading to a prevalence figure of 0.265% (265 per 100,000). The authors concluded that this prevalence is very close to that reported from Western countries and there seems to be no difference between the races.

Likewise, a true population-based study was also reported from Korea [22]. A geographically stratified random sample of female adults 18–71 years old was interviewed by telephone calls using ICSI. The survey conducted 52,625 telephone calls and 2,323 women were contacted, 2,300 of these being included in the analysis. The mean composite ICSI score for this group was 4.6, the mean symptom score was 3.6 and problem score was 1.0. Only 8 women reported severe symptoms (12 or greater) and severe problems. Of them, six fulfilled the criteria for "probable PBS/IC" representing 0.26% of the whole study population. Thus the estimated prevalence of PBS/IC was 261 per 100,000 South Korean women, which is almost identical to the respective figure in Japan.

Overall, the lowest reported prevalence of IC is 4.5 per 100,000 [13] and the highest is 12,600 [17]. The truth most often lies in between the extremes. Considering all studies together, the correct figure might well be in the range of 500 per 100,000.

Little is known about racial and ethnic differences in the prevalence of PBS/IC. The only population-based study dealing with these aspects from the United States

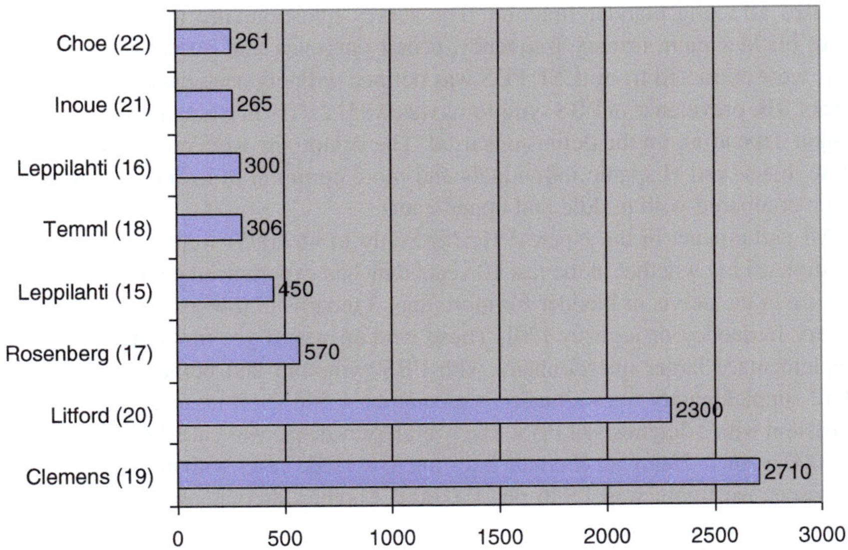

Fig. 2.1 Prevalence/100,000 in population-based epidemiological studies on PBS/IC. *Asia*: Choe, Inoue; *Europe*: Leppilahti, Temml; *USA*: Rosenberg, Litford, Clemens

reported no differences between white, black or Hispanic individuals [19]. Most studies concern white Caucasian or at least do not mention anything about possible other races in the surveys. The new reports from Japan and Korea do not show any marked difference with data from Western countries (Fig. 2.1).

Associated Diseases

It has been known for quite a long time that patients with PBS/IC symptoms have an increased number of certain other diseases or conditions compared with normal population. Hand observed already in 1949 an association of allergies [23], and Sant and Theoharides reported that IC patients suffered often of allergies, migraines and some autoimmune diseases [24]. Alagiri reported in 1997 that patients with IC were 100 times more likely to have inflammatory bowel disease and 30 times more likely to have systemic lupus erythematosus [25]. This surprising finding was detected in a questionnaire-based study evaluating 12 different disease processes among 6,783 individuals in the national database of the Interstitial Cystitis Association (ICA). After calculations among responders and nonresponders and comparisons with population-based prevalence figures of the various diseases, it was estimated that 45.4% of the database individuals had symptoms of allergy and 41.5% had been diagnosed with that disorder. The respective figures for irritable bowel syndrome were 37.7 and 30.2%. Other associated diseases were not that common but their prevalence was clearly greater than that in normal population.

Table 2.3 List of diseases/conditions with increased prevalence among patients with PBS/IC compared with normal population

Different allergies (rhinitis, hay fever, skin rashes, food allergy)
Asthma
Irritable bowel syndrome
Fibromyalgia
Chronic fatigue syndrome
[a]Inflammatory bowel disease (ulcerative colitis, Crohn's disease)
[a]Rheumatoid arthritis
[a]Sjögren's syndrome
[a]Lupus erythematosus
Vulvodynia
Endometriosis
Migraine headache
Tension headache
Temporomandibular disorder
Low back pain
Sensitive skin

[a] Eventual autoimmune diseases

These conditions included fibromyalgia, sensitive skin, vulvodynia, migraine and endometriosis.

Speculations on the possible autoimmune aetiology of IC led to an investigation among patients with Sjögren's syndrome (SS) in Finland [26]. All women aged 18–71 years in the Finnish SS patients' organisation ($n = 1{,}214$) were sent the ICSI questionnaire. The reference group consisted of 2,000 randomly selected women from national population registry. The response rate was 81.5% among the SS patients and 67.2% in the reference group. Subjects with high symptom and problem scores (12 or greater) and nocturia ≥2 times and pain ≥2, without urinary infection or pregnancy, were regarded as probable IC patients. According to these criteria, 5% of the SS patients and 0.3% of the control group fulfilled the criteria for probable IC. Thus the prevalence of IC was 17 times higher among SS patients compared with normal population.

Recently, Nickel reported on a questionnaire survey among 205 patients with PBS/IC and 117 controls matched for age [27]. Percentages for the self-reported diagnoses or symptoms were 38.6% for irritable bowel syndrome in PBS/IC group compared with 5.2% in controls, 17.7% for fibromyalgia versus 2.6% in controls, 9.5% for chronic fatigue syndrome versus 1.7% and 17% for vulvodynia versus 0.9%. Also migraine headache, tension headache, temporomandibular disorder and low back pain were statistically significantly more common in the patient group with PBS/IC compared with the controls. Considerable number of PBS/IC patients had more than one associated condition and with increasing number of these, the well-being measured by several psychosocial parameters decreased. The various diseases and conditions with increased prevalence in patients with PBS/IC are seen in Table 2.3.

Genetic Aspects

Reports on an increased occurrence of IC in twins or close family members [28–30] have suggested genetic susceptibility for the disease. Warren published a survey [31] among members of the ICA inquiring by mail about the existence of IC or respective symptoms in first-degree (parents, siblings, children) family members and came to the conclusion that in these female relatives of patients with NIDDK-confirmed IC, the prevalence of IC with similar criteria may be as high as 995 per 100,000. Despite many laboratory-based genetic innovations we are still missing large-scale population-based genetic studies on IC/PBS.

Future

The methodological problems associated with epidemiological studies on the prevalence of IC/PBS have been recently addressed by Berry and associates [32]. They pointed out that no information exists about the ability of various questionnaires to accurately identify women with IC/PBS (sensitivity) or distinguish them from women diagnosed with other similar conditions (specificity). To solve these problems, a rather large case definition panel was established and validation studies carried out. Two epidemiological definitions were developed, one with high sensitivity (81%) and low specificity (54%), and the other with converse figures (48% sensitivity and 83% specificity). The authors concluded that for reliable prevalence studies two definitions may have to be used. Hopefully, there will be more international co-operation to establish common epidemiological criteria which can be used worldwide to gain comparable figures for analysis.

References

1. Gillenwater JY, Wein AJ. Summary of the National Institute of arthritis, diabetes, digestive and kidney diseases workshop on interstitial cystitis, National Institutes of Health, Bethesda, Maryland, August 28–29, 1987. J Urol. 1988;140:203–6.
2. Hanno PM, Landis JR, Matthews-Cook Y, et al. The diagnosis of interstitial cystitis revisited; lessons learned from the National Institutes of Health Interstitial Cystitis Database study. J Urol. 1999;161:553–7.
3. O'Leary MP, Sant GR, Fowler Jr FJ, et al. The interstitial cystitis symptom index and problem index. Urology. 1997;49:58–63.
4. Lubeck DP, Whitmore K, Sant GR, et al. Psychometric validation of the O'Leary-Sant interstitial cystitis symptom index in a clinical trial of pentosan polysulfate sodium. Urology. 2001;57:62–6.
5. Parsons CL, Dell J, Stanford EJ, et al. Increased prevalence of interstitial cystitis: previously unrecognized urologic and gynecologic cases identified using a new symptom questionnaire and intravesical potassium sensitivity. Urology. 2002;60:573–8.
6. Kushner L, Moldwin RM, Kushner L, et al. Efficiency of questionnaires used to screen for interstitial cystitis. J Urol. 2006;176:587–92.

7. van de Merwe JP, Nordling J, Bouchelouche P, et al. Diagnostic criteria, classification and nomenclature for painful bladder syndrome/interstitial cystitis: an ESSIC proposal. Eur Urol. 2008;53:60–7.
8. Oravisto KJ. Epidemiology of interstitial cystitis. Ann Chir Gynaecol Fenn. 1975;64:75–7.
9. Held PJ, Hanno PM, Wein AJ, et al. Epidemiology of interstitial cystitis: 2. In: Hanno PM, Staskin DR, Krane RJ, Wein AJ, editors. Interstitial cystitis. New York: Springer; 1990. p. 29–48.
10. Jones CA, Harris MA, Nyberg L. Prevalence of interstitial cystitis in the United States. J Urol. 1994;151:423A. Abstract 781.
11. Curhan GC, Speizer FE, Hunter DJ, et al. Epidemiology of interstitial cystitis: a population based study. J Urol. 1999;161:549–52.
12. Bade JJ, Rijcken B, Mensink HJ. Interstitial cystitis in The Netherlands: prevalence, diagnostic criteria and therapeutic preferences. J Urol. 1995;154:2035–7. Discussion 2037–8.
13. Miki M, Yamada T. Interstitial cystitis in Japan. BJU Int. 2000;86:634–7.
14. Nickel JC, Teichman JMH, Gregoire M, et al. Prevalence, diagnosis, characterization and treatment of prostatitis, interstitial cystitis and epididymitis in outpatient urological practice: the Canadian PIE study. Urology. 2005;66:935–40.
15. Leppilahti M, Tammela TLJ, Huhtala H, Auvinen A. Prevalence of symptoms related to interstitial cystitis in women: a population based study in Finland. J Urol. 2002;168:139–43.
16. Leppilahti M, Sairanen J, Tammela TLJ, et al. Prevalence of clinically confirmed interstitial cystitis in women: a population based study in Finland. J Urol. 2005;174:581–3.
17. Rosenberg MT, Hazzard M. Prevalence of interstitial cystitis symptoms in women: a population based study in the primary care office. J Urol. 2005;174:2231–4.
18. Temml C, Wehrberger C, Riedl C, et al. Prevalence and correlates for interstitial cystitis symptoms in women participating in a health screening project. Eur Urol. 2007;51:803–9.
19. Clemens JQ, Link CL, Eggers PW, et al. Prevalence of painful bladder symptoms and effect on quality of life in black, hispanic and white men and women. J Urol. 2007;177:1390–4.
20. Litford KL, Curhan GC. Prevalence of painful bladder syndrome in older women. Urology. 2009;73:494–8.
21. Inoue Y, Mita K, Kakehashi M, et al Prevalence of painful bladder syndrome (PBS) symptoms in adult women in general population in Japan. Neurourol Urodyn. 2009;28:214–8.
22. Choe JH, Son H, Song YS, et al. Prevalence of painful bladder syndrome/interstitial cystitis-like symptoms in women: a population-based study in Korea. World J Urol. 2010. doi: 10.1007/s00345-010-0536-4
23. Hand JR. Interstitial cystitis: report of 223 cases (204 women and 19 men). J Urol. 1949;61:291–310.
24. GR S, Theoharides TC. The role of mast cell in interstitial cystitis. Urol Clin North Am. 1994;21:41–53.
25. Alagiri M, Chottiner S, Ratner V, et al. Interstitial cystitis: unexplained associations with other chronic disease and pain syndromes. Urology. 1997;49:52–7.
26. Leppilahti M, Tammela TLJ, Huhtala H, et al. Interstitial cystitis-like urinary symptoms among patients with Sjögren's syndrome – a population-based study in Finland. Am J Med. 2003;115:62–5.
27. Nickel JC, Tripp DA, Pontari M, et al. Interstitial cystitis/painful bladder syndrome and associated medical conditions with an emphasis on irritable bowel syndrome, fibromyalgia and chronic fatigue syndrome. J Urol. 2010;184:1358–63.
28. Oravisto KJ. Interstitial cystitis as an autoimmune disease: review. Eur Urol. 1980;6:10–3.
29. Warren JW, Keay SK, Meyers D, Xu J Concordance of interstitial cystitis in monozygotic and dizygotic twin pairs. Urology. 2001;57:22–5.
30. Dimitrakov JD. A case of familial clustering of interstitial cystitis and chronic pelvic pain syndrome. Urology. 2001;58:281–3.
31. Warren JW, Jackson TL, Langenberg P, et al. Prevalence of interstitial cystitis in first-degree relatives of patients with interstitial cystitis. Urology. 2004;63:17–21.
32. Berry SH, Bogart LM, Pham C, et al. Development, validation and testing of an epidemiological case definition of interstitial cystitis/painful bladder syndrome. J Urol. 2010;183:1848–52.

Chapter 3
Diagnostic Criteria, Classification and Nomenclature for Bladder Pain Syndrome

Joop P. van de Merwe, Jørgen Nordling, Pierre Bouchelouche, Mauro Cervigni, Magnus Fall, and Jean-Jacques Wyndaele

Introduction

The National Institute of Diabetes and Digestive and Kidney Disease (NIDDK) formulated criteria for a diagnosis of interstitial cystitis (IC) in 1987 [1, 2]. These criteria were meant for scientific studies but by time there has been varying understanding of the substance of these criteria causing a lot of confusion. An illustration

---

The text of this chapter is partly based on a paper published previously: Van de Merwe JP, Nordling J, Bouchelouche P, et al., European Urology 2008;53:60–7.

J.P. van de Merwe, MD, PhD
Departments of Immunology and Internal Medicine, Erasmus MC, University Medical Center Rotterdam, Rotterdam, The Netherlands
e-mail: email@jpvandemerwe.nl

J. Nordling, MD, Dr.med.Sci, FEBU (✉)
Department of Urology, Herlev Hospital, University of Copenhagen, Kurvej 11, Bagsvaerd 2880, Denmark
jnordling@dadlnet.dk

P. Bouchelouche, MD
Department of Clinical Biochemistry, Koege Hospital, University of Copenhagen, Lykkebaek vej 1, Copenhagen 4600, Denmark
e-mail: pnb@regionsjaelland.dk

M. Cervigni, MD
Department of Urogynecology, S. Carlo-IDI, Rome, Italy

Department Obstetrics and Gynecology, Catholic University, Rome, Italy

M. Fall, MD, PhD
Department of Urology, Institute of Clinical Sciences, Sahlgrens Academy at University of Gothenburg, Bruna straket 11B, Göteborg 41345, Sweden

J.-J. Wyndaele, MD, DSci, PhD
Department of Urology, University Hospital Antwerp and Antwerp University, 10 Wilrijkstraat, Edegem 2650, Belgium

J. Nordling et al. (eds.), *Bladder Pain Syndrome: A Guide for Clinicians*,
DOI 10.1007/978-1-4419-6929-3_3, © Springer Science+Business Media New York 2013

Table 3.1 Overview of mandatory features in publications for the diagnosis of interstitial cystitis (IC), painful bladder syndrome (PBS), bladder pain syndrome (BPS) and hypersensitive bladder syndrome (HSB, HBS)

		Mandatory feature			
Source	Name	Pain	Urgency	Frequency	Other
NIDDK, 1988 [1]	IC	No	No	No	Pain *or* urgency, glomerulations, Hunner's ulcer, other
Holm–Bentzen et al., 1987 [4]	IC is a subgroup of PB disease	Yes	No	No	
Witherow et al., 1989 [5]	PBS	Yes	No	Yes	
ICS, 2002 [6]	PBS	Yes	No	No	
	IC	Yes	No	No	IC = PBS + cystoscopic and histological features
EAU, 2010 [7]	PBS/BPS	Yes	No	No	
ICI, 2004 [8]	PBS/IC	Yes	No	No	
ESSIC, 2006, 2008 [9, 10]	BPS types	Yes	No	No	
ARHP, 2007 [11]	IC/PBS	Yes	No	No	Urgency *or* frequency
Homma, 2007, 2009 [12, 13]	HSB/HBS	No	No	No	
	PBS	Yes	No	No	
	IC	No	No	No	

of that fact is that the criteria were fulfilled by only one-third of patients thought to have IC by experts [3]. Moreover, pain is not a mandatory feature for the diagnosis. This is in contrast to all definitions published after 1987 [4–11] with the exception of the Japanese guideline (Table 3.1) [12, 13]. This guideline distinguishes hypersensitive bladder syndrome, painful bladder syndrome and interstitial cystitis and pain is only mandatory for the diagnosis of painful bladder syndrome (PBS). The International Continence Society (ICS) defined the term "PBS" as "the complaint of suprapubic pain related to bladder filling, accompanied by other symptoms such as increased daytime and night-time frequency, in the absence of proven urinary infection or other obvious pathology"[6]. The name IC was reserved for PBS with typical cystoscopic and histologic features. Logically IC should include some form of inflammation in the deeper layers of the bladder wall, whereas PBS should include pain in the region of the bladder. At the International Consultation on Interstitial Cystitis in Japan (ICICJ) in 2003, it became clear that the evaluation and diagnosis of patients differed enormously among centres in Europe, North America and Japan [14] and that a new approach was urgently needed.

Criteria for the diagnosis of a disease are needed if the target disease may be confused with other diseases (confusable diseases) because of overlapping features [15]. Symptoms and signs for use in diagnostic criteria do not need to be specific for the target disease. On the contrary, if a specific symptom or sign existed for the target disease, a diagnosis would only require the presence of the specific feature

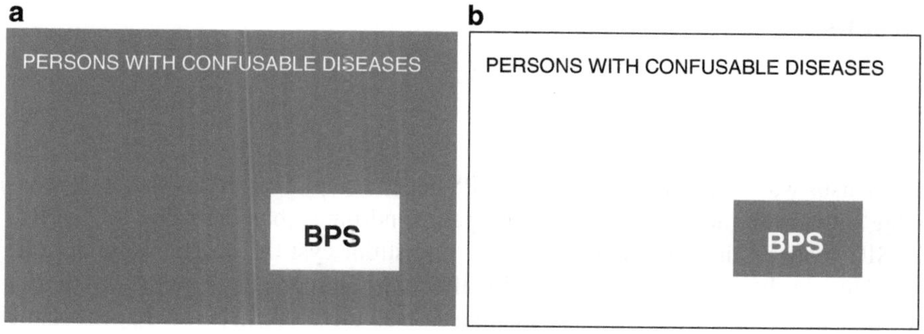

Fig. 3.1 Schematic representation by *grey* areas of a diagnosis of BPS by exclusion of all confusable diseases (**a**) or by recognition of a typical combination of features of BPS (**b**)

and diagnostic criteria would not be necessary. For a diagnosis, the target disease has to be recognized in a pool of confusable diseases by exclusion of (all) confusable diseases or by recognition of a typical combination of features of the target disease (Fig. 3.1). For the diagnosis of bladder pain syndrome (BPS), the name we prefer for IC and PBS (see below), ideally both methods should be used because:

- Confusable diseases are more common than BPS, so recognition of a confusable disease is mandatory because many can be treated.
- Failure to diagnose a confusable disease if present would automatically incorrectly yield a diagnosis of BPS.
- Patients may have two diseases at the same time, a confusable disease and BPS.

The diagnosis of BPS is thus made on the basis of exclusion of confusable diseases in addition to the presence of a typical combination of symptoms and signs of BPS. If the main urinary symptoms are not explained by a single diagnosis (confusable disease or BPS), the presence of a second diagnosis should be considered.

Methods

ESSIC held meetings in 2003 and 2004 (Copenhagen, Denmark) on standardization of medical history, physical examination, laboratory tests, symptoms evaluation, urodynamics and technique and classification of cystoscopic and histologic findings [16]. Briefly, glomerulations represent submucosal bleedings at cystoscopy with hydrodistention, with grade 2 being large submucosal bleeding (ecchymosis) and grade 3 diffuse global mucosal bleeding. Detrusor mastocytosis is defined as mast cell counts exceeding 28 mast cells/mm^2 [16]. At ESSIC meetings in 2005 in Baden and 2006 in London, the following approach to the diagnosis of BPS was discussed:

- Selection of patients who need further evaluation for the presence of BPS.
- Definition of confusable diseases that may cause urinary symptoms.
- Classification of BPS.

Results

Name

Consensus was obtained that the name BPS better complies with our present knowledge and current nomenclature of other pain syndromes than the name IC or PBS. ESSIC realized that omitting the name “interstitial cystitis” might cause serious problems in different health systems by affecting reimbursement or the possibility for patients to gain disability benefits, and it was therefore decided that the name bladder pain syndrome/interstitial cystitis (BPS/IC) could be used parallel with BPS for the time being.

Selection of Patients

It was agreed that BPS would be diagnosed on the basis of chronic (>6 months) [7] pelvic pain, pressure or discomfort perceived to be related to the urinary bladder accompanied by at least one other urinary symptom such as persistent urge to void or frequency. Confusable diseases as the cause of the symptoms must be excluded. Further documentation and classification of BPS might be performed according to findings at cystoscopy with hydrodistention and morphologic findings in bladder biopsies. The presence of other organ symptoms as well as cognitive, behavioural, emotional and sexual symptoms should be addressed.

Confusable Diseases

Diseases that were discussed and accepted as confusable diseases for BPS are listed in Table 3.2 with an indication on how they can be recognized or excluded.

Classification of BPS

Consensus was obtained that for the documentation of positive but not mandatory signs for the diagnosis of BPS, hydrodistention at cystoscopy was a prerequisite and if indicated also a biopsy to document histologic details of BPS. Cystoscopic features that were accepted as positive signs of BPS were glomerulations grade 2–3 or Hunner’s lesions, or both (see below). Histologic findings that were accepted as positive signs of BPS were inflammatory infiltrates, granulation tissue, detrusor mastocytosis and/or intrafascicular fibrosis.

Table 3.2 Confusable diseases for bladder pain syndrome (BPS)

Confusable disease	Excluded or diagnosed by *
Carcinoma and carcinoma in situ	Cystoscopy and biopsy
Infection with	
Common intestinal bacteria	Routine bacterial culture
Chlamydia trachomatis, Ureaplasma urealyticum, Mycoplasma hominis, Mycoplasma genitalium, Corynebacterium urealyticum, Candida species	Special cultures
Mycobacterium tuberculosis	Dipstick; if "sterile" pyuria culture for *M. tuberculosis*
Herpes simplex and *Human Papilloma Virus*	Physical examination
Radiation	Medical history
Chemotherapy, including immunotherapy with cyclophosphamide	Medical history
Anti-inflammatory therapy with tiaprofenic acid	Medical history
Bladder neck obstruction and neurogenic outlet obstruction	Uroflowmetry and ultrasound
Bladder stone	Imaging or cystoscopy
Lower ureteric stone	Medical history and/or haematuria: Upper urinary tract imaging such as CT or IVP
Urethral diverticulum	Medical history and physical examination
Urogenital prolapse	Medical history and physical examination
Endometriosis	Medical history and physical examination
Vaginal candidiasis	Medical history and physical examination
Cervical, uterine and ovarian cancer	Physical examination
Incomplete bladder emptying (retention)	Post-void residual urine volume measured by ultrasound scanning
Overactive bladder	Medical history and urodynamics
Prostate cancer	Physical examination and PSA
Benign prostatic obstruction	Uroflowmetry and pressure-flow studies
Chronic bacterial prostatitis	Medical history, physical examination, culture
Chronic non-bacterial	Prostatitis medical history, physical examination, culture
Pudendal nerve entrapment	Medical history, physical examination, nerve block may prove diagnosis
Pelvic floor muscle related pain	Medical history, physical examination

CT = computed tomography; IVP = intravenous pyelogram; PSA = prostate-specific antigen.
* The diagnosis of a confusable disease does not necessarily exclude a diagnosis of BPS

Hunner's Lesion

Hunner's "ulcer" is not a chronic ulcer but rather a distinctive inflammatory lesion presenting a characteristic deep rupture through the mucosa and submucosa provoked by bladder distension. The word "ulcer" suggests that it can be seen at cystoscopy without hydrodistention. Consequently, the name Hunner's ulcer was replaced by Hunner's lesion. The following definition by M. Fall was accepted: "The Hunner's lesion typically presents as a circumscript, reddened mucosal area with small vessels radiating towards a central scar, with a fibrin deposit or coagulum attached to this area. This site ruptures with increasing bladder distension, with petechial oozing of blood from the lesion and the mucosal margins in a waterfall manner. A rather typical, slightly bullous edema develops post-distension with varying peripheral extension". Despite the fact that cystoscopy with hydrodistension is not mandatory as part of the clinical evaluation for a diagnosis of BPS, it is highly recommended as it is virtually the best way to diagnose a Hunner's lesion with major therapeutic implications.

Types of BPS

BPS shows large variations among patients in clinical presentation, complaints, quality of life, cystoscopic and biopsy findings, response to treatment, clinical course and prognosis. It was generally appreciated that these characteristics may be correlated only to some extent. Diagnostic criteria and disease classification should facilitate future studies on these relationships. Consequently, types of BPS were defined based on the findings used to document positive signs for the diagnosis of BPS. The name BPS will be followed by a type indication that consists of two symbols: Symbols 1, 2 or 3 indicate findings at cystoscopy with hydrodistention and symbols A, B or C of biopsy findings. X indicates that no cystoscopy with hydrodistention (first symbol) or no biopsy (second symbol) was done (Table 3.3). BPS types thus also allow classification of patients with normal findings at cystoscopy with hydrodistention and normal biopsies as long as they fulfil the patient selection criteria and also confusable diseases are excluded (BPS type 1A; see Fig. 3.2 and Table 3.3).

Table 3.3 Classification of types of bladder pain syndrome on the basis of findings at cystoscopy with hydrodistension and of biopsies

		Cystoscopy with hydrodistension			
		Not done	Normal	Glomerulations[a]	Hunner's lesion[b]
Biopsy	Not done	XX	1X	2X	3X
	Normal	XA	1A	2A	3A
	Inconclusive	XB	1B	2B	3B
	Positive[c]	XC	1C	2C	3C

[a]Cystoscopy: Glomerulations grade 2–3

[b]With or without glomerulations

[c]Histology showing inflammatory infiltrates, detrusor mastocytosis, granulation tissue and/or intrafascicular fibrosis

Discussion

Why Do We Need New Criteria?

The NIDDK criteria for the diagnosis of IC were intended for use in scientific studies. These criteria, however, did not comprise more than one-third of patients considered to have IC by experts [3]. Pain was not a mandatory feature for the diagnosis in contrast to almost all definitions published after 1987 [4–10]. Moreover, patients under the age of 18 years were excluded as were those with voided volumes of more than 350 ml, thus making it difficult to study early stages of the disease. These considerations made the NIDDK criteria less useful in clinical situations and limited their value in scientific studies because the criteria only recognized a biased minority of the patient population. The need for the design of new diagnostic criteria is obvious. To avoid unacceptable discrepancies between scientific studies and clinical practice, it was considered essential that new diagnostic criteria could be used in both situations.

Why Is Pain a Prerequisite?

BPS is characterized by urinary bladder pain [4–10, 17, 18]. A recent study, however, demonstrated a correlation between pain bother in the IC problem index (burning, discomfort, pain or pressure) and the presence of pain in the IC symptom index of only 0.7 [19]. This finding underscores that many patients report a sensation of pressure or discomfort in the bladder/pelvic area and do not report this sensation as pain but rather as urgency (see below). The International Association for the Study of Pain (IASP; http://www.iasp-pain.org) definition of pain is: “An unpleasant sensory and emotional experience associated with actual or potential tissue damage, or described in terms of such damage” [20]. Patients having microwave treatment for benign prostatic obstruction producing tissue damage at the bladder neck report the same sensation of pressure and discomfort in the bladder region [21–23]. The sensation is therefore by definition a pain sensation, but not described as such by the patient. Pain or the equivalent pressure, discomfort perceived to be related to the bladder, was, therefore, considered to be a prerequisite for the description of symptoms on the basis of which patients should undergo further investigations for BPS. The increase of pain on bladder filling was left out of the description because this association is not always present [18, 24, 25].

Why Is Urgency Not Included in the Description of Patients Who Need Further Evaluation for BPS?

Urgency is defined by the ICS as the complaint of a sudden compelling desire to pass urine, which is difficult to defer [6]. BPS is commonly mistaken for overactive bladder (OAB) and vice versa because the term “urgency” is used to describe

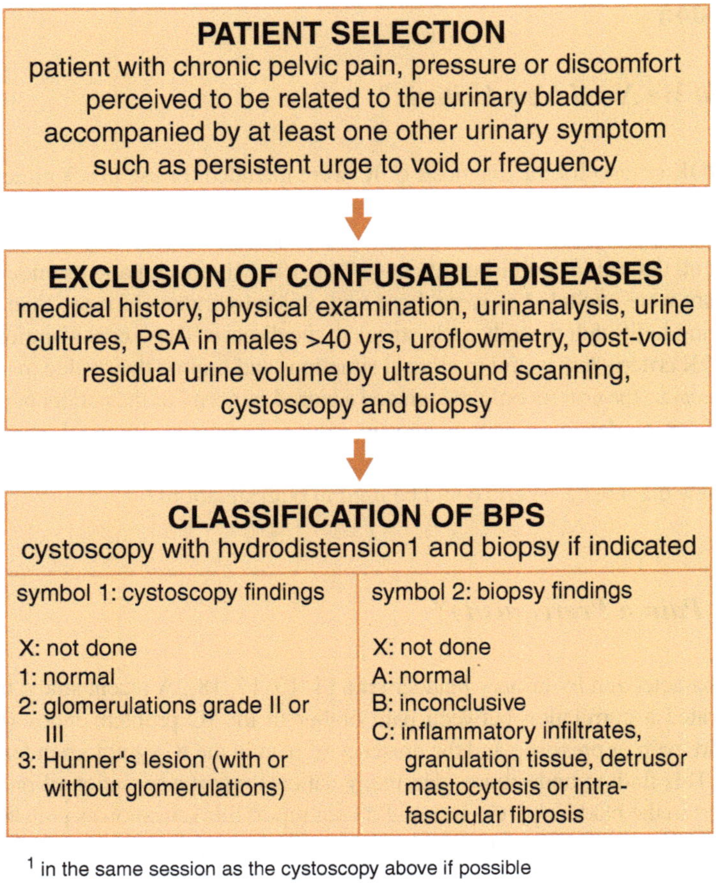

Fig. 3.2 Schematic representation of the proposed approach for the diagnosis of bladder pain syndrome (BPS)

the symptoms of both disorders. For some women, urgency is used to indicate the heightened need to make it to a toilet quickly to avoid getting wet, whereas other women consider urgency to mean a need to void as a way of avoiding intensifying pain, pressure or discomfort. The first group is most likely to have OAB, and the latter group can be expected to have BPS [18]. Urinary urgency was left out of the description of patients who need further evaluation for the presence of BPS for several reasons. First, urgency is the key symptom of OAB [17, 24], a major confusable disease for BPS, that is ten times more common than BPS [18]. Second, the clinical aspects of urgency are complex [6, 18, 24, 26–29]. At a meeting arranged by the Association of Reproductive Health Professionals in the United States in February 2007 involving 33 urologists, gynaecologists and nurses it was proposed to use the term "persistent urge" instead of urgency to avoid confusion with OAB [11]. Many patients find the strong, unpleasant urge to void the most dominant and disabling part of their symptoms, so patients (and doctors) are often confused because, with the present terminology, a patient is not allowed to use the word urge to describe complaints. In the Oxford Advanced Learner's Dictionary of Current English urge is defined as "a strong desire", whereas urgency is defined as "needing prompt decision or action" [30]. So the words urgency and urge describe very well the difference between the sensation felt by the patient with OAB and the patient with BPS. Persistent urge was therefore included in the definition as a typical symptom, such as frequency. It must be stressed that the presence of these symptoms is not necessary to suspect or diagnose BPS.

Why is the Potassium Sensitivity Test Not Used as a Diagnostic Tool?

The potassium sensitivity test (PST) is based on the hypothesis that instilled potassium provokes symptoms such as pain and urgency when the bladder epithelium is abnormally permeable. The PST has been found positive in 66–83% of patients with BPS but also in similar proportions of patients with cystitis due to radiation and other causes, prostatitis and bladder cancer and even in one-third of healthy subjects [31–35]. The low sensitivity and specificity make the PST unsuitable as a diagnostic tool [36].

Why is the APF Test Not Used as a Diagnostic Tool?

The antiproliferative factor (APF) is a peptide secreted by bladder epithelial cells from patients with BPS [37]. APF inhibits bladder cell proliferation by means of regulation of cell adhesion protein and growth factor production. It has been detected in 86% of women with BPS, compared with 8% of asymptomatic control women, 12% of women with bacterial cystitis and 0% of women with vulvovaginitis, yielding sensitivity and specificity values of 91.4 and 90.6%, respectively. The test is advocated as a useful non-invasive means for diagnosing BPS in women [38]. However, no data on the clinical value of the APF test for the diagnosis of BPS are available to support this claim. Moreover, the test is not yet widely available, so the APF test cannot be recommended as a diagnostic tool to date.

Why Should Confusable Diseases Be Excluded?

In evidence-based medicine, diagnoses are based on medical history, physical examination and appropriate clinical investigations to eliminate diseases from the list of differential diagnoses (confusable diseases) and to confirm the final diagnosis.

BPS may occur together with confusable diseases such as chronic or remitting urinary infections or endometriosis.

Cystoscopy with hydrodistention and biopsies might in this situation document positive signs of BPS, thereby making a double diagnosis more probable. For therapeutic studies it makes sense to exclude patients who also have a confusable disease because symptoms and signs may be caused by BPS, the confusable disease or both. For prevalence studies of BPS, on the other hand, all cases with BPS should be included, also those with a confusable disease. This approach eliminates the need for separate diagnostic criteria for clinical practice and scientific studies.

Why Do We Need Various BPS Types?

Unravelling the cause of a disease usually begins with grouping patients with similar symptoms and signs. The hypothesis is that these patients have a disease with the same aetiology and pathogenesis that is better recognized in homogeneous than in heterogeneous groups. This has been the reason for dividing BPS patients into subgroups (types) based on positive signs. It is worth noting that the Hunner type of disease stands out as a specific type not only cystoscopically but also with reference to histopathology, response to treatment and complications [7, 39].

Why Do We Propose to Change the Name of IC?

Hanno recently stated that the term IC was not descriptive of the clinical syndrome or the pathologic findings in many cases. Moreover, the term IC is misleading because it directs attention only to the urinary bladder and inflammation [40]. The name IC excludes patients with typical IC symptoms but normal cystoscopic and histologic findings from disease classification in many countries around the world. The inability to classify these patients might have severe negative consequences for the patients, for example, in therapeutic, personal, social and many other aspects. IC, originally considered a bladder disease, is now considered a chronic pain syndrome [41]. These perceptions have led to the current effort to reconsider the name of the disorder [7, 40, 42, 43]. It is also the contention of the ESSIC that the existing terminology of IC hampers development in this area.

Why Do We Propose to Choose BPS as the New Name?

For some time now there has been much work going on in international organizations to create a logical and workable terminology for chronic (persistent) pain conditions. For background information we refer to the 2010 Guidelines on Chronic Pelvic Pain issued by the European Association of Urology (EAU) [7]. The EAU definitions are in line with recent recommendations for terminology from the ICS [6] and use the axial structure of the IASP classification [20]. This implies a taxonomy-like approach under the umbrella term of chronic pelvic pain syndrome. Further identification is based on the primary organ that appears to be affected on clinical grounds. Urologic pelvic pain syndromes are divided into bladder pain syndrome, urethral pain syndrome, penile pain syndrome, prostate pain syndrome and others. More specific terminology is based on the identification of, for example, inflammation or infection [42, 44]. The classification system of chronic pelvic pain syndromes aims to draw together the expertise of many specialist groups. The impact of the classification of chronic pelvic pain syndromes thus goes far beyond the scope of IC. Another essential feature is that the nomenclature and knowledge of pathophysiologic mechanisms do not conflict with each other. In this context, the name bladder pain syndrome was considered the best new name for IC to date, because the name is in line with the other chronic pelvic pain syndromes and is in balance with the clinical presentation of the syndrome and the level of knowledge of its pathophysiology. We realize that changing the name of IC into BPS may have emotional implications, understandably for patients, but also for patient organizations with a scope limited to IC and for insurance and reimbursement in different health systems around the world. Considering these consequences, although BPS is the name of choice, ESSIC agrees that including IC in the overall term (BPS/IC) could be used in parallel to BPS during a transition period. In this context, it is worth remembering that a subgroup of BPS patients (representing the Hunner type of disease) presents interstitial inflammation and thus fulfils the requirements of the original term of IC.

References

1. Gillenwater JY, Wein AJ. Summary of the National Institute of Arthritis, Diabetes, Digestive and Kidney Diseases Workshop on Interstitial Cystitis, National Institutes of Health, Bethesda, Maryland, August 28–29, 1987. J Urol. 1988;140:203–6.
2. Wein AJ, Hanno P, Gillenwater JY. An introduction to the problem. In: Hanno P, Staskin DR, Krane RJ, Wein AJ, editors. Interstitial cystitis. London: Springer-Verlag; 1990. pp. 3–15.
3. Hanno PM, Landis JR, Matthews-Cook Y, Kusek J, Nyberg Jr L. The diagnosis of interstitial cystitis revisited: lessons learned from the National Institutes of Health Interstitial Cystitis Database study. J Urol. 1999;161:553–7.
4. Holm-Bentzen M, Jacobsen F, Nerstrom B, Lose G, Kristensen JK, Pedersen RH, Krarup T, Feggetter J, Bates P, Barnard R, et al. Painful bladder disease: clinical and pathoanatomical differences in 115 patients. J Urol. 1987;138:500–2.
5. Witherow RO, Gillespie L, McMullen L, Goldin RD, Walker MM. Painful bladder syndrome – a clinical and immunopathological study. Br J Urol. 1989;64:158–61.
6. Abrams P, Cardozo L, Fall M, Griffiths D, Rosier P, Ulmsten U, van Kerrebroeck P, Victor A, Wein A. The standardisation of terminology of lower urinary tract function: report from the Standardisation Sub-committee of the International Continence Society. Neurourol Urodyn. 2002;21:167–78.
7. Fall M, Baranowski AP, Elneil S, Engeler D, Huges J, Messelink EJ, et al. EAU guidelines on chronic pelvic pain. Eur Urol. 2010;57(1):35–48.

8. Abrams P, Andersson KE, Brubaker L, Cardozo L, Cottenden A, Denis L, Donovan J, Fonda D, Fry C, Griffiths D, et al. Recommendations of the International Scientific Committee: evaluation and treatment of urinary incontinence, pelvic organ prolapse and faecal incontinence. In: Abrams P, Cardozo L, Khoury S, Wein A, editors. Incontinence. Paris: Health Publications Ltd; 2005. p. 1589–630.
9. van de Merwe JP, Nordling J: Interstitial cystitis: definitions and confusable diseases. Essic Meeting 2005 Baden. European Urology Today. 2006;18:6, 7, 16, 17.
10. van de Merwe JP, Nordling J, Bouchelouche P, Bouchelouche K, Cervigni M, Daha LK, Elneil S, Fall M, Hohlbrugger G, Irwin P, et al. Diagnostic criteria, classification, and nomenclature for painful bladder syndrome/interstitial cystitis: an ESSIC proposal. Eur Urol. 2008;53:60–7.
11. ARHP. Definition and nomenclature of interstitial cystitis/painful bladder syndrome (IC/PBS). In: Screening, treatment, and management of interstitial cystitis/painful bladder syndrome; Washington, DC. Association of Reproductive Health Professionals; 2007.p. 5–7.
12. Homma Y. Disease name, definition, diagnosis and evaluation. In: 2nd ICICJ International Consultation on Interstitial Cystitis; 2007; Kyoto, Japan.
13. Homma Y, Ueda T, Tomoe H, Lin AT, Kuo HC, Lee MH, Lee JG, Kim DY, Lee KS. Clinical guidelines for interstitial cystitis and hypersensitive bladder syndrome. Int J Urol. 2009;16:597–615.
14. Ueda T, Sant GR, Hanno PM, Yoshimura N. Proceedings of the International Consultation on Interstitial Cystitis. March 28–30, 2003. Kyoto, Japan. Int J Urol. 2003;10(Suppl i–iv):S1–70.
15. Fries JF, Hochberg MC, Medsger Jr TA, Hunder GG, Bombardier C. Criteria for rheumatic disease. Different types and different functions. The American College of Rheumatology Diagnostic and Therapeutic Criteria Committee. Arthritis Rheum. 1994;37:454–62.
16. Nordling J, Anjum FH, Bade JJ, Bouchelouche K, Bouchelouche P, Cervigni M, Elneil S, Fall M, Hald T, Hanus T, et al. Primary evaluation of patients suspected of having interstitial cystitis (IC). Eur Urol. 2004;45:662–9.
17. Abrams P. Urgency: the key to defining the overactive bladder. BJU Int. 2005;96 Suppl 1:1–3.
18. Hanno P. Toward optimal health: Philip Hanno, M.D., M.P.H., discusses improved management of painful bladder syndrome (interstitial cystitis). Interview by Jodi R. Godfrey. J Womens Health (Larchmt). 2007;16(1):3–8.
19. Sirinian E, Azevedo K, Payne CK. Correlation between 2 interstitial cystitis symptom instruments. J Urol. 2005;173:835–40.
20. Merskey H, Bogduk N. Classification of chronic pain, descriptions of chronic pain syndromes and definitions of pain terms. Seattle: IASP Press; 2002.
21. Trachtenberg J, Roehrborn CG. Updated results of a randomized, double-blind, multicenter sham-controlled trial of microwave thermotherapy with the Dornier Urowave in patients with symptomatic benign prostatic hyperplasia. Urowave Investigators Group. World J Urol. 1998;16:102–8.
22. Tsai YS, Lin JS, Tong YC, Tzai TS, Yang WH, Chang CC, Cheng HL, Lin YM, Jou YC. Transurethral microwave thermotherapy for symptomatic benign prostatic hyperplasia: short-term experience with Prostcare. Urol Int. 2000;65:89–94.
23. Wagrell L, Schelin S, Nordling J, Richthoff J, Magnusson B, Schain M, Larson T, Boyle E, Duelund J, Kroyer K, et al. Three-year follow-up of feedback microwave thermotherapy versus TURP for clinical BPH: a prospective randomized multicenter study. Urology. 2004;64:698–702.
24. Abrams P, Hanno P, Wein A. Overactive bladder and painful bladder syndrome: there need not be confusion. Neurourol Urodyn. 2005;24:149–50.
25. Warren JW, Meyer WA, Greenberg P, Horne L, Diggs C, Tracy JK. Using the International Continence Society's definition of painful bladder syndrome. Urology. 2006;67:1138–42. discussion 1142–1133.

26. Blaivas JG, Panagopoulos G, Weiss JP, Somaroo C, Chaikin DC. The urgency perception score: validation and test-retest. J Urol. 2007;177:199–202.
27. Chambers GK, Fenster HN, Cripps S, Jens M, Taylor D. An assessment of the use of intravesical potassium in the diagnosis of interstitial cystitis. J Urol. 1999;162:699–701.
28. Diggs C, Meyer WA, Langenberg P, Greenberg P, Horne L, Warren JW. Assessing urgency in interstitial cystitis/painful bladder syndrome. Urology. 2007;69:210–4.
29. Parsons CL, Greenberger M, Gabal L, Bidair M, Barme G. The role of urinary potassium in the pathogenesis and diagnosis of interstitial cystitis. J Urol. 1998;159:1862–6. discussion 1866–1867.
30. Hornby AS, Cowie AP, editors. Oxford advanced learner's dictionary of current English. Oxford: University Press; 1985: 946
31. Parsons CL, Stein PC, Bidair M, Lebow D. Abnormal sensitivity to intravesical potassium in interstitial cystitis and radiation cystitis. Neurourol Urodyn. 1994;13:515–20.
32. Parsons CL, Albo M. Intravesical potassium sensitivity in patients with prostatitis. J Urol. 2002;168:1054–7.
33. Yilmaz U, Liu YW, Rothman I, Lee JC, Yang CC, Berger RE. Intravesical potassium chloride sensitivity test in men with chronic pelvic pain syndrome. J Urol. 2004;172:548–50.
34. Hanno P. Is the potassium sensitivity test a valid and useful test for the diagnosis of interstitial cystitis? Against. Int Urogynecol J Pelvic Floor Dysfunct. 2005;16:428–9.
35. Parsons CL, Rosenberg MT, Sassani P, Ebrahimi K, Koziol JA, Zupkas P. Quantifying symptoms in men with interstitial cystitis/prostatitis, and its correlation with potassium-sensitivity testing. BJU Int. 2005;95:86–90.
36. Fall M, Baranowski A, Fowler CJ, Hughes J, Lepinard V, Malone-Lee JG, Messelink EJ, Oberpenning F, Osborne JL, Schumacher S. Guidelines on chronic pelvic pain. European Association of Urology Guidelines 2007;1–70
37. Keay SK, Szekely Z, Conrads TP, Veenstra TD, Barchi Jr JJ, Zhang CO, Koch KR, Michejda CJ. An antiproliferative factor from interstitial cystitis patients is a frizzled 8 protein-related sialoglycopeptide. Proc Natl Acad Sci U S A. 2004;101:11803–8.
38. Keay S, Zhang CO, Hise MK, Hebel JR, Jacobs SC, Gordon D, Whitmore K, Bodison S, Gordon N, Warren JW. A diagnostic in vitro urine assay for interstitial cystitis. Urology. 1998;52:974–8.
39. Peeker R, Fall M. Toward a precise definition of interstitial cystitis: further evidence of differences in classic and nonulcer disease. J Urol. 2002;167:2470–2.
40. Hanno PM. Painful bladder syndrome/interstitial cystitis and related disorders. In: Wein AJ, editor. Campbell-Walsh Urology. 9th ed. Philadelphia: Saunders; 2007. pp. 330–70.
41. Janicki TI. Chronic pelvic pain as a form of complex regional pain syndrome. Clin Obstet Gynecol. 2003;46:797–803.
42. Abrams P, Baranowski A, Berger RE, Fall M, Hanno P, Wesselmann U. A new classification is needed for pelvic pain syndromes–are existing terminologies of spurious diagnostic authority bad for patients? J Urol. 2006;175:1989–90.
43. Hanno P, Keay S, Moldwin R, Van Ophoven A. International consultation on IC – Rome, September 2004/forging an international consensus: progress in painful bladder syndrome/interstitial cystitis. Report and abstracts. Int Urogynecol J Pelvic Floor Dysfunct. 2005;16 Suppl 1:S2–34.
44. Habermacher GM, Chason JT, Schaeffer AJ. Prostatitis/chronic pelvic pain syndrome. Annu Rev Med. 2006;57:195–206.

Part I
Pathophysiology

Chapter 4
Clinical Pathophysiology and Molecular Biology of the Urothelium and the GAG Layer

Gianfranco Tajana and Mauro Cervigni

Background

In an organism, epithelia are sophisticated semipermeable barriers dividing the external environment from the internal one. Their function is an accurate selection of any molecule they encounter. If harmful or useless, molecules can be neutralized or eliminated or absorbed and transformed in ways which make them usable. Other than analyzing the microenvironment they surround, it should be noted that epithelia are an integral part of the "sensory web," the system regulating the overall functioning of the organ they are part of.

In particular, the urothelium can synthesize and release into urine molecules performing significant homeostatic functions [1], as well as act as an efficient mechanosensor [2]. Receptors [3] functionally related to ion channels allow the urothelium to respond to mechanical inputs by generating chemical outputs which stimulate nerve endings, either acutely and/or chronically (Fig. 4.1) [4].

By knocking out one or more genes regulating the synthesis of urothelial receptors, pathological conditions may develop: vesicoureteral reflux, hydronephrosis, renal failure, or pictures caused by some congenital urinary abnormalities and, in particular, by bladder pain syndrome/interstitial cystitis [5]. This has led to suggest a possible involvement of the urothelium in several urological diseases. Aim of this monograph is to define, through a molecular pathophysiological analysis, the actual role played by the urothelium in the "natural history" of such disorders: "passive bystander or active participant?" [6]

G. Tajana, M.D.
Department of Pharmaceutical and Biomedical Sciences (FARMABIOMED),
University of Salerno, Salerno, Italy

M. Cervigni (✉)
Viale Glorioso 13, 00153, Rome, Italy
e-mail: m.cervigni@idi.it

J. Nordling et al. (eds.), *Bladder Pain Syndrome: A Guide for Clinicians*,
DOI 10.1007/978-1-4419-6929-3_4, © Springer Science+Business Media New York 2013

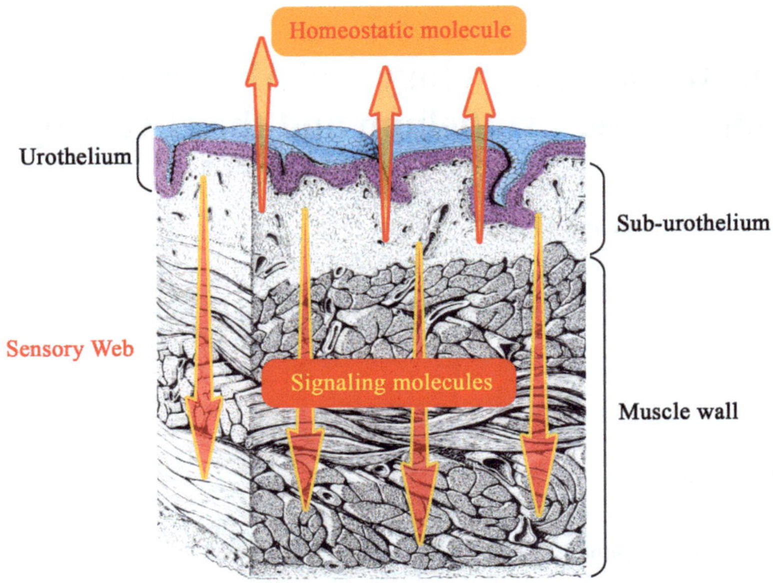

Fig. 4.1 The urothelium releases homeostatic molecules into urine (tissue-type plasminogen activator, urokinase, PP5); through its receptors (vanilloids, purinergic P2X3), it produces "signaling molecules" (ATP, acetylcholine, nitric oxide) regulating the urinary tract physiology through the "sensory web." From Tajana G. Fisiopatologia clinica e biologia molecolare dell'urotelio. Minerva Urol Nefrol 2009; 61(3 suppl 1):1–29. Reprinted with permission from Edizioni Minerva Medica

Urothelium

Molecular Bases of Impermeability and Distensibility

The mucosa lining the urinary tract is impermeable and distensible: this is due to the structural and molecular arrangement of its lining epithelium, termed urothelium.

The urothelium consists of three layers of epithelial cells (urothelial cells): a line of small, irregularly discoidal or polyedrical basal cells; several lines of intermediate cells, and pyriform or clavate cells, with a surface-bound swollen end and a thin extremity between basal cells; and one line of superficial umbrella cells; the latter have a polygonal contour, are very bulky, and, sometimes, binuclear (Fig. 4.2) [7]. Their convex, apical surface protrudes into the lumen and is coated by a thin PAS/Alcian-positive lining (coating); their basal surface exhibits some pits matching with the swollen ends of intermediate cells. Urothelial cells can be typified according to the type of keratin they synthesize: basal cells express keratins 5, 3, 14, 17 and superficial cells express keratins 7, 8, 18, 20 [8].

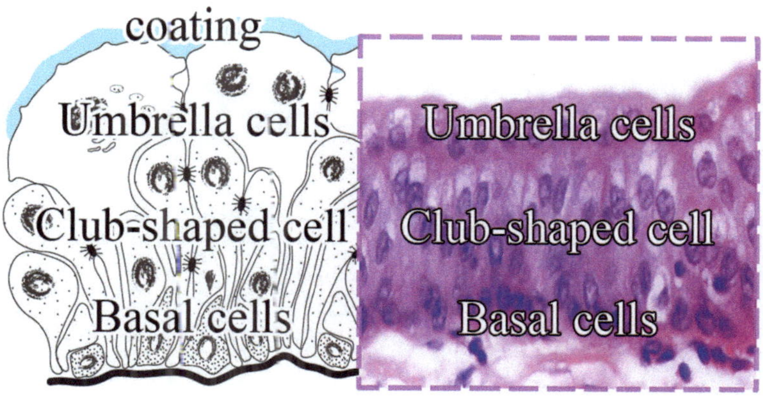

Fig. 4.2 Urothelium cell populations: Urothelial cells. From Tajana G. Fisiopatologia clinica e biologia molecolare dell'urotelio. Minerva Urol Nefrol 2009; 61(3 suppl 1):1–29. Reprinted with permission from Edizioni Minerva Medica

Selective Impermeability: The Three Urothelial Barriers

The urothelium is interfaced not only with urine but also with the sub-urothelium blood microcirculation. Therefore, it must possess efficient systems to guarantee impermeability as well as selective permeability. This mechanism is regulated by the synchronized action of three barriers in the apical, lateral, and basal regions (Fig. 4.3) [9, 10].

The apical barrier prevents the passage of small molecules, neutralizes toxic substances, inhibits the formation of microcrystals, and hinders uropathogen adhesion. It consists of an "umbrella" cell coating and some classes of membrane proteins from the uroplakin family.

Lateral barriers prevent the intercellular percolation of urine thanks to the sequential arrangement of desmosomes, leaky and tight junctions [11]. These junction systems are regulated by at least one hundred genes producing over forty proteins which in turn form a complex molecular "mastic." Junctional proteins belong to three classes: cadherins, claudins, and occludins.

Cadherins (desmoplakin, cadherin-E) are typically found in desmosomes; their functioning depends on calcium levels; calcium chelation makes their adhesive capacity less potent. There exist different isoforms of claudins (1, 2, 4, 5, 7, 8, 12, 14, 16). Of these, a key role is played by 4, 8, 12 which connect "umbrella" cells to clavate and basal cells [12]; a major role is also played by occludins (ZO-1, ZO-2, ZO-3, cingulin) [13, 14]. Some of them, along with laminin, make up the basal barrier, which mediates adhesion to the basal lamina regulating the electrostatic balance of the entire urothelium. Urothelial junction systems provide for intercellular adhesion (gate function) and largely determine the polarity of urothelial cells by preventing the diffusion of phospholipids or the migration of proteins inside the plasma membrane (fence function). Their synthesis is regulated by several factors: EGF, PPAR-gamma, and RAS gene; in particular, a RAS gene mutation

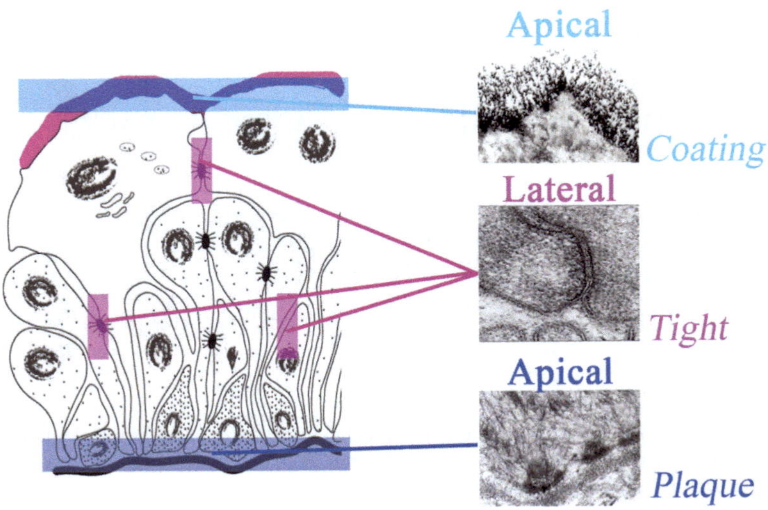

Fig. 4.3 Urothelium impermeability results from cooperation among three barriers: apical, lateral, basal. From Tajana G. Fisiopatologia clinica e biologia molecolare dell'urotelio. Minerva Urol Nefrol 2009; 61(3 suppl 1):1–29. Reprinted with permission from Edizioni Minerva Medica

alters the urothelial tridimensional structure [15]. Finally, the three barriers play an active role in controlling the urothelial phenotype: through the cytoskeleton, barriers can communicate any plasticity changes to the genome. Such changes may affect the whole urothelium during the micturition cycle. Changes are switched into "regulatory signals" of the urothelium gene expression [16].

In the early 1980s, it was shown that during the micturition cycle, urothelial cells go through a deep plastic remodeling aimed at adapting their tridimensional shape to any bladder volumetric change (Fig. 4.4).

Club-shaped cells decrease in height and wedge themselves into basal cells; "umbrella" cells get flat and change their shape from cuboidal to squamous cells with a +22 % increase of their apical surface [17]. Overall, these cytoskeleton-regulated changes [18] are associated to an increase of intracellular calcium and a tenfold greater ATP production [17].

Urothelium distensibility results from an expansion of its apical surface. Discoidal vesicles, present in cytoplasm, merge and integrate with the apical membrane increasing the surface of this latter.

Discoidal vesicles are flattened membrane sacculi; they originate from the Golgi apparatus. When the bladder wall is stretched, they migrate from Golgi apparatus to reach and merge with specific portions of the membrane called attachment plaques; in this way, the cell surface is amplified and the bladder is distended. Discoidal vesicles, other than integrating their phospholipids with those of the umbrella cell plasma membrane, transfer a number of proteins into their bilayer (uroplakins, synaptobrevin, SNAP23, syntaxin) regulating exo-endocytosis mechanisms [19]. The fine-tuning of such mechanisms depends on the alignment between attachment plaques, cytoskeleton, and cytokeratins 7 and 20 forming a kind of "migration

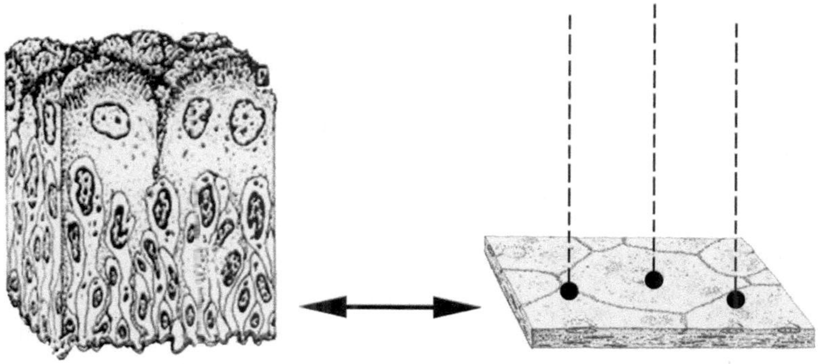

Fig. 4.4 The urothelium is heavily modified through the reversible distension of its urothelial cells. From Tajana G. Fisiopatologia clinica e biologia molecolare dell'urotelio. Minerva Urol Nefrol 2009; 61(3 suppl 1):1–29. Reprinted with permission from Edizioni Minerva Medica

tracks" for discoidal vesicles. Plasma membrane fusion increases the luminal surface by 50 %, from 2,900 to 4,300 μm² [20].

An increased apical surface is associated to a matching endocytosis counter-mechanism, which begins within 5 min. By then, the plasma membrane curbs its expansion by producing endocytosis vesicles; these move into the inside of the cell where they are partially destroyed by lysosomes and, finally, by proteosomes. This establishes an "exocytosis–endocytosis cycle" which adapts the "umbrella" cell surface to the macroscopic changes affecting the bladder during the micturition cycle [21].

Interestingly, the stretch exerted on the apical portion is accompanied by the activation of sodium channels which remain open throughout exocytosis. When the stretch is transferred to the basolateral portions of the cell, potassium channels regulating endocytosis are activated [22]. Hence, the alternate operation of sodium/potassium channels "synchronizes" urothelial distensibility. An alteration of ion flow (elevated potassium levels) may interfere with the exo/endocytosis cycle.

The Role of Dynamin in the Regulation of Vesicular Traffic in the Urothelium

Vesicular traffic is regulated by a cyclic AMP-dependent protein kinase mechanism. However, the "engine" of this cycle starts from a specific molecule: dynamin, a 100-kDa GTP ase [23] which can direct "exo/endocytosis" mechanisms [24].

Dynamin is found in the Golgi apparatus and in other cellular districts [25]. Its close interactions with actin, on the cytoplasmic side of the membrane, makes it a possible "propellant" of vesicular traffic [26]. It has two isoforms (dynamin 1 and 2), directly interacting with the clathrin transport system; both contribute to the structural stabilization of centrosome [27]. Moreover, it is an important transducer and can induce P53 synthesis, decrease the cell proliferation rate, and activate apoptosis through caspase 3 [25]. While dynamin activity is sterically specialized, COOH-terminus regulates endocytosis mechanisms and NH (2)- triggers apoptotic mechanisms [28].

Dynamin activity can be reversibly blocked by Dynasore, a fast-acting small molecule; it was isolated after screening over 16,000 compounds. It acts as a noncompetitive inhibitor and can reversibly block dynamin-dependent endocytosis mechanisms [29].

Attachment Plaques: Molecular Composition

Attachment plaques play a crucial role in the "exo/endocytosis mechanism." Also called Asymmetric Unit Membranes (AUMs), they consist of uroplakins, a set of four protein species (Ia, Ib, II, III). Cryo-electron microscopy shows their crystalline hexamer arrangement; they are 135 nm thick and protrude by 2 nm into the membrane: they have close functional interactions with the cytoskeleton inside and with coating components on the outside.

These complexes are not mere structural stabilizers; they play a crucial role in controlling apical permeability. Uroplakins are found in discoidal vesicles, travel through the Golgi apparatus, and, from here, through the cytoskeleton, are sorted at plaque level where they merge with the plasma membrane [30].

The quali-quantitative assortment of uroplakins varies across various urothelial regions and is affected by the mechanical activity exerted vby the pressure–stretch combination [31]. The assembly of uroplakins implies their partial structural change. This is handled by a set of molecules called maturation-facilitators, consisting of coating components and specific glycosyltransferases [32]. Uroplakins position themselves in specific regions of the phospholipid bilayer, called "rafts," i.e., plasma membrane micro-domains formed by a specific lipid subset (phosphatydilcholine, phosphatydilethanolamine, cerebrosides, sulfatides, and cholesterol) and by a number of coating-related glycophospholipids. The composition of "rafts" can change with the diet and metabolism; they can interfere with the uroplakin function [33]. If damaged, "rafts" may prevent uropathogens from adhering to specific receptors, thus suggesting their paradoxical protective role [34].

The same lipid membrane composition can influence the urothelium exo/endocytosis mechanisms [35].

Urothelial Coating

Urothelial "Coating" Is the Carbohydrate Coating of "Umbrella" Cells

The urothelial lumen is lined by a soft, flexible coating (cell coat, glycocalix, fuzz), a constituent of the apical membrane of "umbrella" cells. This thin layer is all but compact: it is made from a material resembling a frayed "down," under electron microscopy; as to optical microscopy, special fixation techniques should be employed to avoid its solubilization. Histochemistry and immunocytochemistry techniques can detect and identify its molecular components [36].

Coating can be easily identified with Alcian Blue (AB), in a sodium acetate buffer (pH 5.8 or 0.6 M/0.8 M $MgCl_2$). Under transmission electron microscopy, coating can be seen through specific probes like ferritin or ruthenium red. The use of EDX (Energy-dispersive X-ray spectrometry) does confirm its mucopolysaccharide nature [37]. A combination of specific antibodies shows a good correlation between the coating ultrastructural appearance and its molecular composition [38]. The tridimensional morphology of coating, urothelium, and sub-urothelium can be explored in vivo thanks to confocal microscopy and coating-binding fluorescent probes (SYTO 179) [39]; other options include confocal laser endomicroscopy [40] or ultrahigh resolution optical coherence tomography (UHR-OCT): these techniques yield high-resolution morphological images like conventional microscopy [41].

Coating acts as a barrier against small molecules (urea), prevents the formation of microcrystals in urine (nucleation), and provides a significant antibacterial protection by interfering with uropathogen adhesion. A decreased efficiency and/or loss of these properties can modify the overall function of the urothelium and promote the onset of a urothelial dysfunction [42].

The Coating Molecular Components

Urothelial coating can be roughly subdivided into a deep and a superficial portion. The deep portion consists of carbohydrate termini of glycoproteins, proteoglycans, and glycolipids; the superficial portion consists of glycosaminoglycans (GAGs) with a stable and/or labile interaction with the deep-layer molecular component (Fig. 4.5).

Coating Glycoproteins

Functional Glycoproteins

Integral membrane proteins carrying 1 to 15 poorly ramified oligosaccharide chains into the extremity protruding outside the cell. They occupy the deep portion of coating where they play a co-receptor function, synergizing the action of growth factors or hormones.

Structural Glycoproteins

Similar to the previous ones, their highly ramified chains can establish dynamic interactions with the different molecular components of coating.

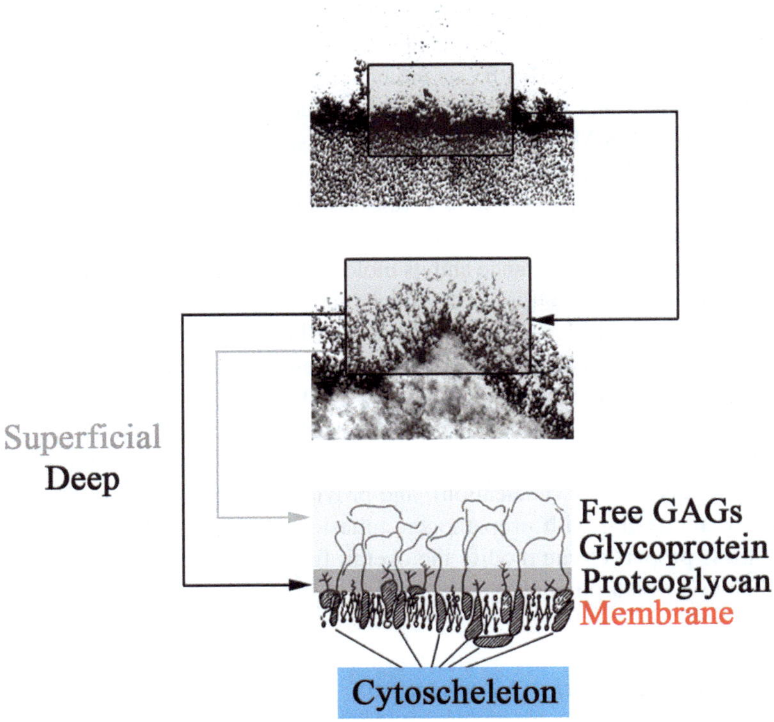

Fig. 4.5 Special techniques (celylpyridinium chloride and ruthenium red) preserve and detect the presence of coating as a fine "black precipitate" (**a**). On a larger magnification (**b**), coating shows its specific arrangement: a superficial layer largely consisting of glycoprotein carbohydrate chains and "free" GAGs and a deep layer where the largest share is represented by proteoglycans. From Tajana G. Fisiopatologia clinica e biologia molecolare dell'urotelio. Minerva Urol Nefrol 2009; 61(3 suppl 1):1–29. Reprinted with permission from Edizioni Minerva Medica

Polyfunctional Glycoproteins: HB-EGF

Heparin-binding epidermal growth factor-like growth factor (HB-EGF) is a glycoprotein of the Epidermal Growth Factor (EGF) family performing several functions.

These proteins exist in two molecular versions: 27 kDa proHB-EGF and 19 kDa sHBEGF [43, 44].

proHB-EGF is localized in the plasma membrane where it interacts with integrin and alpha3beta1 [45, 46]. It performs a paracrine mitogenic function, since it acts directly on EGF receptor [47]. Moreover, HB-EGF can stabilize the coating [48] structure by specifically and unspecifically binding to heparan sulfate as well as to various classes of GAGs and some coating-specific glucosides (D-mannose, D-galactose, L-fucose, *N*-acetyl-D-glucosamine) [49].

Calcium-depending binding efficiency can be [50] analyzed by evaluating the labeled-radioligand binding. HB-EGF has two binding areas in its structure. The largest area has approximately 1,000,000 cell/binding sites and a 6.1 nM–44 nM affinity constant K(d); the smaller one has 23,000 cell/binding sites [51].

Once protein kinase has been activated, HB-EGF structure cleaves 74 aminoacids; in this way, 27 kDa proHB-EGF is transformed into 19 kDa sHB-EGF and, by shedding, is expelled from the membrane; yet, its EGF receptor mitogenic stimulatory role remains intact [52, 53].

Anti-lithiasis Glycoproteins: THP

THP (Tamm–Horsfall glycoprotein 68 kDa) or uromodulin (UMOD) is a sialoglycoprotein capable of neutralizing the potential formation of microcrystals [54], thanks to the combined action of its sialic acid residues with albumin [55]. Alike renal "nephron units," the urothelium synthesizes THP and places it into its coating [56]; here, it can neutralize potentially harmful low-molecular-weight polyamines and cathiones [57] by means of the electrostatic action of sialic acid residues [58].

THP is the most abundant urinary glycoprotein. Mostly produced by the thick ascending limb of Henle's loop and distal convoluted tubule cells, it is found in the membrane apical portion through a glycolipid portion called GPI (Glycosyl Phosphatidylinositol-anchored) and SPd1 antigen, thanks to specific glycosyltransferase-regulated binding. This generates a coating regulating water impermeability in the nephron diluting segments. Its involvement in calcium-containing kidney stones is still unclear; its role in other pathophysiological conditions (medullary cystic kidney disease-2, MCKD2; familial juvenile hyperuricemic nephropathy, FJHN; juvenile hyperuricemia) is poorly understood, even though its possible immunopathogenetic role in chronic interstitial nephritis has raised a remarkable interest [59].

Anti-pathogen Glycoproteins: GP51

GP51 is a 51 kDa glycoprotein: when placed in the coating, it creates a "strategic" defense mechanism against gram-positive and -negative uropathogens.

Escherichia coli, Enterobacter cloacae, Klebsiella pneumoniae, Proteus vulgaris, Pseudomonas aeruginosa, Serratia marcescens, Staphylococcus aureus, S. epidermidis, Streptococcus faecalis.

It is produced by the entire urothelium and especially by the bladder; its concentration rises during both tissue and urinary infections [60, 61].

Epitectin (MUC-1 Glycoprotein)

It is a membrane protein with a typical 20 amino acid sequence subject to a varying degree of glycosylation (20- to 120-fold). It significantly protects against pathogens; moreover, it can bind and transduce "signals." Its increased synthesis and

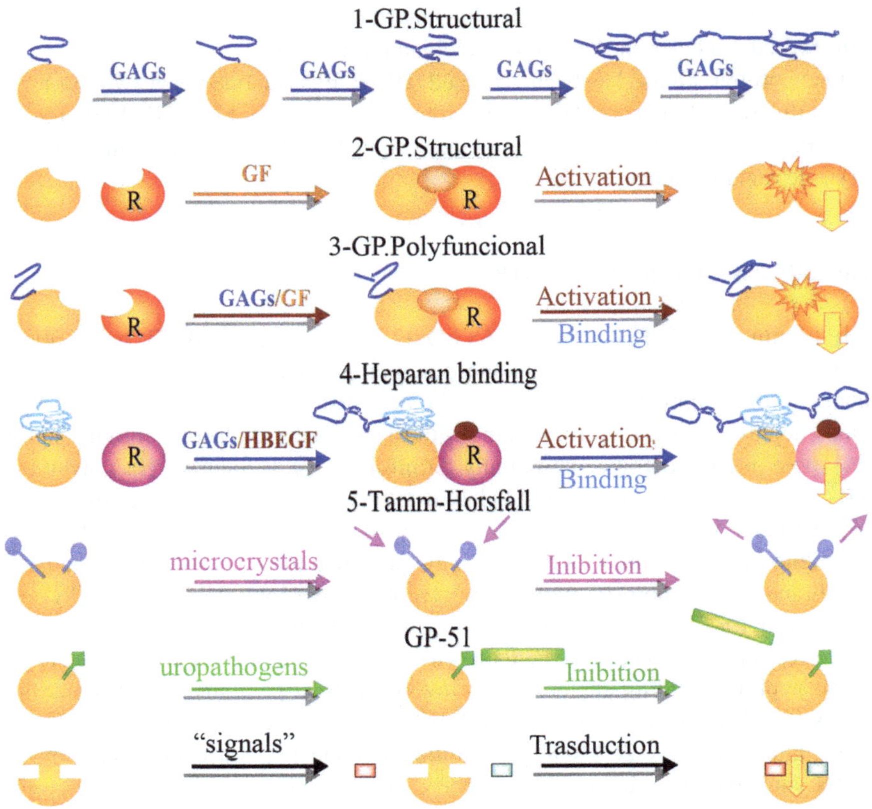

Fig. 4.6 Coating glycoproteins (GP): Functions: (1) Structural GPs: interact with PGs and bind GAGs; (2) functional GPs: activate growth factor receptors (R); (3) polyfunctional GPs: interact with PGs, bind GAGs, and activate growth factor receptors; (4) HB-EGF: bind GAGs and activate EGF receptor; (5) THP: scavenging action, prevents formation of crystals; (6) GP-51: inhibits uropathogen adhesion; (7) epitectin: "signal" transduction. From Tajana G. Fisiopatologia clinica e biologia molecolare dell'urotelio. Minerva Urol Nefrol 2009; 61(3 suppl 1):1–29. Reprinted with permission from Edizioni Minerva Medica

glycosylation have been associated with the onset of cancer. Its expression is stable throughout the menstrual cycle and can generally be assayed in urine (epitectin >4 μg/ml) (Fig. 4.6) [62].

Proteoglycans

Unlike glycoproteins where proteins prevail, proteoglycans comprise a main protein (core protein) and a large series of heteropolysaccharide chains called GAGs. The latter interact with each other or with other coating components to form "molecular sieves": these have a variable selectivity, according to the diameter of porosities and the final net charge. These "dynamic filters" (they are continuously formed and destroyed) can bind to signal transduction molecules; action of these is prevented through sequestration or enhanced when their local concentration is increased [63].

In urothelial coating, four classes of proteoglycans with different molecular weights have been identified [64].

Low-Molecular-Weight Proteoglycans

Biglycan

Type I proteoglycan I (PG-I) is also known as biglycan, because it consists of two molecules of chondroitin sulfate joined at one end by a leucin-rich polypeptide.

Decorin

TypeII proteoglycan (PG-II): Alike PG-I, it comprises a protein portion joined to just one chondroitin sulfate molecule.

High-Molecular-Weight Proteoglycans

Perlecan

Markedly polyanionic, it interacts with GAGs to form an efficient electrostatic barrier.

Sindecan

Its "protein core" acts as a transmembrane protein and/or as a co-receptor for some growth factors (Fig. 4.7).

Glycosaminoglycans

Long, linear heteropolysaccharide chains mostly comprising heparan sulfate, chondroitin sulfate, dermatan sulfate, and hyaluronic acid; they can complement with proteoglycans or create a "free pool" interacting through weak bindings (hydrogen bindings, Van der Walls, Coulomb forces) with coating structural GAGs so as to lengthen them; also, they can fill any electrostatically empty areas. Chondroitin sulfate is the most commonly observed GAG [65].

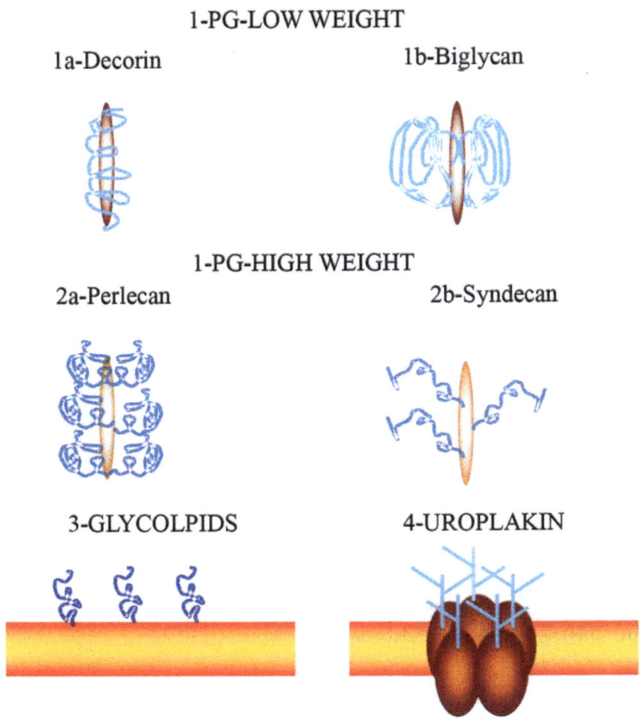

Fig. 4.7 Proteoglycans, glycolipids, and uroplakins; high- and low-molecular-weight PGs form selective filters together with GPs. Glycolipids demarcate GP and PG position in coating; they also interact with uroplakins to perform their barrier function. From Tajana G. Fisiopatologia clinica e biologia molecolare dell'urotelio. Minerva Urol Nefrol 2009; 61(3 suppl 1):1–29. Reprinted with permission from Edizioni Minerva Medica

Colorimetric techniques allow to define the overall amount of sulfated GAGs, not found in the urothelium. While non-sulfated GAGs (hyaluronic acid) have a 2.15×10^{-4}–5.50×10^{-4} mmol/kg dry weight, sulfated GAGs' dry weight varies between 2.00×10^{-1} and 7.40×10^{-1} mmol/kg. These values match those obtained through different methods (gel electrophoresis) [66, 67].

Balanced mixtures of GAGs employed in bladder instillation come together in this "free pool" where they can integrate with the various coating components.

Glycolipids

Structural lipids enclosed in membrane "rafts"; they bind the polar heads of carbohydrates and can therefore interact with glycoproteins and GAGs; they play a key role in the formation of the coating filtering portion and can influence the uroplakin function.

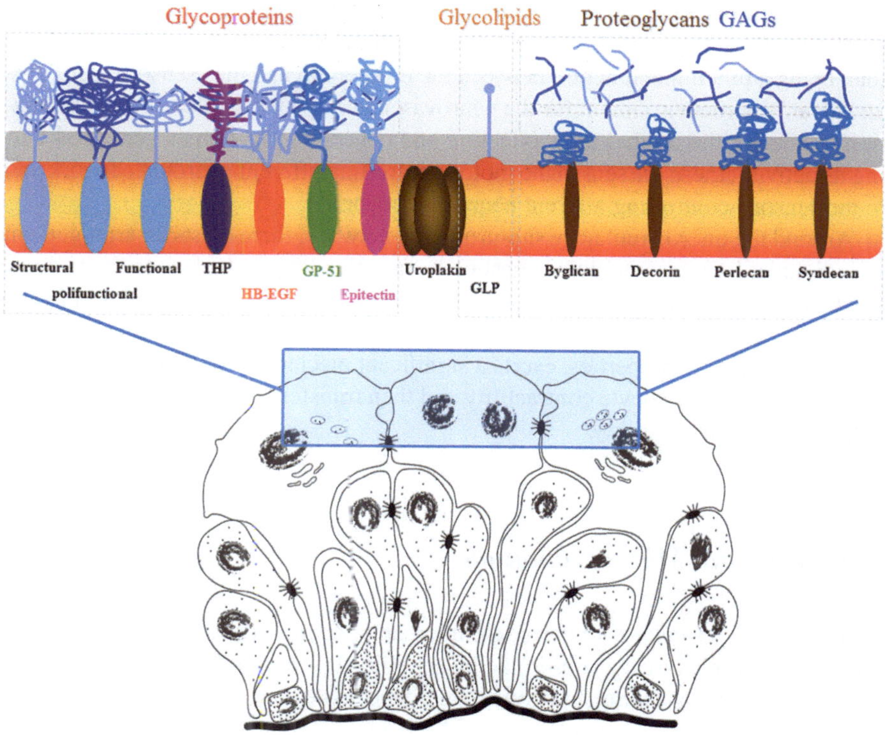

Fig. 4.8 Reconstruction of coating molecular components: Glycoproteins, proteoglycans, glycolipids, free GAGs, and uroplakins. From Tajana G. Fisiopatologia clinica e biologia molecolare dell'urotelio. Minerva Urol Nefrol 2009; 61(3 suppl 1):1–29. Reprinted with permission from Edizioni Minerva Medica

Basolateral Barriers

Chondroitin sulfate is found not only in coating but also particularly in the basal portions where it might be involved in the regulation of differentiation mechanisms and, more specifically, of ion channel efficiency; hyaluronic acid is involved in maintaining urothelial differentiation (Fig. 4.8) [65].

Sub-urothelium

Sub-urothelial Interstitium: Cell Populations and Formations

The sub-urothelial region (lamina propria) is the interstitial tissue extending from the basal lamina, where it adheres to the urothelium, to the muscle wall. It is a deformable and flexible connective matrix, given its molecular composition: elastin complex (elastin; fibrillin-1; microfibril-associated glycoprotein, MAGP) and type I, III, and IV collagen [68, 69], stabilized by fibronectin and laminin [70]. Other than being a functional junction between the urothelium and the "sensory web," it is an "ideal" microenvironment for the neurovascular network: it allows microcirculation to nourish the urothelium, collecting and concentrating signals generated during its activity; these are sent to the motor-controlling efferent neuronal network and to the sensory-controlling afferent neuronal network.

Around the microcirculatory sub-urothelial network, there exists an arrangement of individual lymphatic nodules, mast cells, fat cell islets, and, close to the trigone, small, aberrant urethral glands. These cell populations establish connections of various types with afferent and efferent nerve endings. Finally, the sub-urothelium, thanks to its elastic properties, exerts a significant mechanical action: it absorbs the tone generated by myocyte contractility and then transfers it to the urothelium, thus amplifying its distensibility.

Sub-urothelial Microcirculation

A study of the vascular tridimensional microarchitecture of the bladder shows two major vascular plexuses: a sub-urothelial superficial plexus and a deep one, in close contact with myocytes. Such plexuses are connected through a series of capillaries which, depending on the distension of the bladder wall, change their shape from helicoidal to rectilinear: they act as pressure shock absorbers regulating the supply of blood in the bladder wall to prevent the onset of local hypertension (Fig. 4.9) [71].

The sub-urothelium begins to develop during the embryo-fetal period and is fully formed by the early years of life. It is regulated by the urothelium itself through soluble factors which can guide the differentiation of resident mesenchymal cells into myocytes: a low concentration level inhibits differentiation whereas a high concentration level promotes the formation of myoblasts both before and afterwards, other than regulating the myogenesis of complex muscle wall systems [72]. Likewise, the sub-urothelium produces factors capable of directing the differentiation of the urothelium and its barriers [73].

The Urothelial Pacemaker

The bladder expresses a series of spontaneous rhythmic contractions (SRCs). This auto-rhythmicity is regulated by a sophisticated "impulse generator," located in the sub-urothelium.

Similar to the heart, where the atrial sinus node generates a basic or sinus rhythm, which can vary and spread through the conduction tissue, the bladder is provided with a sophisticated "pacemaker" generating and sending autonomous electric impulses.

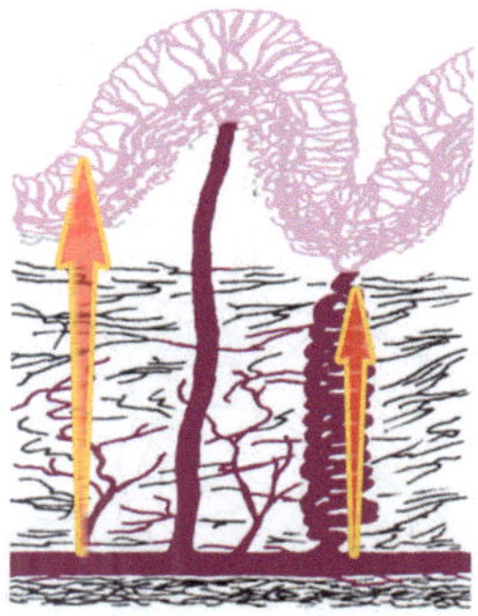

Fig. 4.9 Sub-urothelium microcirculation. From Tajana G. Fisiopatologia clinica e biologia molecolare dell'urotelio. Minerva Urol Nefrol 2009; 61(3 suppl 1):1–29. Reprinted with permission from Edizioni Minerva Medica

The bladder "rhythmic section" consists of interstitial or Cajal cells, which can be visualized as Kit 67 and vimentin-positive cells [74]. These star-shaped cells connect to each other or to myocytes through the gap junction (connexins 40, 43, 45) [75]; at the same time, they can establish functional connections with the bladder intramural nerve endings [76]. Thanks to M3 muscarinic receptor [77], such cells are functionally related with the autonomic nervous system; they respond to NO by releasing intracellular cGMP [78]. Moreover, they are provided with an efficient cycloxigenase-producing prostaglandins, essential to confer a specific pace to spontaneous rhythmic contractions [79].

Urinary Cajal cells have a similar morphology and activity as intestinal Cajal cells involved in the generation of peristaltic waves. With their marked bioelectric features, these cells are found in the urinary tract of every mammal and play a central role in bladder pathophysiology (Fig. 4.10) [80].

Sui's group analyzed Cajal cells' electrophysiological properties in vitro. After a "mechanical stretch" or an "electrical stimulation of the urothelium" with a subsequent ATP production and release, Cajal cells can (by means of intracellular calcium increase) establish an efficient "sensory feedback" with the urothelium [75]. Imaging techniques monitoring the intracellular calcium flux showed that Cajal cells are not phenotypically homogenous; there exist at least two subtypes generating high/low frequencies which stabilize/change the rhythm, respectively, thus modulating the signal transmission [81].

Functional Significance of the Bladder Impulse Generator

According to Lang, two distinct, synchronous pacemakers seem to coexist in the bladder: the bladder and the urethral pacemakers; the latter seems to generate a "rudimentary" peristalsis [82].

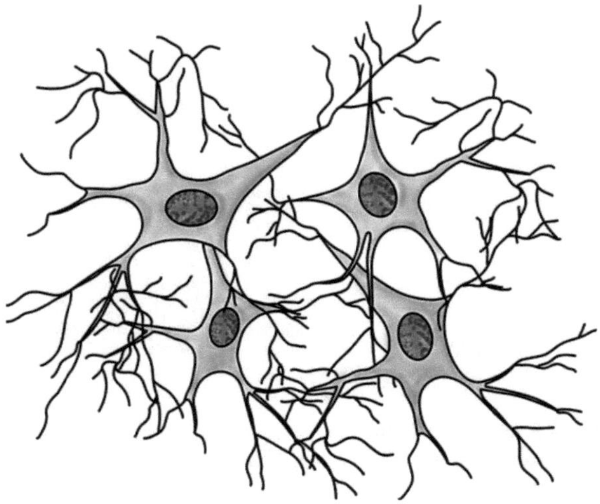

Fig. 4.10 Cajal cells. From Tajana G. Fisiopatologia clinica e biologia molecolare delleprinted with permission from Edizioni Minerva Medica

Seemingly, their functional role consists of promoting, through a basic rhythm, local contractions generating stresses which, once spread, quickly activate stretching receptors or, alternatively, induce the synthesis and release of urothelial derived factors. In this way, the whole system would avail itself of a "perceptive system" which can be continuously modulated [83].

This hypothesis was demonstrated by J Gillespie's group in a number of animal models: the administration of various exogenous substances was shown to modify basal RMCs. In the lack of stimulation, spontaneous elevations of mechanical tension occur. Muscarinic and nicotinic agonists cause an increase of contractile width and synchronicity. Adrenergic agonists, CGRP, or an elevated AMPc level reduce the width and frequency of contractions; on the other hand, ATP and P substance analogues cause an increased frequency [84–86].

Capsaicin exerts a complex effect on spontaneous contractions: it induces CGRP and P substance release from afferent nerve endings [87]. This observation suggests that local reflex can modulate the generation of spontaneous contractions.

In conclusion, Cajal cells and their receptors constitute a potential target for a pharmacological approach aimed at reducing detrusor spontaneous contractions without interfering with its function.

Myofibroblasts as a "Conduction Tissue"

The bladder pacemaker action on the muscle wall contraction is not direct: it is mediated by interstitial myofibroblasts (Fig. 4.11). These play a significant liaison and modulation role. In many ways, they resemble the cardiac conduction tissue; myofibroblasts communicate with each other and with Cajal cells and myocytes through a set of gap-junctions showing a sophisticated arrangement. This creates an

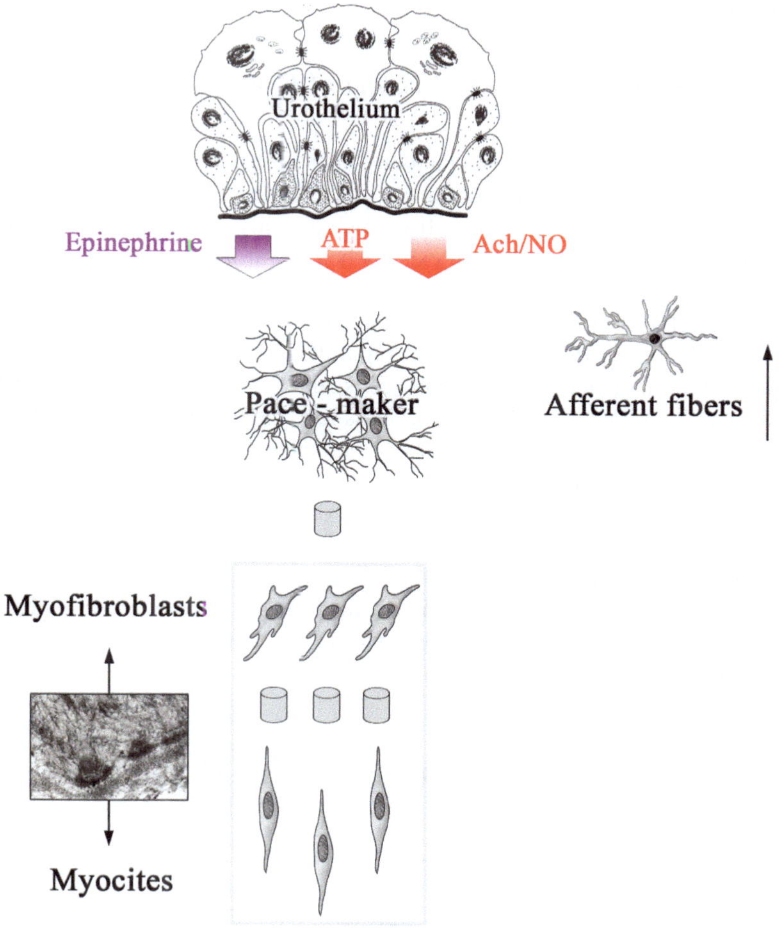

Fig. 4.11 The "sensory web" structure. Activity of the urothelium generates chemical signals (ATP, adrenaline, acetylcholine, NO) regulating Cajal cell function; Cajal cells interact with afferent and efferent fibers. Through myofibroblasts and the "gap-junctions" system, myocyte contraction as well as control of muscle wall are activated. From Tajana G. Fisiopatologia clinica e biologia molecolare dell'urotelio. Minerva Urol Nefrol 2009; 61(3 suppl 1):1–29. Reprinted with permission from Edizioni Minerva Medica

extremely efficient cyto-electric syncytium having a synergistic function with the local nervous network [88].

The network efficiency is due to the gap-junction molecular characteristics. Their structure contains, other than conventional connexins (26, 43, 45), cadherin 11 which can enhance the transmission efficacy [89, 90]. Since myofibroblasts have their own muscarinic receptors (M2 and M3), they can be directly stimulated. Although alterations of the myofibroblast network have been related with bladder overactivity, their role in the onset and maintenance of clinical pictures is thought to be limited and/or minor [91–93].

Urothelial Dysfunction

From Urothelial Function to Urothelial Dysfunction

A "dysfunction" is the quantitative/qualitative alteration of a function (hyper- or hypofunction). This generic pathophysiological term, however, lends itself pretty well to defining a complex set of symptoms, from both a clinical and molecular standpoint. As to the urothelium, a dysfunction exists when the urothelium cannot perform its normal physiological activity, determining an abnormal sensory web function.

A urothelial dysfunction can be experimentally induced by protamine, a polycationic protein. This action determines a rapid disappearance of coating, alters the cytoskeleton arrangement of "umbrella" cells, and destabilizes the basolateral barriers with a direct impact on junction proteins (occludins, claudins, ZO-1) [94].

A comparative microarray study of control and "cloned" urothelial cells from patients diagnosed with urothelial dysfunction has led to quantify 302 involved genes: 162 genes were shown to be "up-regulated," and 140 were "down-regulated" (Table 4.1) [95].

Hence, the identification of a specific etiology is quite difficult in the natural history of urothelial dysfunction. Table 4.2, based on data available in the literature, shows conditions which can determine a dysfunction. These are thought to be urothelial barrier alterations or a consequence of the altered function of urothelium basic "activities" or are caused by exogenous factors.

Dysfunctions Induced by Urothelial "Barrier" Alterations

Coating Deterioration

Quali-quantitative alterations of the coating molecular components can impair the urothelium function.

Given the complexity and high interaction levels established by these macromolecules, it is extremely difficult to define a time sequence or a priority order in the deterioration of the coating molecular components. The initial analysis of coating residues or "remnant" identified significant changes in the amount of glycoproteins rather than proteoglycans [96]. In particular, according to Moskowitz study, GP-1 epitectin dramatically dropped in 61 % of patients or was totally absent in 35 % of them [97]. As to GAGs, chondroitin sulfate levels appeared to be markedly reduced [65]. More sensitive methods showed that all molecular components of coating were affected. In the absence of flogosis, coating suffers from a structural collapse mostly due to a loss of low- and high-molecular-weight proteoglycans (biglycan and perlecan) [64]. Such finding correlates with the increased excretion of these urinary components.

Even free GAGs could hardly integrate into coating because of a decrease of binding structures (HB-EGF) and the presence of THP with low sialic acid levels. After the coating deterioration, the apical membrane shows numerous pleomorphic microvilli lined with "remnants" [98].

Table 4.1 Profile of genes activated during bladder inflammation [124]

Up-regulated genes
– Phosphodiesterase 1C
– cAMP-dependent protein kinase
– iNOS
– Beta-NGF
– Proenkephalin B and orphanin
– Corticotrophin-releasing factor (CRF) R
– Estrogen R
– PAI2
– Protease inhibitor 17
– NFkB p105
– c-fos
– fos-B
– Basic transcription factors
– Cytoskeleton and motility proteins
Down-regulated genes
– HSF2
– NF-kappa B p65
– ICE
– IGF-II and FGF-7
– MMP2
– MMP14
– Presenilin 2

Permeability Changes

Coating modifications can induce an increased potassium flow in urothelial cells [56, 99] and influence the activity of other functionally related membrane proteins. In particular, uroplakins II and IIIa in normal conditions are assembled into heterodimers thanks to a series of structural rearrangements regulated by specific "maturation-facilitators."

Since coating facilitates the self-assembly of uroplakins, a coating deterioration quite plausibly may disassemble uroplakins, thus compromising the permeability of the "umbrella" cell apical portions [32, 100].

Alterations in Junctional Structures

Coating and apical barrier modifications are associated with a progressive new synthesis of ICAM class adhesion molecules, capable of activating flogosis. These molecules do not only induce cell de-adhesion but also interfere with the "information flow" reaching the genome from tight junctions.

ICAM synthesis (regulated by activated mast cells) [101] is directly linked to the onset of typical symptoms of cystitis [10].

Table 4.2 Conditions determining a urothelial dysfunction

(A) Dysfunction induced by "urothelial barrier" alteration
a1. Urothelial coating deterioration
a2. Modifications of apical permeability in "umbrella cells"
a3. Alterations of junctional structures in the basolateral portions
(B) Dysfunction due to urothelial activity alterations
b1. Proliferation control
b2. Deficient cellular repair mechanisms
b3. Modification of differentiation-maintaining genes
(C) Dysfunction induced by exogenous factors
c1. Cytotoxic action of urothelium-injuring molecules
c2. Activation of flogistic reactions
c3. Production of autoantibodies towards molecules associated with urothelial physiological functions
(D) Conditions determining typical dysfunctional symptoms
d1. Increased intracellular potassium flow
d2. Altered purinergic transmission
d3. Abnormal detrusor regulation
d4. Sensory sprouting

Adhesion molecules are proteins found in the plasma membrane. Their expression can be constitutive or induced by appropriate stimuli. During an allergic reaction, they play a fundamental role in recruiting inflammatory cells. More specifically, they direct migration from blood. ICAM-1 is mostly expressed by the epithelium of allergic subjects; it is considered an allergic flogosis marker accounting for the sub-urothelium lymphocytic infiltration, since it is the ligand of LFA-1 and Mac1, integrins expressed by leukocytes.

Basal Lamina

A change in the molecular composition (decrease of type IV collagen) has been identified; in theory, this can affect the electrostatic stability of the urothelium [102].

Functional Alterations

Proliferation Control

Urothelium proliferation stems from a complex synergy between growth factors and hormones (estrogens and progesterone) [103]. More specifically, these latter act through two receptors (Er-a and Er-b) regulating the activity of D1 and E cyclins [104].

In experimental animals, castration modifies coating GAGs' profile with a pronounced decrease of hyaluronic acid; such loss can be offset by an appropriate supplementation with either individual GAGs or a combination of them [105].

A crucial element in the coating deterioration is the drastic reduction of GAG-binding functional glycoproteins. A less efficient conversion of proHB-EGF into HB-EGFs reduces the urothelium proliferation rate and the capacity to bind GAGs to coating. This is mostly due to the inhibitory activity of urothelium-impairing molecules on pro HB-EGF synthesis through the MAP kinase system inhibition [106]. Finally, peroxisome proliferator-activated receptor (PPAR)'s actual regulatory capacity in terms of urothelium gene expression is unclear; PPARs are involved in the synthesis of essential urothelial proteins (cytokeratins 13 and 20, claudin 3, uroplakins 1 and 2) [14].

Urothelial Repair Mechanism Deficiency

The urothelium takes care of its own "ordinary maintenance" through multiple repair mechanisms controlled by some stress proteins (72 kDa), the synthesis of which is induced by the same toxic factors. The activation of such mechanisms depends on the execution of one or more apoptosis-related desquamation cycles [107]. Failure to control such mechanisms may progressively lead the urothelium to become dysfunctional [108].

Differentiated State Maintenance

The urothelial differentiated state is regulated by a family of genes (Polycomb group genes) involved with tissue repair mechanisms. These can act only after removing inhibitory histones (H3 lysine 27 trimethylation H3K27me3) thanks to a specific demethylase which in turn can be activated by a JMJD3 factor increased expression [109, 110].

Expression of this factor during Bladder Pain Syndrome (BPS) suggests that a urothelial dysfunction may be an alternative differentiation state of the urothelium, i.e., an epigenetic reprogramming related to the activation of repair processes [111]. It should be noted, however, that in a state of dysfunction the phenotypic expression of some differentiation keratin markers (usually expressed by different classes of urothelial cells) undergoes certain modifications (7, 8, 14, 17, 18, 20).

Exogenous Factors

Urothelium-Injuring Molecules

A loss of the coating barrier effect can be due to cytotoxic factors in urine, not sufficiently neutralized [112].

A marked inhibition of urothelial proliferation can be induced by anti-proliferative Factor (APF), a 3,000 kDa sialoglycopeptide (frizzled-8-related peptide) produced by the urothelium: it can bind to coating and interfere with mitotic triggering mechanisms [113–116].

APF has one hydrophobic terminus which may interfere with urothelial proliferation mechanisms [117] by blocking G2 cells and increasing p53 levels [118].

This effect occurs at picomolar concentration levels in urothelial cells from interstitial cystitis patients [115, 119].

APF determines quali-quantitative modifications in the molecular composition of coating, as proven by a microarray analysis highlighting a "down regulation" of several genes affecting the coating structure and function [120].

The APF can diminish the coating barrier effect and induce the synthesis of specific cytokines inhibiting the production of glycoproteins, GAGs receptors, and ligands. Quite plausibly, this inhibition causes their urinary buildup [121].

Activation of Flogistic Mechanisms

APF promotion of NFkB activation in the urothelium and sub-urothelium suggests that this could be a pathway to release flogosis mediators (TNF-alpha, IL-1beta, IL-6, and IL-8) (see Table 4.1) [122–124].

Autoantibody Production

Although urine of patients with BPS may contain anti-urothelium antibodies (anti-THP), these do not seem to be the primary cause of the disease [125].

Conditions Determining Symptoms

Potassium Flow and Bladder Overactivity

The lack of a coating barrier effect and an altered uroplakin system cause a loss of impermeability of the apical membrane with an excessive inflow of potassium. This builds up in the cytoplasm and interferes with urothelial "exo/endocytosis" mechanisms. Once it is spread across the sub-urothelium, potassium depolarizes nerve endings inducing bladder overactivity and pain [126].

Purinergic Transmission

When subject to mechanical and/or osmotic stretching, the urothelium increases ATP production by approximately tenfold. This ATP "surplus" can either be utilized by the urothelium or released outside, where it activates specific purinic receptors in the sub-urothelium.

The urothelium expresses four different ATP receptors (A1, A2a, A2b, and A3). These are localized mostly in the apical region of "umbrella" cells. A2a, A2b, and A3 receptors are localized in the intracellular and/or basolateral regions; they are involved in the exo/endocytosis cycle management (see Table 4.2) [127].

Detrusor Abnormal Regulation

The detrusor is a relatively fast muscle expressing myosin isoforms of smooth muscle cells. Its contractile system, in response to different pathophysiological conditions, exhibits remarkable adaptive properties. Its cells are organized in the form of "functional units"; thanks to a thick net of gap-junctions, these cells can synchronize and amplify contractions by modifying calcium intracellular concentration and the subsequent phosphorylation of myosin light chains.

Their contraction can be modulated by a complex set of signals sent from nerve endings (adrenergic and cholinergic) or locally generated by NANC system (nonadrenergic and noncholinergic); the detrusor receives and processes these signals through a series of specific receptors. A key role in activating contraction is played by muscarinic M3 and purinergic P2X receptors 1.

Sprouting

A urothelial dysfunction can be associated to a considerable increase of nerve fibers in the sub-urothelium. Interestingly, cystolysis induces a massive depletion of mediators and a downsizing of nerve endings; however, these modifications do not affect the detrusor [128]. Since the number of nerve endings, histamine levels, and mast cell count are mutually related, their possible interaction during BPS has been hypothesized [129].

Sub-urothelium

A partial impairment of the sub-urothelium and vascular network is observed in over 70 % of BPS patients. In particular, the elastin component shows marked signs of deterioration [130]. Endothelial cells tend to lose adherence; in the newly formed spaces, platelets and polymorphonuclear cells are commonly observed. The endothelium exhibits cytoskeleton alterations with a progressive increase of "granulations," suggesting a cell injury, along with an increased expression of P substance receptors, causing painful symptoms (Figs. 4.12 and 4.13) [131].

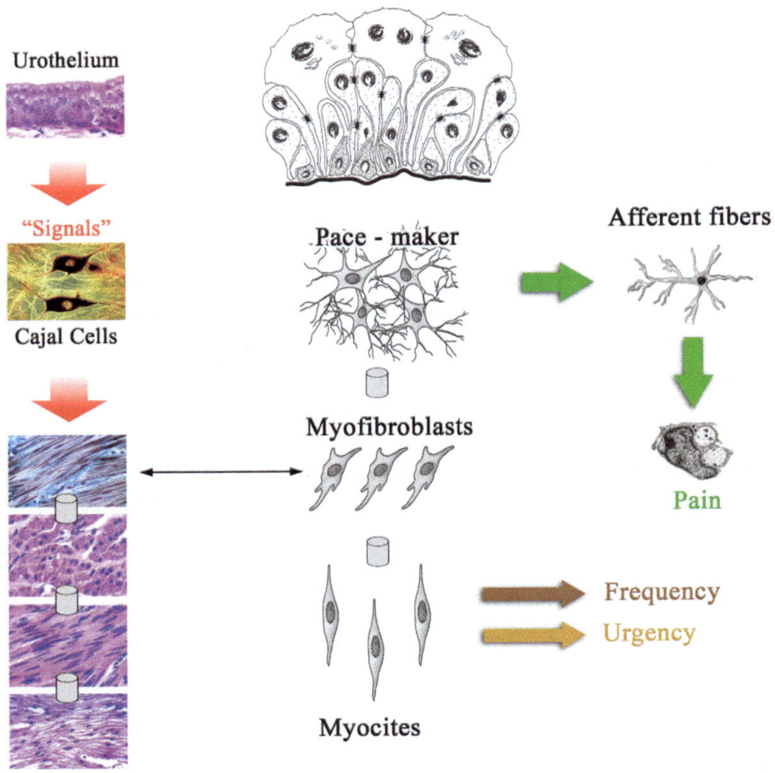

Fig. 4.12 A proper urothelial function gives rise to "chemical signals" responsible for an accurate control of the micturition cycle. The collapse of urothelial barriers induces a dysfunctional state with the production of "abnormal chemical signals" altering contraction kinetics with the subsequent frequency and urgency symptoms. The involvement of C fibers determines the onset of pain. From Tajana G. Fisiopatologia clinica e biologia molecolare dell'urotelio. Minerva Urol Nefrol 2009; 61(3 suppl 1):1–29. Reprinted with permission from Edizioni Minerva Medica

The Theoretical Foundations of "Coating Repair"

A direct action on the urothelium and sub-urothelium can be achieved through instillation therapy, aimed at coating repair and barrier restoration with the help of either individual or combined GAGs. The urothelium is provided with its own, efficient self-repair system. Following an experimental injury (protamine sulfate, 10 mg/ml), "umbrella" cells recover their control of apical permeability within 72 h; apical permeability is related to the uroplakin system, whereas a gradual restoration of basolateral barriers is completed by day 5.

Interestingly, urothelial cells and, more specifically, "umbrella" cells, at the end of the process, are smaller in volume and show a decreased trophism; as to the urothelium, a reduced thickness and minimal changes in the coating molecular composition are observed [10]. Sound theoretical foundations allow to plan a

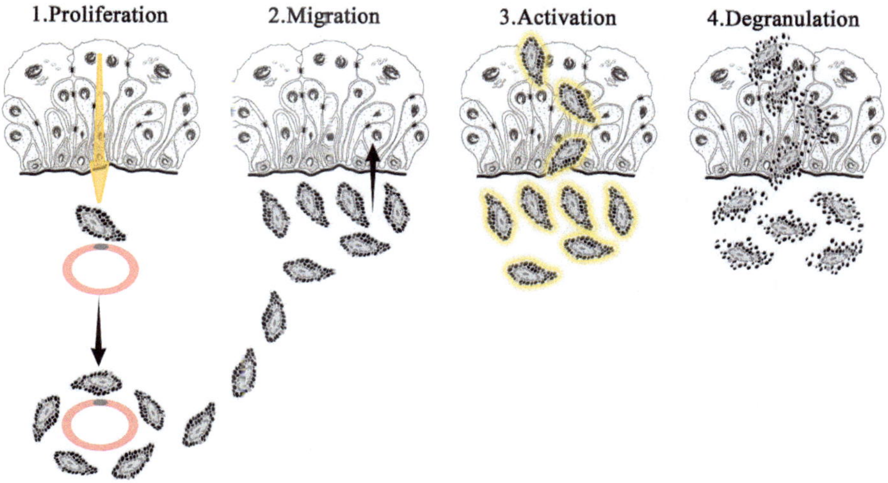

Fig. 4.13 Deterioration of coating and urothelial barriers causes the passage of potentially allergenic molecules; these initiate mast cell proliferation and their migration from the sub-urothelium to the urothelium. The effects of activation and degranulation are largely related with most BPS symptoms. From Tajana G. Fisiopatologia clinica e biologia molecolare dell'urotelio. Minerva Urol Nefrol 2009; 61(3 suppl 1):1–29. Reprinted with permission from Edizioni Minerva Medica

therapy aimed at enhancing the urothelium self-repair, through a direct action on coating for restoring the urothelial function and the overall activity of the sensory web. The coating repair can activate a sequence of events leading to the functional restoration of basolateral barriers, a stabilization of the neuro-immune-endocrine components of the sub-urothelium, and a significantly improved clinical picture. Based on literature data, Table 4.3 illustrates a possible sequence of mechanisms following GAG instillation.

First, their administration determines an increased concentration of free GAGs, with a more efficient binding to glycoproteins and proteoglycans in the "remnant" [132]. Heparin, pentosan polysulfate, and hyaluronic acid were shown to be able to integrate into the structure of injured coatings and block the penetration of labeled urea (14C) [132, 133]. Exogenous GAGs establish a series of secondary interactions which can slow down/stop the sequence of coating deterioration processes; the latter promote the formation (autopoiesis) of complex intercatenary bindings generating domains that give rise to a rudimentary neo-coating, as visualized through atomic force microscopy [134]. This would allow "umbrella" cells to reactivate the exo/endocytosis cycle: through the latter, they recover their selective permeability, as proven by a negative PST test and a significantly improved bladder function [134–138].

Urothelial cells gradually restore their defense and repair mechanisms [139] and activate the binding protein synthesis of basolateral junctions [140].

Hyaluronic acid can neutralize the destabilizing effect of ICAM-1 on the barrier structure; it sterically interferes with ICAM-1 ecotaxic action [140], exerting a

Table 4.3 Possible sequence of mechanisms induced by GAG instillation

Increased share of free GAGs [148]
Interaction and binding with GP, binding function [132, 133]
Interaction and binding with PG [132, 133]
Restoration of primary filter [134, 135]
Recovery of selective apical permeability [136]
Normalization of K flow [136–138]
Normalization of endo/exocytosis cycle [148]
Restoration of defense mechanisms [148]
Induction of repair mechanisms [139]
Recovery of basolateral barriers [140]
Mast cell deactivation [141, 142]
Inhibition of pre-inflammatory processes [140]
Inhibition of fibrosis [143]
Normalization of bladder tone [137]
Action on sub-urothelial microcirculation [145]
Disappearance of pain [136, 146]

major anti-inflammatory action. In summary, coating restoration seems to allow the urothelium to gain back its two fundamental functions (impermeability and distensibility), stimulate urothelial proliferation, and restore molecular mechanisms maintaining a state of differentiation [139].

Exogenous GAGs are quickly disseminated in the sub-urothelium where they deactivate mast cells by means of various mechanisms [141]. Hyaluronic acid binds to mast cell CD44; in this way, it deeply affects their function by inhibiting the release of histamine and the production of pro-inflammatory mediators [142] with a marked inhibition of fibrosis [143]. Pentosan polysulfate exerts its pro-urothelium (antiflogistic) action by interfering with molecules rather than through a direct NFkB inhibition [144]. Normalization of the bladder tone [137, 138] and the simultaneous effect on sub-urothelium microcirculation are thought to be due to the hypotension induced by protamine and heparin–protamine complexes through the release of NO (produced via NOS) [145]. No experimental data are available [146] to explain the disappearance and/or attenuation of pain assessed through visual analogue scale (VAS) and O'Leary–Saint Symptom and Problem Index (OSPI) [136].

As to GAGs, the hyaluronic acid–chondroitin sulfate combination was shown to significantly reduce pro-inflammatory cytokines (interleukin-6) [147] in vitro (urothelial cell line T24).

Conclusions

The urothelium is a special, somehow unique, epithelium. Starting from its basic functions (impermeability and distensibility), it can generate "signaling molecules" which, through the "sensory web," contribute to the regulation of the urinary function. The knowledge of its molecular basis is getting increasingly detailed in disclosing its "complex mechanisms"; control of the latter, through a targeted therapy, represents an exciting challenge for basic research as well as for urology.

The urothelial dysfunction seems to represent a mandatory pathogenetic pathway; it can originate diverse clinical conditions, ranging from idiopathic detrusor overactivity (IDO) to Stress Urinary Incontinence (SUI) or complex clinical presentations epitomized by IC, although this is not the only one [148].

Interestingly, some analogies with endothelial dysfunction can be observed.

HB-EGF, produced by the urothelium and subsequently sent to myocytes as a function of mechanical stretch, is equally synthesized by endothelial cells undergoing shear stress. HB-EGF stimulates the proliferation of the vessel muscle component, thus balancing out any flow abnormalities [149, 150].

During physical exercise, skeletal muscle synthesizes HB-EGF, too. It promotes the peripheral utilization of glucose, facilitates the action of insulin, and prevents obesity [151]. These findings call for a thorough review of the interactions existing in several urogenital districts between endothelium and urothelium, and of their functional meaning relative to general clinical conditions such as the multimetabolic syndrome.

In the future, thanks to the confocal microscopic analysis of urothelium function in vivo and to the identification of molecules controlling barriers and the sensory web regulation, research may provide information to single out the "prime mover" of urothelial dysfunction. A more widespread use of instillation therapy can be promoted through "engineered GAG" delivery vectors like liposomes [152] or nanoemulsions [153], an essential support for a gene therapy of urothelial dysfunction.

References

1. Deng FM, Ding M, Lavker RM, Sun TT. Urothelial function reconsidered: a role in urinary protein secretion. Proc Natl Acad Sci U S A. 2001;98:154–9.
2. Khandelwal P, Ruiz WG, Balestreire-Hawryluk E, Weisz OA, Goldenring JR, Apodaca G. Rab11a-dependent exocytosis of discoidal/fusiform vesicles in bladder umbrella cells. Proc Natl Acad Sci U S A. 2008;105:15773–8.
3. Birder L. Role of the urothelium in bladder function. Scand J Urol Nephrol Suppl. 2004;215:48–53.
4. Birder L. Urinary bladder urothelium: molecular sensors of chemical/thermal/mechanical stimuli. Vascul Pharmacol. 2006;45:221–6.
5. Wu XR, Kong XP, Pellicer A, Kreibich G, Sun TT. Uroplakins in urothelial biology, function, and disease. Kidney Int. 2009;75:1153–65.
6. de Groat WC. The urothelium in overactive bladder: passive bystander or active participant? Urology. 2004;64(6 Suppl 1):7–11.
7. Jost SP, Gosling JA, Dixon JS. The morphology of normal human bladder urothelium. J Anat. 1989;167:103–15.
8. Laguna P, Smedts F, Nordling J, Horn T, Bouchelouche K, Hopman A, et al. Keratin expression profiling of transitional epithelium in the painful bladder syndrome/interstitial cystitis. Am J Clin Pathol. 2006;125:105–10.
9. Negrete HO, Lavelle JP, Berg J, Lewis SA, Zeidel ML. Permeability properties of the intact mammalian bladder epithelium. Am J Physiol. 1996;271:F886–94.

10. Lavelle J, Meyers S, Ramage R, Bastacky S, Doty D, Apodaca G, et al. Bladder permeability barrier: recovery from selective injury of surface epithelial cells. Am J Physiol Renal Physiol. 2002;283:F242–53.
11. Eldrup J, Thorup J, Nielsen SL, Hald T, Hainau B. Permeability and ultrastructure of human bladder epithelium. Br J Urol. 1983;55:488–92.
12. Acharya P, Beckel J, Ruiz WG, Wang E, Rojas R, Birder L, et al. Distribution of the tight junction proteins ZO-1, occludin, and claudin-4, -8, and -12 in bladder epithelium. Am J Physiol Renal Physiol. 2004;287:F305–18.
13. D'Atri F, Nadalutti F, Citi S. Evidence for a functional interaction between cingulin and ZO-1 in cultured cells. J Biol Chem. 2002;277:27757–64.
14. Varley CL, Southgate J. Effects of PPAR agonists on proliferation and differentiation in human urothelium. Exp Toxicol Pathol. 2008;60:435–41.
15. Varley CL, Garthwaite MA, Cross W, Hinley J, Trejdosiewicz LK, Southgate J. PPAR gamma-regulated tight junction development during human urothelial cytodifferentiation. J Cell Physiol. 2006;208:407–17.
16. Mullin JM, Leatherman JM, Valenzano MC, Huerta ER, Verrechio J, Smith DM, et al. Ras mutation impairs epithelial barrier function to a wide range of non electrolytes. Mol Biol Cell. 2005;16:5538–50.
17. Wang E, Truschel S, Apodaca G. Analysis of hydrostatic pressure-induced changes in umbrella cell surfacearea. Methods. 2003;30:207–17.
18. Lewis SA, de Moura JL. Apical membrane area of rabbit urinary bladder increases by fusion of intracellular vesicles: an electrophysiological study. J Membr Biol. 1984;82:123–36.
19. Born M, Pahner I, Ahnert-Hilger G, Jöns T. The maintenance of the permeability barrier of bladder facet cells requires a continuous fusion of discoid vesicles with the apical plasma membrane. Mol Biol Cell. 2002;13:830–46.
20. Veranic P, Romih R, Jezernik K. What determines differentiation of urothelial umbrella cells? Eur J Cell Biol. 2004;83:27–34.
21. Truschel ST, Wang E, Ruiz WG, Leung SM, Rojas R, Lavelle J, et al. Stretch-regulated exocytosis/endocytosis in bladder umbrella cells. Mol Biol Cell. 2002;13:830–46.
22. Kreft ME, Jezernik K, Kreft M, Romih R. Apical plasma membrane traffic in superficial cells of bladder urothelium. Ann N Y Acad Sci. 2009;1152:18–29.
23. Cao H, Chen J, Awoniyi M, Henley JR, McNiven MA. Dynamin 2 mediates fluid-phase micropinocytosis in epithelial cells. J Cell Sci. 2007;120(Pt 23):4167–77.
24. Terada N, Ohno N, Saitoh S, Saitoh Y, Fujii Y, Kondo T, et al. Involvement of dynamin-2 in formation of discoid vesicles in urinary bladder umbrella cells. Cell Tissue Res. 2009;337:91–102.
25. Henley JR, Cao H, McNiven MA. Participation of dynamin in the biogenesis of cytoplasmic vesicles. FASEB J. 1999;13 Suppl 2:S243–7.
26. Lee E, De Camilli P. Dynamin at actin tails. Proc Natl Acad Sci U S A. 2002;99:161–6.
27. Thompson HM, Cao H, Chen J, Euteneuer U, McNiven MA. Dynamin 2 binds gamma-tubulin and participates in centrosome cohesion. Nat Cell Biol. 2004;6:335–42.
28. Fish KN, Schmid SL, Damke H. Evidence that dynamin- 2 functions as a signal-transducing GTPase. J Cell Biol. 2000;150:145–54.
29. Kirchhausen T, Macia E, Pelish HE. Use of dynasore, the small molecule inhibitor of dynamin, in the regulation of endocytosis. Methods Enzymol. 2008;438:77–93.
30. Hudoklin S, Zupancic D, Romih R. Maturation of the Golgi apparatus in urothelial cells. Cell Tissue Res. 2009;336:453–63.
31. Riedel I, Liang FX, Deng FM, Tu L, Kreibich G, Wu XR, et al. Urothelial umbrella cells of human ureter are heterogeneous with respect to their uroplakin composition: different degrees of urothelial maturity in ureter and bladder? Eur J Cell Biol. 2005;84:393–405.
32. Hu CC, Liang FX, Zhou G, Tu L, Tang CH, Zhou J, et al. Assembly of urothelial plaques: tetraspanin function in membrane protein trafficking. Mol Biol Cell. 2005;16:3937–50.
33. Bongiovanni GA, Eynard AR, Calderón RO. Altered lipid profile and changes in uroplakin properties of rat urothelial plasma membrane with diets of different lipid composition. Mol Cell Biochem. 2005;271:69–75.

34. Duncan MJ, Li G, Shin JS, Carson JL, Abraham SN. Bacterial penetration of bladder epithelium through lipid rafts. J Biol Chem. 2004;279:18944–51.
35. Grasso EJ, Calderón RO. Urinary bladder membrane permeability differentially induced by membrane lipid composition. Mol Cell Biochem. 2009;330(1–2):163–9.
36. Grist M, Chakraborty J. Identification of a mucin layer in the urinary bladder. Urology. 1994;44:26–33.
37. Alm P, Colleen S. A histochemical and ultrastructural study of human urethral uroepithelium. Acta Pathol Microbiol Immunol Scand A. 1982;90:103–11.
38. Nickel JC, Cornish J. Ultrastructural study of an antibody- stabilized bladder surface: a new perspective on the elusive glycosaminoglycan layer. World J Urol. 1994;12:11–4.
39. Koenig F, Knittel J, Schnieder L, George M, Lein M, Schnorr D. Confocal laser scanning microscopy of urinary bladder after intravesical instillation of a fluorescent dye. Urology. 2003;62:158–61.
40. Sonn GA, Jones SN, Tarin TV, Du CB, Mach KE, Jensen KC, et al. Optical biopsy of human bladder neoplasia with in vivo confocal laser endomicroscopy. J Urol. 2009;182(4):1299–305.
41. Hermes B, Spöler F, Naami A, Bornemann J, Först M, Grosse J, et al. Visualization of the basement membrane zone of the bladder by optical coherence tomography: feasibility of non-invasive evaluation of tumor invasion. Urology. 2008;72:677–81.
42. Hurst RE. Structure, function, and pathology of proteoglycans and glycosaminoglycans in the urinary tract. World J Urol. 1994;12:3–10.
43. Higashiyama S, Lau K, Besner GE, Abraham JA, Klagsbrun M. Structure of heparin-binding EGF-like growth factor. Multiple forms, primary structure, and glycosylation of the mature protein. J Biol Chem. 1992;267:6205–12.
44. Shin SY, Takenouchi T, Yokoyama T, Ohtaki T, Munekata E. Chemical synthesis and biological activity of the EGF-like domain of heparin-binding epidermal growth factor-like growth factor (HB-EGF). Int J Pept Protein Res. 1994;44:485–90.
45. Nakagawa T, Higashiyama S, Mitamura T, Mekada E, Taniguchi N. Amino-terminal processing of cell surface heparin-binding epidermal growth factor-like growth factor up-regulates its juxtacrine but not its paracrine growth factor activity. J Biol Chem. 1996;271:30858–63.
46. Nakamura Y, Handa K, Iwamoto R, Tsukamoto T, Takahasi M, Mekada E. Immunohistochemical distribution of CD9, heparin binding epidermal growth factor- like growth factor, and integrin alpha3beta1 in normal human tissues. J Histochem Cytochem. 2001;49:439–44.
47. Iwamoto R, Handa K, Mekada E. Contact-dependent growth inhibition and apoptosis of epidermal growth factor (EGF) receptor-expressing cells by the membrane- anchored form of heparin-binding EGF-like growth factor. J Biol Chem. 1999;274:25906–12.
48. Nishi E, Klagsbrun M. Heparin-binding epidermal growth factor-like growth factor (HB-EGF) is a mediator of multiple physiological and pathological pathways. Growth Factors. 2004;22:253–60.
49. Friedrich MV, Göhring W, Mörgelin M, Brancaccio A, David G, Timpl R. Structural basis of glycosaminoglycan modification and of heterotypic interactions of perlecan domain V. J Mol Biol. 1999;294:259–70.
50. Ujita M, Shinomura T, Ito K, Kitagawa Y, Kimata K. Expression and binding activity of the carboxyl-terminal portion of the core protein of PG-M, a large chondroitin sulfate proteoglycan. J Biol Chem. 1994;269:2760.
51. Chu CL, Goerges AL, Nugent MA. Identification of common and specific growth factor binding sites in heparin sulfate proteoglycans. Biochemistry. 2005;44:12203–13.
52. Harding PA, Davis-Fleischer KM, Crissman-Combs MA, Miller MT, Brigstock DR, Besner GE. Induction of anchorage independent growth by heparin-binding EGF-like growth factor (HB-EGF). Growth Factors. 1999;17:49–61.
53. Takemura T, Hino S, Kuwajima H, Yanagida H, Okada M, Nagata M, et al. Induction of collecting duct morphogenesis in vitro by heparin-binding epidermal growth factor-like growth factor. J Am Soc Nephrol. 2001;12:964–72.
54. Kumar V, Peña de la Vega L, Farell G, Lieske JC. Urinary macromolecular inhibition of crystal adhesion to renal epithelial cells is impaired in male stone formers. Kidney Int. 2005;68:1784–92.

55. Chen WC, Lin HS, Chen HY, Shih CH, Li CW. Effects of Tamm-Horsfall protein and albumin on calcium oxalate crystallization and importance of sialic acids. Mol Urol. 2001;5:1–5.
56. Neal Jr DE, Dilworth JP, Kaack MB. Tamm-Horsfall autoantibodies in interstitial cystitis. J Urol. 1991;145:37–9.
57. Akiyama A, Stein PC, Houshiar A, Parsons CL. Urothelial cytoprotective activity of Tamm-Horsfall protein isolated from the urine of healthy subjects and patients with interstitial cystitis. Am J Physiol Renal Physiol. 2004;287:F305–18.
58. Parsons CL, Rajasekaran M, Arsanjani AH, Chenoweth M, Stein P. Role of sialic acid in urinary cytoprotective activity of Tamm-Horsfall protein. Urology. 2007;69:577–81.
59. Bachmann S, Mutig K, Bates J, Welker P, Geist B, Gross V, et al. Renal effects of Tamm-Horsfall protein (uromodulin) deficiency in mice. Am J Physiol Renal Physiol. 2005;288:F559–67.
60. Byrne DS, Sedor JF, Estojak J, Fitzpatrick KJ, Chiura AN, Mulholland SG. The urinary glycoprotein GP51 as a clinical marker for interstitial cystitis. J Urol. 1999;161:1786–90.
61. Shupp Byrne DE, Sedor JF, Soroush M, McCue PA, Mulholland SG. Interaction of bladder glycoprotein GP51 with uropathogenic bacteria. J Urol. 2001;165:1342–6.
62. Erickson DR, Mast S, Ordille S, Bhavanandan VP. Urinary epitectin (MUC-1 glycoprotein) in the menstrual cycle and interstitial cystitis. J Urol. 1996;156:938–42.
63. Hurst RE, Rhodes SW, Adamson PB, Parsons CL, Roy JB. Functional and structural characteristics of the glycosaminoglycans of the bladder luminal surface. J Urol. 1987;138:433–7.
64. Hauser PJ, Dozmorov MG, Bane BL, Slobodov G, Culkin DJ, Hurst RE. Abnormal expression of differentiation related proteins and proteoglycan core proteins in the urothelium of patients with interstitial cystitis. J Urol. 2008;179:764–9.
65. Hurst RE, Roy JB, Min KW, Veltri RW, Marley G, Patton K, et al. A deficit of chondroitin sulfate proteoglycans on the bladder uroepithelium in interstitial cystitis. Urology. 1996;48:817–21.
66. Parsons CL, Stauffer C, Schmidt JD. Bladder-surface glycosaminoglycans: an efficient mechanism of environmental adaptation. Science. 1980;208:605–7.
67. Poggi MM, Johnstone PA, Conner RJ. Glycosaminoglycan content of human bladders: a method of analysis using cold-cup biopsies. Urol Oncol. 2000;5:234–7.
68. Ewalt DH, Howard PS, Blyth B, Snyder 3rd HM, Duckett JW, Levin RM, et al. Is lamina propria matrix responsible for normal bladder compliance? J Urol. 1992;148(2 Pt 2):544–9.
69. Koo HP, Macarak EJ, Chang SL, Rosenbloom J, Howard PS. Temporal expression of elastic fiber components in bladder development. Connect Tissue Res. 1998;37:1–11.
70. Smeulders N, Woolf AS, Wilcox DT. Extracellular matrix protein expression during mouse detrusor development. J Pediatr Surg. 2003;38:1–12.
71. Miodosky M, Abdul-Hai A, Tsirigotis P, Or R, Bitan M, Resnick IB, et al. Treatment of post-hematopoietic stem cell transplantation hemorrhagic cystitis with intravesicular sodium hyaluronate. Bone Marrow Transplant. 2006;38:507–11.
72. Cao M, Liu B, Cunha G, Baskin L. Urothelium patterns bladder smooth muscle location. Pediatr Res. 2008;64:352–7.
73. Erdani Kreft M, Sterle M. The effect of lamina propria on the growth and differentiation of urothelial cells in vitro. Pflugers Arch. 2000;440(5 Suppl):R181–2.
74. Davidson RA, McCloskey KD. Morphology and localization of interstitial cells in the guinea pig bladder: structural relationships with smooth muscle and neurons. J Urol. 2005;173:1385–90.
75. Sui GP, Rothery S, Dupont E, Fry CH, Severs NJ. Gap junctions and connexin expression in human suburothelial interstitial cells. BJU Int. 2002;90:118–29.
76. Fang Q, Yang J, Pan JH, Li WB, Shen WH, Li LK, et al. Morphological study on the role of ICC like cells in detrusor neuro-modulation of rat urinary bladder. Zhonghua Wai Ke Za Zhi. 2008;46:1542–5.
77. Grol S, Essers PB, van Koeveringe GA, Martinez-Martinez P, de Vente J, Gillespie JI. M(3) muscarinic receptor expression on suburothelial interstitial cells. BJU Int. 2009;104:398–405.

78. Gillespie JI, Harvey IJ, Drake MJ. Agonist- and nerve induced phasic activity in the isolated whole bladder of the guinea pig: evidence for two types of bladder activity. Exp Physiol. 2003;88:343–57.
79. Collins C, Klausner AP, Herrick B, Koo HP, Miner AS, Henderson SC, et al. Potential for control of detrusor smooth muscle spontaneous rhythmic contraction by cyclooxygenase products released by interstitial cells of Cajal. J Cell Mol Med. 2009;13(9):3236–50.
80. Metzger R, Schuster T, Till H, Franke FE, Dietz HG. Cajal-like cells in the upper urinary tract: comparative study in various species. Pediatr Surg Int. 2005;21:169–74.
81. Hashitani H, Yanai Y, Suzuki H. Role of interstitial cells and gap junctions in the transmission of spontaneousCa2+ signals in detrusor smooth muscles of the guinea-pig urinary bladder. J Physiol. 2004;559(Pt 2):567–81.
82. Lang RJ, Klemm MF. Interstitial cell of Cajal-like cells in the upper urinary tract. J Cell Mol Med. 2005;9:543–56.
83. Gillespie JI. The autonomous bladder: a view of the origin of bladder overactivity and sensory urge. BJU Int. 2004;93:478–83.
84. Gillespie JI. Phosphodiesterase-linked inhibition of nonmicturition activity in the isolated bladder. BJU Int. 2004;93:1325–32.
85. Gillespie JI. Noradrenaline inhibits autonomous activity in the isolated guinea pig bladder. BJU Int. 2004;93:401–9.
86. Gillespie JI, Drake MJ. The actions of sodium nitroprusside and the phosphodiesterase inhibitor dipyridamole on phasic activity in the isolated guinea-pig bladder. BJU Int. 2004;93:851–8.
87. Gillespie JI. Modulation of autonomous contractile activity in the isolated whole bladder of the guinea pig. BJU Int. 2004;93:393–400.
88. Fry CH, Hussain M, McCarthy C, Ikeda Y, Sui GP, Wu C. Recent advances in detrusor muscle function. Scand J Urol Nephrol 2004;(215 Suppl):20–5.
89. Neuhaus J, Pfeiffer F, Wolburg H, Horn LC, Dorschner W. Alterations in connexin expression in the bladder of patients with urge symptoms. BJU Int. 2005;96:670–6.
90. Kuijpers KA, Heesakkers JP, Jansen CF, Schalken JA. Cadherin-11 is expressed in detrusor smooth muscle cells and myofibroblasts of normal human bladder. Eur Urol. 2007;52:1213–21.
91. Drake MJ, Hedlund P, Andersson KE, Brading AF, Hussain I, Fowler C, et al. Morphology, phenotype and ultrastructure of fibroblastic cells from normal and neuropathic human detrusor: absence of myofibroblast characteristics. J Urol. 2003;169:1573–6.
92. Drake MJ, Gardner BP, Brading AF. Innervation of the detrusor muscle bundle in neurogenic detrusor overactivity. BJU Int. 2003;91:702–10.
93. Drake MJ, Hedlund P, Harvey IJ, Pandita RK, Andersson KE, Gillespie JI. Partial outlet obstruction enhances modular autonomous activity in the isolated rat bladder. J Urol. 2003;170:276–9.
94. Peixoto EB, Collares-Buzato CB. Protamine-induced epithelial barrier disruption involves rearrangement of cytoskeleton and decreased tight junction-associated protein expression in cultured MDCK strains. Cell Struct Funct. 2005;29:165–78.
95. Erickson DR, Schwarze SR, Dixon JK, Clark CJ, Hersh MA. Differentiation associated changes in gene expression profiles of interstitial cystitis and control urothelial cells. J Urol. 2008;180:2681–7.
96. Bhavanandan VP, Erickson DR. An investigation of the nature of bladder mucosal glycoconjugates and their role in interstitial cystitis. Indian J Biochem Biophys. 1997;34:205–11.
97. Moskowitz MO, Byrne DS, Callahan HJ, Parsons CL, Valderrama E, Moldwin RM. Decreased expression of a glycoprotein component of bladder surface mucin (GP1) in interstitial cystitis. J Urol. 1994;151:343–5.
98. Anderström CR, Fall M, Johansson SL. Scanning electron microscopic findings in interstitial cystitis. Br J Urol. 1989;63:270–5.
99. Stein P, Rajasekaran M, Parsons CL. Tamm-Horsfall protein protects urothelial permeability barrier. Urology. 2005;66:903–7.

100. Graham E, Chai TC. Dysfunction of bladder urothelium and bladder urothelial cells in interstitial cystitis. Curr Urol Rep. 2006;7:440–6.
101. Green M, Filippou A, Sant G, Theoharides TC. Expression of intercellular adhesion molecules in the bladder of patients with interstitial cystitis. Urology. 2004;63:688–93.
102. Wilson CB, Leopard J, Nakamura RM, Cheresh DA, Stein PC, Parsons CL. Selective type IV collagen defects in the urothelial basement membrane in interstitial cystitis. J Urol. 1995;154:1222–6.
103. Bassuk JA. Positive and negative regulators of human urothelial cell proliferation. Urology. 2001;57(6 Suppl 1):104–5.
104. Teng J, Wang ZY, Jarrard DF, Bjorling DE. Roles of estrogen receptor alpha and beta in modulating urothelial cell proliferation. Endocr Relat Cancer. 2008;15:351–64.
105. de Deus JM, Girão MJ, Sartori MG, Baracat EC, Rodrigues de Lima G, Nader HB, et al. Glycosaminoglycan profile in bladder and urethra of castrated rats treated with estrogen, progestogen, and raloxifene. Am J Obstet Gynecol. 2003;189:1654–9.
106. Kim J, Keay SK, Freeman MR. Heparin-binding epidermal growth factor-like growth factor functionally antagonizes interstitial cystitis antiproliferative factor via mitogen-activated protein kinase pathway activation. BJU Int. 2009;103:541–6.
107. Erman A, Zupancic D, Jezernik K. Apoptosis and desquamation of urothelial cells in tissue remodeling during rat postnatal development. J Histochem Cytochem. 2009;57:721–30.
108. Ito T, Stein PC, Parsons CL, Schmidt JD. Elevated stress protein in transitional cells exposed to urine from interstitial cystitis patients. Int J Urol. 1998;5:444–8.
109. Sen GL, Webster DE, Barragan DI, Chang HY, Khavari PA. Control of differentiation in a self-renewing mammalian tissue by the histone demethylase JMJD3. Genes Dev. 2008;22:1865–70.
110. Lan F, Shi Y. Epigenetic regulation: methylation of histone and non-histone proteins. Sci China C Life Sci. 2009;52:311–22.
111. Shaw T, Martin P. Epigenetic reprogramming during wound healing: loss of polycomb-mediated silencing may enable upregulation of repair genes. EMBO Rep. 2009;10:881–6.
112. Rajasekaran M, Stein P, Parsons CL. Toxic factors in human urine that injure urothelium. Int J Urol. 2006;13:409–14.
113. Saitoh T, Hirai M, Katoh M. Molecular cloning and characterization of human Frizzled-8 gene on chromosome 10p11.2. Int J Oncol. 2001;18:991–6.
114. Erickson DR, Sheykhnazari M, Ordille S, Bhavanandan VP. Increased urinary hyaluronic acid and interstitial cystitis. J Urol. 1998;160:1282–4.
115. Keay S, Szekely Z, Conrads TP, Veenstra TD, Barchi Jr JJ, Zhang C-O, et al. An antiproliferative factor from interstitial cystitis patients is a frizzled 8 protein-related sialoglycopeptide. Proc Natl Acad Sci U S A. 2004;101:11803–8.
116. Barchi Jr JJ, Kaczmarek P. Short and sweet: evolution of a small glycopeptide from a bladder disorder to an anticancer lead. Mol Interv. 2009;9:14–7.
117. Sharifi BG, Johnson TC. Affinity labeling of the sialoglycopeptide antimitogen receptor. J Biol Chem. 1987;262:15752–5.
118. Kim J, Keay SK, Dimitrakov JD, Freeman MR. p53 mediates interstitial cystitis antiproliferative factor (APF)-induced growth inhibition of human urothelial cells. FEBS Lett. 2007;581:3795–9.
119. O'Leary MP, Sant GR, Fowler FJ, Whitmore KE, Spolarich-Kroll J. The interstitial cystitis symptom index and problem index. Urology. 1997;49:58–63.
120. Keay S, Takeda M, Tamaki M, Hanno P. Current and future directions in diagnostic markers in interstitial cystitis. Int J Urol. 2003;10:S27–30.
121. Tomaszewski JE, Landis JR, Russack V, Williams TM, Wang LP, Hardy C, et al. Biopsy features are associated with primary symptoms in interstitial cystitis: results from the interstitial cystitis database study. Urology. 2001;57:67–81.
122. Abdel-Mageed AB, Ghoniem GM. Potential role of rel/nuclear factor-kappaB in the pathogenesis of interstitial cystitis. J Urol. 1998;160(6 Pt 1):2000–3.

123. Abdel-Mageed AB, Bajwa A, Shenassa BB, Human L, Ghoniem GM. NF-kappaB-dependent gene expression of proinflammatory cytokines in T24 cells: possible role in interstitial cystitis. Urol Res. 2003;31:300–5.
124. Saban MR, Nguyen NB, Hammond TG, Saban R. Gene expression profiling of mouse bladder inflammatory responses to LPS, substance P, and antigen-stimulation. Am J Pathol. 2002;160:2095–110.
125. Keay S, Zhang CO, Trifillis AL, Hebel JR, Jacobs SC, Warren JW. Urine autoantibodies in interstitial cystitis. J Urol. 1997;157:1083–7.
126. Parsons CL, Greene RA, Chung M, Stanford EJ, Singh G. Abnormal urinary potassium metabolism in patients with interstitial cystitis. J Urol. 2005;173:1182–5.
127. Yu W, Zacharia LC, Jackson EK, Apodaca G. Adenosine receptor expression and function in bladder uroepithelium. Am J Physiol Cell Physiol. 2006;291:C254–65.
128. Christmas TJ, Rode J, Chapple CR, Milroy EJ, Turner-Warwick RT. Nerve fibre proliferation in interstitial cystitis. Virchows Arch A Pathol Anat Histopathol. 1990;416:447–51.
129. Lundeberg T, Liedberg H, Nordling L, Theodorsson E, Owzarski A, Ekman P. Interstitial cystitis: correlation with nerve fibres, mast cells and histamine. Br J Urol. 1993;71:427–9.
130. Mattila J, Pitkänen R, Vaalasti T, Seppänen J. Finestructural evidence for vascular injury in patients with interstitial cystitis. Virchows Arch A Pathol Anat Histopathol. 1983;398:347–55.
131. Marchand JE, Sant GR, Kream RM. Increased expression of substance P receptor-encoding mRNA in bladder biopsies from patients with interstitial cystitis. Br J Urol. 1998;81:224–8.
132. Kyker KD, Coffman J, Hurst RE. Exogenous glycosaminoglycans coat damaged bladder surfaces in experimentally damaged mouse bladder. BMC Urol. 2005;5:4.
133. Nickel JC, Downey J, Morales A, Emerson L, Clark J. Relative efficacy of various exogenous glycosaminoglycans in providing a bladder surface permeability barrier. J Urol. 1998;160:612–4.
134. Lee DG, Cho JJ, Park HK, Kim DK, Kim JI, Chang SG, et al. Preventive effects of hyaluronic acid on Escherichia coli-induced urinary tract infection in rat. Urology. 2010;75(4):949–54.
135. Parsons CL, Boychuk D, Jones S, Hurst R, Callahan H. Bladder surface glycosaminoglycans: an epithelial permeability barrier. J Urol. 1990;143:139–42.
136. Daha LK, Lazar D, Simak R, Pflüger H. Is there a relation between urinary interleukin-6 levels and symptoms before and after intra-vesical glycosaminoglycan substitution therapy in patients with bladder pain syndrome/interstitial cystitis? Int Urogynecol J Pelvic Floor Dysfunct. 2007;18:1449–52.
137. Daha LK, Riedl CR, Lazar D, Simak R, Pflüger H. Effect of intravesical glycosaminoglycan substitution therapy on bladder pain syndrome/interstitial cystitis, bladder capacity and potassium sensitivity. Scand J Urol Nephrol. 2008;42:369–72.
138. Daha LK, Lazar D, Simak R, Pflüger H. The effects of intravesical pentosanpolysulfate treatment on the symptoms of patients with bladder pain syndrome/interstitial cystitis: preliminary results. Int Urogynecol J Pelvic Floor Dysfunct. 2008;19:987–90.
139. Alho AM, Underhill CB. The hyaluronate receptor is preferentially expressed on proliferating epithelial cells. J Cell Biol. 1989;108:1557–65.
140. Leppilahti M, Hellström P, Tammela TL. Effect of diagnostic hydrodistension and four intravesical hyaluronic acid instillations on bladder ICAM-1 intensity and association of ICAM-1 intensity with clinical response in patients with interstitial cystitis. Urology. 2002;60:46–51.
141. Vasiadi M, Kalogeromitros D, Kempuraj D, Clemons A, Zhang B, Chliva C, et al. Rupatadine inhibits proinflammatory mediator secretion from human mast cells triggered by different stimuli. Int Arch Allergy Immunol. 2009;151:38–45.
142. Boucher WS, Letourneau R, Huang M, Kempuraj D, Green M, Sant GR, et al. Intravesical sodium hyaluronate inhibits the rat urinary mast cell mediator increase triggered by acute immobilization stress. J Urol. 2002;167:380–4.
143. Takahashi K, Takeuchi J, Takahashi T, Miyauchi S, Horie K, Uchiyama Y. Effects of sodium hyaluronate on epithelial healing of the vesical mucosa and vesical fibrosis in rabbits with acetic acid induced cystitis. J Urol. 2001;166:710–3.

144. Sadhukhan PC, Tchetgen MB, Rackley RR, Vasavada SP, Liou L, Bandyopadhyay SK. Sodium pentosan polysulfate reduces urothelial responses to inflammatory stimuli via an indirect mechanism. J Urol. 2002;168:289–92.
145. Takakura K, Mizogami M, Fukuda S. Protamine sulfate causes endothelium-independent vasorelaxation via inducible nitric oxide synthase pathway. Can J Anaesth. 2006;53:162–7.
146. Lilly JD, Parsons CL. Bladder surface glycosaminoglycans is a human epithelial permeability barrier. Surg Gynecol Obstet. 1990;171:493–6.
147. Schulz A, Vestweber AM, Dressler D. Anti-inflammatory action of a hyaluronic acid-chondroitin sulfate preparation in an in vitro bladder model. Aktuelle Urol. 2009;40:109–12.
148. Parsons CL. Epithelial coating techniques in the treatment of interstitial cystitis. Urology. 1997;49(5A Suppl):100–4.
149. Southgate J, Varley CL, Garthwaite MA, Hinley J, Marsh F, Stahlschmidt J, et al. Differentiation potential of urothelium from patients with benign bladder dysfunction. BJU Int. 2007;99:1506–16.
150. Zhang H, Sunnarborg SW, McNaughton KK, Johns TG, Lee DC, Faber JE. Heparin-binding epidermal growth factor-like growth factor signaling in flowinduced arterial remodeling. Circ Res. 2008;102:1275–85.
151. Fukatsu Y, Noguchi T, Hosooka T, Ogura T, Kotani K, Abe T, et al. Muscle-specific overexpression of heparinbinding epidermal growth factor-like growth factor increases peripheral glucose disposal and insulin sensitivity. Endocrinology. 2009;150:2683–91.
152. Tyagi P, Hsieh VC, Yoshimura N, Kaufman J, Chancellor MB. Instillation of liposomes vs dimethyl sulphoxide or pentosan polysulphate for reducing bladder hyperactivity. BJU Int. 2009;104(11):1689–92.
153. Hwang TL, Fang CL, Chen CH, Fang JY. Permeation enhancer-containing water-in-oil nanoemulsions as carriers for intravesical cisplatin delivery. Pharm Res. 2009;26:2314–23.

Chapter 5
Mast Cell and Bladder Pain Syndrome

Kirsten Bouchelouche and Pierre Bouchelouche

Introduction

The exact etiology of Bladder Pain Syndrome (BPS) is unclear. However, there is general agreement that BPS may have a multifactorial etiology that may act predominantly through one or more pathways resulting in the typical symptom-complex [1]. Among the proposed theories during the years, the two main theories have been those of a defect in bladder cytoprotection and increased mast cells. The "leaky epithelium," mast cell activation, and neurogenic inflammation, or some combination of these and other factors may result in chronic bladder pain and voiding dysfunction. A pathophysiologic role for the mast cells was first suggested by Simmons and Bunce [2]. An increased number of activated mast cells in the bladder lining are thought to play a role in causing the symptoms of BPS, and there is increasing evidence that mast cells play an important role in BPS, at least in a subgroup of the patients [3–8]. The role of mast cells in BPS is the topic for this chapter, and the mast cell, published data on bladder mastocytosis in clinical studies, mast cell mediators in urine, and possible interaction between mast cells, bladder neurons, and detrusor muscle cells are reviewed. Furthermore, the ESSIC recommendations on the evaluation of mast cells in bladder tissue are described.

K. Bouchelouche, M.D., D.M.Sc. (✉) • P. Bouchelouche, M.D.
Smooth Muscle Research Center, Department of Clinical Biochemistry, Koege Hospital,
University of Copenhagen, Lykkebaekvej 1, DK-4600, Koege, Denmark
e-mail: bouchelouche@mail.dk

J. Nordling et al. (eds.), *Bladder Pain Syndrome: A Guide for Clinicians*,
DOI 10.1007/978-1-4419-6929-3_5, © Springer Science+Business Media New York 2013

Mast Cell

Mast Cell Function

Mast cells have classically been related to allergic responses. However, several recent studies indicate that these cells essentially contribute to other common diseases. Their constitutive residence at the border of the body and environment, combined with their array of diverse mediators, suggests that they are strategically situated to innate immune and inflammatory responses. In such locations, including the bladder wall, mast cells are well placed to function in host defense [9]. Mast cells participate in many biological responses including allergic diseases, host responses to parasites and neoplasms, blood vessel formation, acute and chronic inflammatory disorders, fibrotic conditions, tissue modeling, and wound healing [10]. Locally, mast cells may influence many of these processes through the production of a broad spectrum of multifunctional mediators, especially proinflammatory cytokines [10–13]. Their central role in immunological processes is further reflected by the large number of mediators by which mast cells may influence other cells. These mediators allow mast cells to regulate either local tissue functions or host defense by acting as innate immune cells, by interacting with the specific immune system, or by inducing and regulating inflammation. Since mast cells are located at the border of the body and environment, they are perfectly equipped with their mediators to orchestrate the immune system. The same feature that enables mast cells to protect the organism can run out of control resulting in disease instead of host protection.

Mast cells are known to be the primary responders in allergic reactions, orchestrating strong responses to small antigens. Mast cells are coated with antigen-specific IgE, and exposure to specific antigens induces bringing of surface-bound IgE molecules resulting in a rapid release of preformed mediators from granules, as well as the release of the de novo synthesized mediators, which all act on distinct effector cells to produce the symptoms of allergy and anaphylaxis. The broad spectrum of functions of mast cells might explain why mast cells can be involved in so many different pathologies beyond allergy. An increase in mast cells within tissues is observed in many pathological conditions including asthma, atherosclerosis, autoimmune diseases, atopic dermatitis, inflammatory bowel disease, BPS, multiple sclerosis, psoriasis, rheumatoid arthritis, sarcoidosis, and tumor growths [14, 15]. Apart from being prominently involved in immune and inflammatory responses, mast cells are critical for the tissue integrity and function. This correlates with their presence in nearly all tissues.

Mast Cell Origin and Distribution

Mast cells originate from stem cells in the bone marrow, enter the circulation, and differentiate in the microenvironments of various tissues that are rich in fibroblasts and other mesenchymal elements [10]. Mast cells are normally distributed throughout connective tissues, where they may be especially numerous beneath the epithelial surfaces of the skin, in the respiratory system, in the gastrointestinal and genitourinary tracts, adjacent to blood or lymphatic vessels, and near or within peripheral nerves. In these places the mast cells are near parasites, antigens, etc. that come in contact with the skin or mucosal surfaces. Thus, the mast cells are well placed to function as sentinel cells in host defense [9]. Although mast cells are bone marrow-derived hematopoietic cells, committed mast cell progenitors circulate in small numbers in the blood and are thought to migrate to tissues before undergoing the final stages of maturation, including development of mature granules [13]. However, mature resident mast cells have been shown to proliferate locally in some situations [16]. Mast cell population in the tissue is therefore controlled by a combination of recruitment of committed precursors, maturation of resident precursors, and local proliferation [13]. Local differentiation and maturation of mast cells are regulated by tissue environmental factors. The most important factor for human mast cells is stem cell factor (also known as c-kit ligand) which is secreted by fibroblasts, stromal cells, and endothelial cells. In humans, survival and differentiation of tissue mast cells are also enhanced by other cytokines such as interleukin (IL)-4, IL-6, and IL-10. The main in vivo mast cell growth factors are stem cell factor in combination with cytokines [13, 16]. In the tissue the mast cells have a long half-life of at least 40 days.

Mast Cell Heterogeneity

Mast cells in different localizations, and even in a single site, can have substantial differences in mediator content, sensitivity to agents that induce activation and mediator release, and responses to pharmacological agents. Such heterogeneity is regulated by many factors, including certain cytokines, which influence the cells' stage of maturation, differentiation, proliferation, and other characteristics. The phenotype plasticity of mast cell populations may permit these cells to respond to changes in the microenvironment produced by diseases or immunologic responses. Based on their different phenotypical and biochemical properties, two basic populations of mast cells have been identified—known as MC^{T} and MC^{TC}—with the MC^{T} subtype being more commonly found at mucosal sites and the other, MC^{TC}, more commonly in the connective tissue [8, 17]. These subsets are classified on the basis of the protease content of their granules: whether they contain either tryptase (MC^{T}) or tryptase plus chymase (MC^{TC}). Connective tissue mast cells are found in the skin, peritoneal cavities, serosa, and muscularis propria of the intestine. Muccosal mast cells are found primarily in mucosa and in epithelium.

Mast Cell Mediators

Mast cells store an impressive array of preformed compounds (mediators) in their secretory granules, and upon activation mast cells release a broad variety of proinflammatory mediators. Mast cells produce three main classes of mediators: preformed granule-associated mediators (histamine, serotonin, tryptase, chymase, etc.); newly generated lipid mediators (leukotrienes, prostaglandins); and a variety of cytokines (interleukins, etc.), chemokines (monocyte chemoattractant proteins, RANTES, eotaxin, etc.), growth factors, and free radicals (nitric oxide, superoxide) [13]. Table 5.1 illustrates the main classes of mediators released by mast cells [8, 13, 18]. At present, more than 30 different cytokines have been shown to be produced by human mast cells.

When mast cells degranulate, mediators are released and these have a profound impact on any condition in which mast cell degranulation occurs. These mast cell mediators, when released, may contribute to the overall inflammatory process and to the clinical and pathological findings in some patients with BPS characterized with mast cell involvement of the urinary bladder.

Mast Cell Activation

Mast cells participate in allergic type 1 hypersentivity reactions where immunoglobulin E (IgE) attaches to specific surface-binding proteins on mast cells and triggers a cascade of reactions resulting in a degranulation by compound exocytosis [10, 11]. In addition to IgE and antigen, many other substances and non-immunological stimuli are also capable of triggering mast cell secretion: anaphylatoxins, bacteria, chemicals, contrast media (radiology), cytokines, drugs, free radicals, growth factors, hormones, kinins, neuropeptides, neurotransmitters, radiation, toxins, and viruses [11]. Activated preformed mediators within granules can be released by two morphological distinct processes: (1) exocytosis by mast cell degranulation (rapid and massive release, characteristically occurring during IgE-dependent allergic reactions) and (2) differential mediator release (slow release of mediators in a selective fashion).

Analysis of Mast Cell in Tissue

In the evaluation of patients suspected of having BPS it is important to obtain information on mast cell involvement in order to categorize the patients according to the ESSIC criteria [19]. In 2004, ESSIC published recommendations on the primary evaluation of the patients suspected of having BPS [20]. The recommendations included how to evaluate biopsies in a standardized way for mast cell involvement. In 2008, new recommendations on quantifying mast cells in BPS by immunohistochemical analysis were published by Larsen et al. [21]. In brief, the recommendations are the following:

Table 5.1 Selection of mast cell mediators produced by human mast cells

Preformed (stored) mediators	Mediators produced on activation (de novo synthesis)
Biogenic amines:	*Phospholipid metabolites*:
Histamine	Leukotriene B_4 (LTB_4)
Serotonin (5-hydroxy-tryptamine)	Leukotriene C_4 (LTC_4)
	PGD_2, PGE_2
	Platelet-activating factor (PAF)
Enzymes:	*Cytokines*:
Tryptase	IL-1, 3, 4, 5, 6, 8, 9, 10, 12, 13, 14, 16, 18, 25
Chymase	MIP-1α and MIP-1β
Carboxypeptidase A	
Peroxidase	Interferon α, β, γ
β-Hexoaminidase	TNFα (Tumor necrosis factor)
Phospholipases	Leptin
Matrix metalloproteinases	
Proteoglycans:	*Nitric oxide (NO)*
Heparin	
Chondroitin sulfate	
Chemokines:	*Growth factors*:
Interleukin-8 (IL-8)	Stem cell factor (SCF)
MCP-1	Granulocyte monocyte-colony stimulatory factor (GM-CSF)
MCP-3	Vascular endothelial growth factor (VEGF)
MCP-4	Fibroblast growth factor (FGF)
RANTES	Nerve growth factor (NGF)
Eotaxin	Platelet-derived growth factor (PDGF)
Polypeptides:	
Renin	
Substance P	
Corticotropin-releasing hormone (CRH)	
Urocortin	
Vasoactive intestinal polypeptide (VIP)	
Angiogenin	

Biopsies

During cystoscopy the bladder is distended to full capacity. After draining the bladder, bladder biopsies are taken at roughly half full bladder capacity. Biopsy procedures should be performed by using large forceps and include detrusor muscle;

alternatively double-punch biopsies or resections of lesions can be used. At least three biopsies from the two lateral walls and bladder dome should be taken in addition to biopsies from lesional areas. The biopsies are to be immediately fixed in formalin. Biopsies are treated conventionally according to routine procedure at the Department of Pathology, and evaluated preferably by a dedicated pathologist.

Mast Cell Staining

Many studies have been published about the presence of mast cells in BPS. However, the value of mast cell count varies widely depending on which methods were used to cut, stain, and count the mast cells. Often such details are not provided in the published articles, resulting in difficulties in comparing studies. Different staining procedures have been applied, and they vary greatly in their ability to detect mast cells [8, 22]. Metachromatic staining with toluidine blue or Giemsa are two of the previous staining methods, but it is now clear that some types of mast cells fixed in formalin are not stained by toluidine blue [8, 22, 23]. In the ESSIC recommendations [20], it was recommended that enzymatic staining with naphtolesterase was used for mast cell counting in 10 μm sections. However, it has been demonstrated that human mast cells are detected effectively by immunocytochemical staining for tryptase, a unique protease found in both types of mast cells, i.e., MC^{T} and MC^{TC} [8, 24]. Furthermore, tryptase staining is easy with an automatic immunostainer and standard 3 μm sections [21]. In contrast, the enzymatic staining with naphtolesterase implies manual procedures, and is therefore both difficult and time consuming. Mast cell count based on naphtolesterase and tryptase shows good correlation with the clinical score, regardless of section thickness [21]. Thus, for evaluation of mast cells tryptase staining is recommended. The detrusor specimens are fixed in formalin, 3 μm sections are cut, and every seventh is mounted on a specimen slide for tryptase staining according to routine procedures [21].

Mast Cell Counting

The mast cell counting is performed using a grid containing 25 squares, each square measuring 0.21 mm^2 [20]. The counting of mast cells in the detrusor is preferably done in 20 squares but at least 7 squares should be counted. If less than seven squares with detrusor are represented the biopsy is insufficient. Only mast cells containing nucleus are included. At least three biopsies must be the subject of mast cell counting and if possible one including a lesional area (Fig. 5.1).

The total number of mast cells per mm^2 is the total number of mast cells divided by the number of squares included in the counting $\times 0.21$ [20]. If biopsies for mast cell counting do not contain detrusor muscle new biopsies must be obtained.

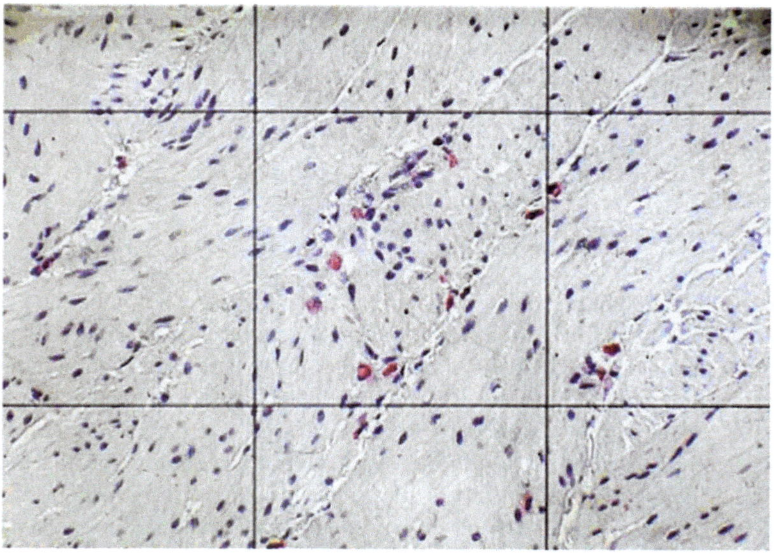

Fig. 5.1 Mast cell counting in detrusor muscle using a standard grid. From Nordling J, et al. Primary evaluation of patients suspected of having interstitial cystitis (IC). Eur Urol. 2004;45:662–9. Reprinted with permission from Elsevier Ltd

The Pathology Report

ESSIC recommends [20] that pathology report should include information about (1) *Epithelium* (not present, present, dysplasia with grading, abnormal but no dysplasia—description); (2) *Propria* (normal, inflammation—description with a grading, other findings are described); (3) *Detrusor muscle* (abnormal muscle cells—describe, intrafascicular fibrosis—present/not present, mast cell count—at least three biopsies should be included in the counting and the biopsy with the highest number of mast cells per mm^2 should be reported); and (4) *Information on detrusor mastocytosis*: (a) less than 20 mast cells/mm^2 = no detrusor mastocytosis; (b) between 20 and 27 = grey zone; and (c) 27 or more mast cells/mm^2 = detrusor mastocytosis [21].

Mast Cells and BPS

Mast cells have frequently been reported to be associated with BPS, and there is increasing evidence that mast cells play a pathophysiological role, at least in a subgroup of patients with BPS. A number of studies have demonstrated increased number of mast cells in the bladder of patients with BPS [2–4, 6, 8, 25–28]. Furthermore, mast cells have been recovered in the bladder washings from patients with classic BPS [26]. Evidence of their importance is mounting, suggesting that they may serve as the final common pathway through which the symptomatic condition is expressed in patients with mast cell involvement of the bladder. Mast cells produce, among other potent compounds, histamine. Histamine release in tissue causes pain, hyperemia, and fibrosis, all notable features of BPS.

Mastocytosis

Several studies in humans have shown an increase in mast cell number and activation in patients with BPS. Simmons and Bunce were the first to suggest that mast cells may play a role in BPS [2]. Larsen et al. demonstrated a highly significant increase in the number of mast cells within the detrusor muscle bundles in patients with BPS as compared to controls [4]. The mast cells were partially or completely degranulated. This mast cell infiltration was widespread throughout the detrusor muscle and was not confined to the ulcerative lesions seen cystoscopically [4]. Aldenborg and associates reported that mast cells are found predominantly in the detrusor muscle in patients with classic BPS with Hunner's lesion, but there is also a secondary population of mast cells in the lamina propria and the bladder epithelium, with staining characteristics distinct from those in the detrusor [23]. None of these epithelial mast cells were found in controls. These findings were interpreted to indicate a transepithelial migration of mast cells in patients with BPS. This epithelial population of mast cells does not appear to be involved in the type of BPS without Hunner's lesion. These epithelial mast cells may also differ from the mast cells found in deeper tissues in physiologic responses and release of secretory products. The "mucosal mast cells" are susceptible to aldehyde fixation and require special fixation and staining techniques for proper demonstration, while detrusor mast cells are not susceptible to fixation techniques [23]. The mast cell expansion in BPS involves both types of mast cells, MC^{T} and MC^{TC} [8, 17, 22]. Yamada et al. demonstrated that MC^{TC} may be the type of mast cells dominantly present in the bladder of BPS, and the MC^{TC} increase with progression of contracted bladder [22]. Figure 5.2 illustrates MC^{T} and MC^{TC} in tissue from BPS. Lynes et al. were the first to suggest that mast cells were highly degranulated in both the submucosal and muscle layer of the bladder in BPS [29]. Mast cell activation is far more pronounced in BPS with Hunner's lesion, which in addition displays prominent inflammation, in contrast to nonulcer BPS, where it is sparse [30]. Peeker et al. showed that redistribution of mast cells into the epithelium and a high mast cell count in the bladder wall distinguish classic BPS from nonulcer BPS [17]. Thus, the basic pathologic processes may differ.

Johansson and Fall reported that mast cells were increased in both lamina propria and detrusor muscle in patients with Hunner's lesion [30]. Patients with classical disease had mucosal ulceration and hemorrhage, granulation tissue, intense inflammatory infiltrate, elevated mast cell counts, and perineural infiltrates. Patients with nonulcer disease, despite the same severe symptoms, had a relatively unaltered mucosa with a sparse inflammatory response, the main feature being multiple, small,

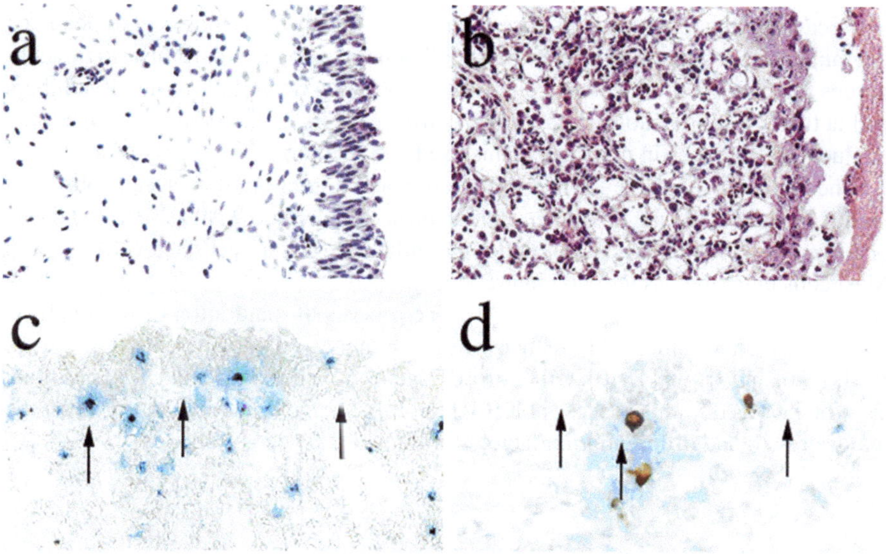

Fig. 5.2 Hematoxylin and eosin staining of (**a**) nonulcer BPS and (**b**) classic BPS with Hunners's lesion. (**c**) shows double labeling of intraepithelial and mucosal stromale tryptase-positive, chymase-negative mast cells (MC^T, *blue*) and (**d**) tryptase-positive, chymase-positive mast cells (MC^{TC}, *brown*) in classic BPS. From Peeker R, et al. Recruitment, distribution and phenotypes of mast cells in interstitial cystitis. J Urol. 2000;163:1009–15. Reprinted with permission from Elsevier Ltd

mucosal ruptures and suburothelial hemorrhages that were noted in a high proportion of the patients. Theoharides et al. demonstrated that mast cells in nonulcer BPS are highly activated by ultrastructural criteria [31]. Furthermore, increased levels of urinary methylhistamine [32] and tryptase [33] support a role of these mast cells.

Feltis et al. proposed the quantification of mast cells in the detrusor as a useful marker in patients with BPS [3]. Kastrup et al. suggested that a mast cell count >28 mast cell/mm^2 in the detrusor (detrusor mastocytosis) is diagnostic for BPS [27]. This was supported by Mortensen et al. who showed that high mast cell counts >28 cells/mm^2 in the detrusor layer of bladder biopsies correlated with clinical outcome [34]. Following the ESSIC recommendations, Wyndaele et al. found a significant correlation between the cystoscopic aspect and inflammatory infiltration, mast cell count in detrusor muscle and stromal edema [35]. Furthermore, maximal bladder capacity was negatively correlated with inflammation, mast cell count, hemorrhages, and the overall cystoscopic findings. Mast cells are more consistently increased in classic BPS with Hunner's lesion. However, mast cell density does not appear to correlate with the duration of symptom amelioration after complete transuretral resection of Hunner's lesion, either in the lamina propria or in the urothelium or the detrusor [36]. However, in another large retrospective study by Richter et al., it was shown that detrusor mastocytosis is associated with multiple treatments and presumed failure of standard urological therapy in patients with BPS, while bladder capacity and glomerulations are not [37].

Because activated mast cells lose their histologically identifiable granules once degranulation occurs, estimates of mast cell density using standard histologic techniques may underestimate mast cell numbers. Varying reports of mast cell numbers and activation in the submucosa versus detrusor layers of the bladder in BPS may be due to differences in mast cell stains used and methods of tissue fixation.

The factors responsible for the proliferation and migration of mast cells observed in the bladder in BPS are unknown. Human mast cells are known to arise from CD34-positive progenitors, particularly under the influence of stem cell factor (SCF) [38]. Mast cells enter the tissues and mature in almost all vascularized tissues, where they can reside for long periods of time [39]. The process of maturation of mast cells is under microenvironmental influences, by SCF, nerve growth factor (NGF), IL-3, IL-4, IL-6, and IL-9 [11, 40]. Other growth factors, chemokines and cytokines, may even be involved in this process [11]. SCF and IL-6 in combination appear to be the major growth and differentiation factors for human mast cells [40].

Ultrastructural Appearance of Mast Cells

It has been demonstrated using electron microscopy that fewer than 30 % of the granules in mast cells from BPS are homogenous, intact, and electron dense as compared to over 70–80 % of mast cells from control patients, indicating mast cell activation with granule release of their content in BPS [31]. The secretory granules of bladder mast cells in BPS contain altered contents and appear empty, and mast cell secretion in BPS appears to be slow and gradual with differential (possible selective) release of secretory mediators, a process shown to involve secretion without exocytosis [41]. Secretion without degranulation as observed in BPS has been termed "piecemeal degranulation" or "intragranular activation" [42, 43]. Mast cells that have totally released their granular contents do not stain with routine histochemistry, thus leading to an underestimating of mast cell number unless electronmicroscopy or measurement of urine mast cell mediators is used concurrently. In an ultrastructural study by Horn et al., a varying number of detrusor smooth muscle cells (SMC) revealed a characteristic oak leaf pattern with protrusion of the sarcolemma [44]. These alterations may express degenerations of SMC secondary to massive exposure to released mast cell mediators. Christmas et al. found that detrusor myopathy is associated with bladder hypocompliance, and patients with detrusor myopathy appear to have more severe disease and are more likely to progress to bladder contracture requiring operation [45].

Mast Cell–Neuron Interactions

It has been proposed that mast cell–neuronal interaction is involved in BPS. Neuroimmune interaction involving mast cells in the bladder may explain the sensory neuronal hyperreactivity and neuropathic pain seen in BPS [5]. A proliferation of sympathetic nerve fibers containing neuropeptide Y and calcitonin gene-related peptide has been demonstrated in BPS [46, 47]. Pang et al. demonstrated increased substance P-containing nerve fibers adjacent to mast cells in the bladder submucosa of BPS patients [48], and a close anatomic relationship between bladder neurons and mast cells has been demonstrated by electron microscopy [43]. Many patients with BPS report that their symptoms are exacerbated by stress [49], and stress has been shown to activate bladder mast cells [50].

Estrogen and Mast Cells

Many patients with BPS report symptom exacerbation perimenstrually or at the time of ovulation [8]. Bladder mast cells in BPS have increased expression of high-affinity estrogen receptors [51] but only few progesterone receptors. In vitro and in vivo studies have shown that estradiol augments mast cell histamine secretion [52, 53]. The effect of female sex hormones on mast cells may contribute to the high incidence of BPC in women and the worsening of symptoms perimenstrually [50].

Mast Cell and Detrusor Muscle

Traditionally, the human detrusor SMC was thought as a passive player in inflammation, contracting in response to inflammatory mediators. Recent studies suggest that SMC may secrete cytokines and chemokines, and express cell adhesion molecules that are important in modulating of the inflammatory process [54–57]. In asthma, mast cell mediators can increase proinflammatory cytokine release from airway SMC, thus interacting directly with inflammatory cell infiltration and activation [58]. This interaction between SMC and mast cells is not only interesting by giving the SMC an active role in inflammation but may also furthermore offer new therapeutic targets in treating this inflammatory lung disorder [59].

Several studies have demonstrated increased number of activated mast cells in the detrusor muscle of patients with BPS [4, 17, 31, 60]. The close relationship of mast cells with detrusor muscle cells in BPS is illustrated in Fig. 5.3. In BPS many of these infiltrating mast cells show signs of activation. Upon activation the mast cells release potent mediators that may interact with the detrusor muscle cells in the bladder wall. Bouchelouche and colleges have demonstrated that mast cell mediators like histamine and LTD_4 induce contraction of human detrusor muscle [61]. Furthermore, it was demonstrated that LTD4 increases human detrusor muscle responsiveness to histamine [62].

The factors responsible for the proliferation and migration of mast cells in the detrusor in BPS are unknown. Stem cell factor and cytokines may be involved in this process. Like in other organs, the detrusor SMC may be an active player in the

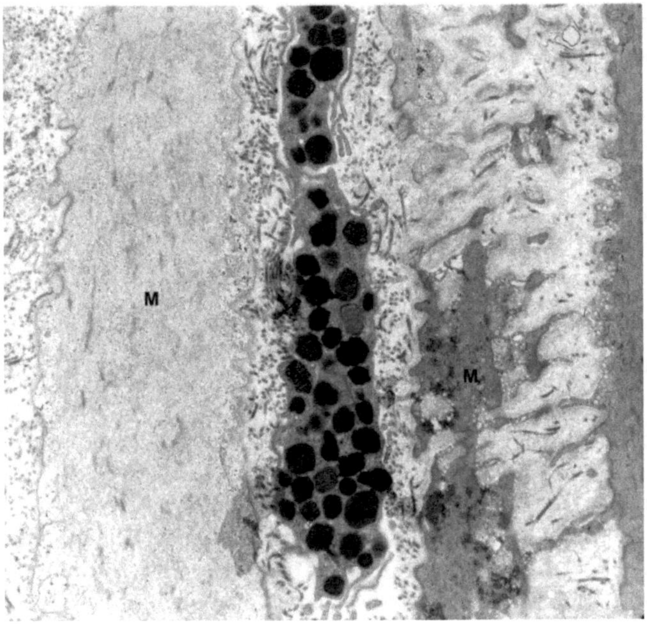

Fig. 5.3 Electron microscopic picture of a mast cell between detrusor muscle cells (*M*)

inflammatory process by producing inflammatory mediators. Until recently, the capacity of the human detrusor SMC to express and release cytokines during bladder inflammation was unknown. Bouchelouche et al. demonstrated that human detrusor SMC are able to express and secrete several cytokines and growth factors including MCP-1, RANTES, eotaxin, IL-8, IL-6, and SCF upon stimulation with proinflammatory mediators [63–65]. Thus, this secretory function of human detrusor muscle is likely to influence mast cell number and activation in a potent and proinflammatory manner, and the detrusor muscle may be an active player in the inflammatory process seen in patients with BPS and mast cell involvement of the bladder.

Urine Mast Cell Mediators

The most compelling support for mast cell involvement without light microscopic evidence of mastocytosis or degranulation is the ability of mast cells to secrete mediators, especially biogenic amines and cytokines. Upon activation bladder mast cells release histamine and other mediators.

In patients with BPS, histamine levels are increased in the bladder wall [27], and urine histamine is elevated after bladder hydrodistention [66]. The major histamine metabolite 1,4-methylimidazole acetic acid is increased in the urine of patients with BPS with detrusor mastocytosis, and methylhistamine is significantly elevated in the urine (24-h urine collection) of patients with nonulcer BPS [32, 67]. Tryptase, the specific human mast cell proteinase enzyme, is also elevated in the urine of patients with BPS [33].

Upon activation mast cells may release IL-6 without concomitant histamine release. Studies have demonstrated increased level of IL-6 in urine from BPS patients, and IL-6-positive cells are present in the mucosal and detrusor layers of their bladders [17, 68]. High urine IL-6 levels are associated with severe inflammation in patients who respond to bladder hydrodistention [69], and IL-6 is also expressed in the urothelium of bladder metaplastic lesions and classic BPS [17].

The finding of increased urinary levels of leukotriene E4 in patients with BPS and detrusor mastocytosis when compared with healthy control subjects [70] suggests that cysteinyl-containing leukotrienes are involved in the inflammatory reaction observed in the urinary bladder of patients with BPS.

Several studies have demonstrated increased urinary excretion of NGF in BPS [71–74]. NGF is expressed in mast cells, and can activate mast cells to degranulate and proliferate. For further details on urinary excretion of mediators in BPS, see Chap. 14 on urinary biomarkers in BPS in this book.

Conclusion

A major theory for BPS is that bladder mast cells are activated, releasing potent mast cell mediators. Current evidence from electron microscopy and immunohistochemical staining techniques confirms a central role for mast cells in the pathogenesis and pathophysiology of BPS, at least in a subgroup of the patients. Urine levels of several mast cell mediators are elevated in patients with BPS supporting a role of mast cells. Identification of patient with BPS and mast cell involvement of the bladder will allow targeted pharmacotherapy with drugs that inhibit mast cell activation and mediator release, or inhibit the effect of released mast cell mediators.

References

1. Hanno P, Nordling J, Fall M. Bladder pain syndrome. Med Clin North Am. 2011;95:55–73.
2. Simmons JL, Bunce PL. On the use of an antihistamine in the treatment of interstitial cystitis. Am Surg. 1958;24:664–7
3. Feltis JT, Perez-Marrero R, Emerson LE. Increased mast cells of the bladder in suspected cases of interstitial cystitis: a possible disease marker. J Urol. 1987;138:42–3.
4. Larsen S, Thompson SA, Hald T, Barnard RJ, Gilpin CJ, Dixon JS, Gosling JA. Mast cells in interstitial cystitis. Br J Urol. 1982;54:283–6.
5. Sant GR, Kempuraj D, Marchand JE, Theoharides TC. The mast cell in interstitial cystitis: role in pathophysiology and pathogenesis. Urology. 2007;69:34–40.
6. Sant GR, Theoharides TC. The role of the mast cell in interstitial cystitis. Urol Clin North Am. 1994;21:41–53.

7. Theoharides TC, Pang X, Letourneau R, Sant GR. Interstitial cystitis: a neuroimmunoendocrine disorder. Ann N Y Acad Sci. 1998;840:619–34.
8. Theoharides TC, Kempuraj D, Sant GR. Mast cell involvement in interstitial cystitis: a review of human and experimental evidence. Urology. 2001;57:47–55.
9. Galli SJ, Maurer M, Lantz CS. Mast cells as sentinels of innate immunity. Curr Opin Immunol. 1999;11:53–9.
10. Galli SJ. New concepts about the mast cell. N Engl J Med. 1993;328:257–65.
11. Galli SJ, Nakae S, Tsai M. Mast cells in the development of adaptive immune responses. Nat Immunol. 2005;6:135–42.
12. Gordon JR, Burd PR, Galli SJ. Mast cells as a source of multifunctional cytokines. Immunol Today. 1990;11:458–64.
13. Marshall JS. Mast-cell responses to pathogens. Nat Rev Immunol. 2004;4:787–99.
14. Theoharides TC, Cochrane DE. Critical role of mast cells in inflammatory diseases and the effect of acute stress. J Neuroimmunol. 2004;146:1–12.
15. Theoharides TC, Conti P. Mast cells: the Jekyll and Hyde of tumor growth. Trends Immunol. 2004;25:235–41.
16. Tsai M, Takeishi T, Thompson H, Langley KE, Zsebo KM, Metcalfe DD, Geissler EN, Galli SJ. Induction of mast cell proliferation, maturation, and heparin synthesis by the rat c-kit ligand, stem cell factor. Proc Natl Acad Sci U S A. 1991;88:6382–6.
17. Peeker R, Enerback L, Fall M, Aldenborg F. Recruitment, distribution and phenotypes of mast cells in interstitial cystitis. J Urol. 2000;163:1009–15.
18. Molderings GJ. Mast cell function in physiology and pathophysiology. Biotrend Rev. 2010;5:1–9.
19. Van De Merwe JP, Nordling J, Bouchelouche P, Bouchelouche K, Cervigni M, Daha LK, Elneil S, Fall M, Hohlbrugger G, Irwin P, Mortensen S, van Ophoven A, Osborne JL, Peeker R, Richter B, Riedl C, Sairanen J, Tinzl M, Wyndaele JJ. Diagnostic criteria, classification, and nomenclature for painful bladder syndrome/interstitial cystitis: an ESSIC proposal. Eur Urol. 2008;53:60–7.
20. Nordling J, Anjum FH, Bade JJ, Bouchelouche K, Bouchelouche P, Cervigni M, Elneil S, Fall M, Hald T, Hanus T, Hedlund H, Hohlbrugger G, Horn T, Larsen S, Leppilahti M, Mortensen S, Nagendra M, Oliveira PD, Osborne J, Riedl C, Sairanen J, Tinzl M, Wyndaele JJ. Primary evaluation of patients suspected of having interstitial cystitis (IC). Eur Urol. 2004;45:662–9.
21. Larsen MS, Mortensen S, Nordling J, Horn T. Quantifying mast cells in bladder pain syndrome by immunohistochemical analysis. BJU Int. 2008;102:204–7.
22. Yamada T, Murayama T, Mita H, Akiyama K. Subtypes of bladder mast cells in interstitial cystitis. Int J Urol. 2000;7:292–7.
23. Aldenborg F, Fall M, Enerback L. Proliferation and transepithelial migration of mucosal mast cells in interstitial cystitis. Immunology. 1986;58:411–6.
24. Li CY. Diagnosis of mastocytosis: value of cytochemistry and immunohistochemistry. Leuk Res. 2001;25:537–41.
25. Bohne AW, Hodson JM, Rebuck JM, Reinhard RE. An abnormal leukocyte response in interstitial cystitis. J Urol. 1962;88:387–91.
26. Enerback L, Fall M, Aldenborg F. Histamine and mucosal mast cells in interstitial cystitis. Agents Actions. 1989;27:113–6.
27. Kastrup J, Hald T, Larsen S, Nielsen VG. Histamine content and mast cell count of detrusor muscle in patients with interstitial cystitis and other types of chronic cystitis. Br J Urol. 1983;55:495–500.
28. Smith BH, Dehner LP. Chronic ulcerating interstitial cystitis (Hunner's ulcer). A study of 28 cases. Arch Pathol. 1972;93:76–81.
29. Lynes WL, Flynn SD, Shortliffe LD, Lemmers M, Zipser R, Roberts LJ, Stamey TA. Mast cell involvement in interstitial cystitis. J Urol. 1987;138:746–52.
30. Johansson SL, Fall M. Clinical features and spectrum of light microscopic changes in interstitial cystitis. J Urol. 1990;143:1118–24.

31. Theoharides TC, Sant GR, El Mansoury M, Letourneau R, Ucci Jr AA, Meares Jr EM. Activation of bladder mast cells in interstitial cystitis: a light and electron microscopic study. J Urol. 1995;153:629–36.
32. El Mansoury M, Boucher W, Sant GR, Theoharides TC. Increased urine histamine and methylhistamine in interstitial cystitis. J Urol. 1994;152:350–3.
33. Boucher W, El Mansoury M, Pang X, Sant GR, Theoharides TC. Elevated mast cell tryptase in the urine of patients with interstitial cystitis. Br J Urol. 1995;76:94–100.
34. Mortensen S, Nordling J, Horn T, Hald T. Interstitial cystitis: a proposal on cardinal symptoms and signs. Urology. 2001;57:122.
35. Wyndaele JJ, Van DJ, Toussaint N. Cystoscopy and bladder biopsies in patients with bladder pain syndrome carried out following ESSIC guidelines. Scand J Urol Nephrol. 2009;43:471–5.
36. Rossberger J, Fall M, Gustafsson CK, Peeker R. Does mast cell density predict the outcome after transurethral resection of Hunner's lesions in patients with type 3C bladder pain syndrome/interstitial cystitis? Scand J Urol Nephrol. 2010;44:433–7.
37. Richter B, Hesse U, Hansen AB, Horn T, Mortensen SO, Nordling J. Bladder pain syndrome/interstitial cystitis in a Danish population: a study using the 2008 criteria of the European Society for the Study of Interstitial Cystitis. BJU Int. 2010;105:660–7.
38. Metcalfe DD, Akin C. Mastocytosis: molecular mechanisms and clinical disease heterogeneity. Leuk Res. 2001;25:577–82.
39. Galli SJ. New insights into "the riddle of the mast cells": microenvironmental regulation of mast cell development and phenotypic heterogeneity. Lab Invest. 1990;62:5–33.
40. Saito H, Ebisawa M, Tachimoto H, Shichijo M, Fukagawa K, Matsumoto K, Iikura Y, Awaji T, Tsujimoto G, Yanagida M, Uzumaki H, Takahashi G, Tsuji K, Nakahata T. Selective growth of human mast cells induced by Steel factor, IL-6, and prostaglandin E2 from cord blood mononuclear cells. J Immunol. 1996;157:343–50.
41. Theoharides TC, Bondy PK, Tsakalos ND, Askenase PW. Differential release of serotonin and histamine from mast cells. Nature. 1982;297:229–31.
42. Dvorak AM, McLeod RS, Onderdonk A, Monahan-Earley RA, Cullen JB, Antonioli DA, Morgan E, Blair JE, Estrella P, Cisneros RL. Ultrastructural evidence for piecemeal and anaphylactic degranulation of human gut mucosal mast cells in vivo. Int Arch Allergy Immunol. 1992;99:74–83.
43. Letourneau R, Pang X, Sant GR, Theoharides TC. Intragranular activation of bladder mast cells and their association with nerve processes in interstitial cystitis. Br J Urol. 1996;77:41–54.
44. Horn T, Holm NR, Hald T. Interstitial cystitis. Ultrastructural observations on detrusor smooth muscle cells. APMIS. 1998;106:909–16.
45. Christmas TJ, Smith GL, Rode J. Detrusor myopathy: an accurate predictor of bladder hypocompliance and contracture in interstitial cystitis. Br J Urol. 1996;78:862–5.
46. Christmas TJ, Rode J, Chapple CR, Milroy EJ, Turner-Warwick RT. Nerve fibre proliferation in interstitial cystitis. Virchows Arch A Pathol Anat Histopathol. 1990;416:447–51.
47. Hohenfellner M, Nunes L, Schmidt RA, Lampel A, Thuroff JW, Tanagho EA. Interstitial cystitis: increased sympathetic innervation and related neuropeptide synthesis. J Urol. 1992;147:587–91.
48. Pang X, Marchand J, Sant GR, Kream RM, Theoharides TC. Increased number of substance P positive nerve fibres in interstitial cystitis. Br J Urol. 1995;75:744–50.
49. Koziol JA, Clark DC, Gittes RF, Tan EM. The natural history of interstitial cystitis: a survey of 374 patients. J Urol. 1993;149:465–9.
50. Spanos C, El Mansoury M, Letourneau R, Minogiannis P, Greenwood J, Siri P, Sant GR, Theoharides TC. Carbachol-induced bladder mast cell activation: augmentation by estradiol and implications for interstitial cystitis. Urology. 1996;48:809–16.
51. Pang X, Cotreau-Bibbo MM, Sant GR, Theoharides TC. Bladder mast cell expression of high affinity oestrogen receptors in patients with interstitial cystitis. Br J Urol. 1995;75:154–61.
52. Conrad MJ, Feigen GA. Sex hormones and kinetics of anphylactic histamine release. Physiol Chem Phys. 1974;6:11–6.

53. Vliagoftis H, Dimitriadou V, Boucher W, Rozniecki JJ, Correia I, Raam S, Theoharides TC. Estradiol augments while tamoxifen inhibits rat mast cell secretion. Int Arch Allergy Immunol. 1992;98:398–409.
54. Howarth PH, Knox AJ, Amrani Y, Tliba O, Panettieri Jr RA, Johnson M. Synthetic responses in airway smooth muscle. J Allergy Clin Immunol. 2004;114:S32–50.
55. Panettieri Jr RA. Airway smooth muscle: an immunomodulatory cell. J Allergy Clin Immunol. 2002;110:S269–74.
56. Panettieri Jr RA. Airway smooth muscle: immunomodulatory cells that modulate airway remodeling? Respir Physiol Neurobiol. 2003;137:277–93.
57. Singer CA, Salinthone S, Baker KJ, Gerthoffer WT. Synthesis of immune modulators by smooth muscles. Bioessays. 2004;26:646–55.
58. Page S, Ammit AJ, Black JL, Armour CL. Human mast cell and airway smooth muscle cell interactions: implications for asthma. Am J Physiol Lung Cell Mol Physiol. 2001;281:L1313–23.
59. Lazaar AL, Panettieri Jr RA. Airway smooth muscle as an immunomodulatory cell: a new target for pharmacotherapy? Curr Opin Pharmacol. 2001;1:259–64.
60. Letourneau R, Sant GR, El Mansoury M, Theoharides TC. Activation of bladder mast cells in interstitial cystitis. Int J Tissue React. 1992;14:307–12.
61. Bouchelouche K, Andersen L, Nordling J, Horn T, Bouchelouche P. The cysteinyl-leukotriene D4 induces cytosolic Ca2+ elevation and contraction of the human detrusor muscle. J Urol. 2003;170:638–44.
62. Bouchelouche K, Bouchelouche P. Cysteinyl leukotriene D4 increases human detrusor muscle responsiveness to histamine. J Urol. 2006;176:361–6.
63. Bouchelouche K, Alvarez S, Andersen L, Nordling J, Horn T, Bouchelouche P. Monocyte chemoattractant protein-1 production by human detrusor smooth muscle cells. J Urol. 2004;171:462–6.
64. Bouchelouche K, Alvarez S, Horn T, Nordling J, Bouchelouche P. Human detrusor smooth muscle cells release interleukin-6, interleukin-8, and RANTES in response to proinflammatory cytokines interleukin-1beta and tumor necrosis factor-alpha. Urology. 2006;67:214–9.
65. Bouchelouche K, Andresen L, Alvarez S, Nordling J, Nielsen OH, Bouchelouche P. Interleukin-4 and 13 induce the expression and release of monocyte chemoattractant protein 1, interleukin-6 and stem cell factor from human detrusor smooth muscle cells: synergy with interleukin-1beta and tumor necrosis factor-alpha. J Urol. 2006;175:760–5.
66. Yun SK, Laub DJ, Weese DL, Lad PM, Leach GE, Zimmern PE. Stimulated release of urine histamine in interstitial cystitis. J Urol. 1992;148:1145–8.
67. Holm-Bentzen M, Sondergaard I, Hald T. Urinary excretion of a metabolite of histamine (1,4-methyl-imidazole- acetic-acid) in painful bladder disease. Br J Urol. 1987;59:230–3.
68. Lotz M, Villiger P, Hugli T, Koziol J, Zuraw BL. Interleukin-6 and interstitial cystitis. J Urol. 1994;152:869–73.
69. Christmas TJ, Rode J. Characteristics of mast cells in normal bladder, bacterial cystitis and interstitial cystitis. Br J Urol. 1991;68:473–8.
70. Bouchelouche K, Kristensen B, Nordling J, Horn T, Bouchelouche P. Increased urinary leukotriene E4 and eosinophil protein X excretion in patients with interstitial cystitis. J Urol. 2001;166:2121–5.
71. Jacobs BL, Smaldone MC, Tyagi V, Philips BJ, Jackman SV, Leng WW, Tyagi P. Increased nerve growth factor in neurogenic overactive bladder and interstitial cystitis patients. Can J Urol. 2010;17:4989–94.
72. Liu HT, Tyagi P, Chancellor MB, Kuo HC. Urinary nerve growth factor level is increased in patients with interstitial cystitis/bladder pain syndrome and decreased in responders to treatment. BJU Int. 2009;104:1476–81.
73. Liu HT, Tyagi P, Chancellor MB, Kuo HC. Urinary nerve growth factor but not prostaglandin E2 increases in patients with interstitial cystitis/bladder pain syndrome and detrusor overactivity. BJU Int. 2010;106:1681–5.
74. Okragly AJ, Niles AL, Saban R, Schmidt D, Hoffman RL, Warner TF, Moon TD, Uehling DT, Haak-Frendscho M. Elevated tryptase, nerve growth factor, neurotrophin-3 and glial cell line-derived neurotrophic factor levels in the urine of interstitial cystitis and bladder cancer patients. J Urol. 1999;161:438–41.

Chapter 6
Neurophysiology of Pelvic Pain Mechanisms

Jean-Jacques Wyndaele and Silvia Malaguti

Introduction

Sensation is a perception made by an individual related to a stimulus that occurs in the body. Neurologically it runs through sensory labeled nervous pathways. Each sensory modality has its own labeled line. Activation of a pathway gives perception of that modality and that type of sensation, regardless of which stimulus activated the pathway. Which sensory perception results from the activation of a pathway will depend on very many different mechanisms such as innervations shared with other structures, modulation in sensory pathways, memory and emotion, attention, and more. Sensation is by definition always subjective and thus special for every single individual.

Nociceptive pain, through direct stimulation of nociceptor sites, is different from neuropathic pain, which results from a direct lesion of the peripheral or central nervous system. Both can be present in chronic pelvic pain and are discussed in this chapter.

J.-J. Wyndaele, M.D., D.Sci., Ph.D.
Department of Urology, University Hospital Antwerp and Antwerp University, Edegem, Belgium

S. Malaguti, M.D. (✉)
Clinical Neurophysiology, Clinical Neurophysiology and Biomechanics of Pelvic Floor Dysfunctions, Milan, Italy
e-mail: smalaguti@malagutilamarche.it

J. Nordling et al. (eds.), *Bladder Pain Syndrome: A Guide for Clinicians*,
DOI 10.1007/978-1-4419-6929-3_6, © Springer Science+Business Media New York 2013

Nociceptive Pain

Nervous Structures Involved in Sensory/Pain Transmission

General Principles

Pain innervation is present throughout the whole body.

As for all sensation it runs through sensory units with different parts: a primary order neuron from receptor/stimulus site to spinal cord or brainstem, a second order neuron towards the thalamus, and a third order neuron towards the sensory cortex.

Primary Order Neurons

Sensors are free nerve endings, activated with tissue damage, inflammation, and compression.

In the urinary bladder of humans and animals, sensory nerves have been identified suburothelially, as well as in the detrusor muscle. Nerve endings that connect to the hypogastric nerves are mainly located in the bladder base and urethra, whereas those connecting via the pelvic nerves are more evenly distributed through the viscus, but with predominance for the bladder body [1]. Suburothelially, the nerves run into a plexus beneath the epithelial lining, with some terminals located within the basal parts of the urothelium [2, 3]. This location makes them extremely sensitive to changes in urine composition, especially if the epithelial barrier is disrupted as would be the case in Bladder Pain Syndrome (BPS) following a glycosaminoglycans layer deficiency or other direct lesion. In addition, a layer of cells with cytologic characteristics of myofibroblasts has been described immediately beneath the epithelial basal lamina in close contact with the afferent nerves [4]. Myofibroblasts express subtypes 2 and 3 muscarinic receptors [5] and purinergic P2X3 and P2Y6 receptors [6]. Detrusor myocytes are spontaneously active during bladder filling and connect via gap junctions and interstitial cells. The spontaneous contractions generate afferent activity via Ad and C-fibers [7]. How this acts in condition of BPS needs to be developed further.

Filling cystometry with inhibition of acetylcholine breakdown by an acetylcholinesterase inhibitor resulted in increased bladder sensation and decreased cystometric capacity in about 80% of overactive bladder patients. This suggests that acetylcholine is released during bladder filling and activates the sensory afferent pathway at least under pathologic conditions [8]. Muscarinic receptors have also been found in the human urothelium [9].

Besides acetylcholine and noradrenaline, a number of nonadrenergic, noncholinergic neurotransmitters are thought to act in the normal neurotransmission in the lower urinary tract (LUT) through specific receptors expressed on afferent nerve terminals. These include adenosine triphosphate (ATP), which binds to purinoceptors; substance P, neurokinin A, and calcitonin gene-related peptide (CGRP), which interact with tachykinin receptors and CGRP receptors, respectively; and prostaglandins, which bind to prostanoid receptors. Nitric oxide, vasoactive intestinal peptide (VIP), and enkephalins may modulate afferent neurotransmission. Vanilloid receptors are also expressed on afferent nerves of the LUT [10–13]. The urothelium by producing mediators serves as a mechanosensor, which can control the activity in afferent nerves.

Recent research has revealed several new data: ATP released from urothelial cells can activate afferent nerves and urothelial cells. The activation of the bladder afferents induced by intravesical application of ATP would be mediated mainly through Capsaicine-insensitive C-fibers [14].

Activation of extracellular signal-regulated kinases (ERKs) enzymes is known to be involved in the development and/or maintenance of the pain associated with, e.g., bladder inflammation. This may be important as these enzymes are increasingly employed as experimental markers of nociceptive processing [15].

Cannabinoid receptor 1 (CB1)-immunoreactive nerve fibers were significantly increased in the suburothelium of BPS specimens, as compared with controls. CB1-immunoreactive suburothelial nerve fiber density correlated significantly with pain scores suggesting that such increased nerve fibers may be related to bladder pain [16].

An increase in nerve growth factor (NGF) has been found by several groups in animal and human studies [17–19].

Upregulating of pituitary adenylate cyclase-activating polypeptide (PACAP), CGRP, and substance P (SP) in micturition reflex pathways after cystitis have been suggested to play a role in altered visceral sensation (allodynia) and/or urinary bladder hyperreflexia in BPS [20, 21].

Increase of the expression and phosphorylation of Trk tyrosine kinase receptor may play a role in decreased urinary tract plasticity as shown in CYP-induced cystitis [22].

A role of NO has been studied recently; results suggest that NO synthase exists in the urinary bladder (rat) and clearly demonstrate that L-arginine, an NO substrate, can inhibit both Aδ (omega) and C mechanosensitive afferent fibers of the bladder. In addition, L-arginine can inhibit the activated responses of both fibers to intravesical acrolein, a metabolite of cyclophosphamide, which causes bladder hypersensitivity [23].

The hypothesis that plasticity in urothelial purinergic receptors and in both pelvic and lumbar splanchnic pathways is linked with the painful bladder symptoms in BPS has been suggested [24, 25].

The nerves involved in sensory information transport are A-delta and C-Fibers. A-delta fibers are thick, myelinated, with fast conduction and the pain sensation related to them is initial, sharp, and localized. C-fibers are thin, nonmyelinated with slow conduction. They relate to diffuse, dull, burning pain.

A-delta fibers synapse in the spinal cord, mount towards the thalamic ventrobasal complex involved in sensation of touch and mount towards the somatosensory cortex.

C-fibers also synapse in the spinal cord and mount to the thalamic middle nucleus and limbic system, regions related to motivation and emotional aspects of pain.

Mucosal afferents consist mostly of unmyelinated fibers, with few myelinated fibers. Closer to the detrusor muscle, the nerves are either myelinated or unmyelinated [26]. Afferents that respond to both distension and contraction of the bladder (i.e., "in series tension receptors") have been identified in the pelvic and hypogastric nerves of cats and rats [27, 28].

Pelvic myelinated A-delta fibers constitute the afferent limb of the normal micturition reflex [29]. Myelinated bladder afferents are silent when the urinary bladder is empty and during the initial phase of slow filling; this can explain why humans do not notice bladder filling until a certain volume has accumulated. However, after exposure to intravesical chemical irritants, as in inflammatory states, pelvic A-delta fibers exhibit ongoing activity and show an altered, more sensitive response to mechanical stimulation. Myelinated mechanoreceptive fibers thus possess chemoreceptive properties and may signal sensory abnormalities arising from pathologically altered tissue [30]. C-fibers appear to be functionally more heterogeneous, with differences in species. In the cat pelvic nerve, most C-fibers are mechano-insensitive [31]. They have no ongoing activity and are not excited by bladder distension even at high pressures. The role of these "silent" receptors during normal bladder filling is questioned. They may, however, become mechanosensitive during inflammation, thereby unmasking a new afferent pathway. The increased afferent input generated by these afferents may provide a substrate for the hypersensitivity (urgency and pain at low bladder contents) seen in various inflammatory bladder diseases [32, 33]. The few unmyelinated units that do show mechanosensitivity do not respond to bladder distension at normal nonpainful pressures, but accurately monitor pressures in the noxious range [34]. They would be the true "nociceptors" and are believed to signal pain [11]. There is some evidence that these units are also sensitive to irritants. In rats, nerve activity of C-fiber afferents that respond only to bladder filling is better correlated to volume than to pressure. They appear to be volume receptors, possibly sensitive to stretch of the mucosa. In the hypogastric nerve, A-delta and C-fibers have also been described, both responding to bladder distension and contraction. Their responses are essentially the same as those of the pelvic nerve afferents. A subpopulation of hypogastric nerve afferents appears to be insensitive for bladder filling but sensitive for the chemical composition of the bladder content. After exposure to chemical solutions, these chemoreceptive fibers become mechanosensitive and respond in an irregular bursting pattern of discharge at some point during bladder filling. Hypogastric afferents may encode nociceptive stimuli differently to normal activity, by a transition from random activity to a bursting pattern of discharge when noxious stimuli are present (i.e., interstitial cystitis and other forms of irritative bladder disorders). One can accept that both A-delta and C-fibers in the pelvic and hypogastric nerve may be able to signal noxious events, giving rise to abnormal sensations such as urgency and pain.

Second Order Neurons

Nociceptive information from different pelvic organs is delivered to the dorsal and anterolateral spinal cord. In the dorsal horn a network of descending pathways projecting from cerebral structures either suppress or potentiate the passage of the nociceptive messages to the brain. Some of the central structures involved in the micturition reflexes and pain modulation are common, e.g., nucleus raphe magnum, nucleus locus coeruleus alpha, periacqueductal gray, etc. Functionally, however, their effects may be similar or contrasting. The central micturition reflexes and descending control pathways of pain also utilize common transmitters and transmitter systems with similar or different effects on micturition and pain, suggesting a certain degree of overlapping between these systems [35]. Direct neurophysiologic evidence has been provided that nociceptive information from the urinary bladder to the ventro-basal group of the thalamus ascends via a dorsal midline pathway [36].

That many changes can occur in the second order neuron pathways has been demonstrated in non-BPS models of chronic pain and a correlation with behavior could be made [37]. Chronic cyclophosphamide (CYP)-induced bladder inflammation can reveal a nociceptive Fos expression pattern in the spinal cord in response to a non-noxious bladder stimulus that is partially mediated by capsaicin-sensitive bladder afferents [38].

In FIC cats at the level of the spinal cord, astrocytic GFAP immuno-intensity was significantly elevated and there was evidence for co-expression of the primitive intermediate filament, nestin, in regions of the S1 cord (superficial and deep dorsal horn, central canal, and laminae V–VII) that receive input from pelvic afferents, both indicative of a reactive state [17].

Third Order Neuron and Brain

Functional imaging studies have been used to show that brain regions implicated in LUT function include the pons (pontine micturition center, PMC), periaqueductal gray (PAG), thalamus, insula, anterior cingulate gyrus, and prefrontal cortices. The PMC and the PAG are thought to be key in the supraspinal control of continence and micturition. Higher centers such as the insula, anterior cingulate gyrus, and prefrontal regions are probably involved in the modulation of the control and cognition of bladder sensations, and in the case of the insula and anterior cingulate, modulation of autonomic function [39]. In subjects with poor bladder control, sensations and brain responses can become exaggerated (with strong sensation) above a certain volume threshold. In abnormal (OAB) responses to bladder filling more is at stake than bladder hypersensitivity. The nature of the afferent signals or the handling of these potentials in the brain is abnormal [40].

Multiple brain regions are involved in pain perception. The limbic, paralimbic, anterior cingulate cortex, insular cortex, prefrontal cortex, and primary and secondary somatosensory cortices are all most probably involved. Central handling of pain permits distinguishing location and quality of pain through a topographic organization in primary somatosensory cortex for nociceptive potentials. Distinction inside of the body is done in the somatosensory cortex. Attention to pain and emotion run through the anterior cingulate cortex.

To explain features often encountered in patients with chronic pelvic pain, such as the presence of multiple pain diagnoses, the frequency of previous abuse, the minimal or discordant pathologic changes of the involved organs, the paradoxical effectiveness of many treatments, and the recurrent nature of the condition, limbic associated pelvic pain is a proposed pathophysiology [41]. This limbic dysfunction is manifest both as an increased sensitivity to pain afferents from pelvic organs and as an abnormal efferent innervation of pelvic musculature, both visceral and somatic. The pelvic musculature undergoes tonic contraction as a result of limbic efferent stimulation, which produces the minimal changes found on pathological examination, and generates a further sensation of pain. The pain afferents from these pelvic organs then follow the medial pain pathway back to the sensitized, hypervigilant limbic system. A cycle installs itself where chronic stimulation of the limbic system by pelvic pain afferents again produces an efferent contraction of the pelvic muscles. Disruption of the cycle can be tried through blocking afferent signals from pelvic organs (anesthesia or muscle manipulation) and/or with psychiatric medication. To prevent recurrence, medical or cognitive treatment targeting the underlying limbic hypervigilance is mandatory.

Clinical observation of hypersensitivity to visceral stimuli in BPS has been studied with potentiating of the eye blink startle reflex under threat which is mediated by output from the amygdala complex and represents a noninvasive marker of responsiveness in this brain circuit [42]. Compared to controls, female patients with BPS showed increased activation of a defensive emotional circuit in the context of a threat of abdominal pain. This supports the hypothesis that the observed abnormality may be involved in the enhanced perception of bladder signals associated with BPS.

Also the positive cotton-tip test for allodynia is now interpreted as evidence of neuroplasticity as a consequence of severe and repeating pain [43].

Central Interpretation of Sensory Potentials

When a sensory stimulus arrives in the perception areas of the brain the interpretation and translating of the stimulus into a sensation are done through different coding mechanisms:

- *Coding for stimulus type*: Relates to the receptor triggered and/or the interpretation by the brain of a combination of potentials if they derive from stimuli for which no specific receptor exists.
- *Coding for stimulus intensity which depends on the* number of receptors activated and the frequency of action potentials.
- *Coding for stimulus location.*

Abdominal viscera are relatively insensitive for mechanical stimuli. But strong distension and spasmodic contractions can produce pain, especially if they involve ischemia. Direct trauma as with cutting, coagulating, and strong electrical stimulation can be perceived as painful. Visceral pain is special that it is often experienced as referred pain, referred to the body surface, because the used second order neurons receive also somatic afferents from superficial regions. Distinguishing between visceral and cutaneous pain is not always easy.

Mainly two types of pain have been described in the bladder [44]: one is a sharp pain, localized in the perineal region or suprapubically, which may be due to inflammation of the bladder, but which can also be felt in conditions causing sacral nerve irritation; second is a painful pressure in the lower abdomen, which may increase during bladder contraction and which can be felt in cases of outlet obstruction and bladder overfilling. Although visceral pain and somatic pain have much in common, they also have important differences [45]. Visceral pain from the bladder can be elicited at various bladder volumes. Pain occurs at high pressures produced by distension, contractions, or combination of the two. Overdistension of the bladder is painful. Bladder contractions can be painful but not during normal voiding, because the afferent firing due to the motor activity and initiated by the central nervous system (CNS) is recognized as such by the CNS.

Wesselman [46] describes three characteristic clinical features of visceral pain: true visceral pain, referred visceral pain, and hyperalgesia associated with visceral pain. Hyperalgesia can present as hyperalgesia at the site of the viscus, at somatic structures, or in other pelvic structures with partially overlapping afferent innervation.

Neuronal Plasticity

Bladder afferents show plasticity; the total number of active primary afferents is not static but critically depends on the state of the tissue. This may account for the changes in bladder sensation as in BPS. Hyperexcitability of C-fiber afferent pathways which are silent in the normal state during bladder filling has been already mentioned above as mechanism for bladder pain and urgency [34]. This hypothesis is supported by the findings that intravesical capsaicin and resiniferatoxin, which selectively suppress C-fiber activity, can improve these symptoms [47, 48]. Antimuscarinic drugs have been shown to lower afferent activity in a rat model [49–51]. Therefore, it is not surprising that in patients with interstitial cystitis, intravesical oxybutynin, e.g., may sometimes be beneficial. Animal experiments have shown neural upregulation of proteinase-activated receptors, tryptase, beta-nerve growth factor, inducible nitric oxide synthase, nuclear transcription factor-kappaB, c-Fos, phosphodiesterase 1C, cyclic adenosine monophosphate (cAMP)-dependent protein kinase, and proenkephalin B with noxious stimuli. After the noxious stimulus has abated, downregulation of genes seems to follow [52].

Peeker et al. [53] found increased density and number of nerve fibers immunoreactive for tyrosine hydroxylase in interstitial cystitis cases compared to controls. Furthermore, there was a difference between classic (ESSIC type 3) and nonulcer (ESSIC type 1 and 2) disease in the overall density of nerves using the antibody mixture, indicating an altered peripheral sympathetic innervation in interstitial cystitis cases. The difference in nerve density observed after incubation with the antibody mixture between classic and nonulcer BPS supports the hypothesis that the two forms represent separate entities.

Mast Cells and Nerves

Mast cell (MC) proliferation has been documented repeatedly in BPS patients. In addition, bladder MCs were shown to be more responsive to a number of secretagogues, such as IgE-antigen, SP, and acetylcholine. Biopsies taken from diseased bladders of BPS patients demonstrated explicit proliferation of neuronal processes, a numerical increase in fibers containing neuropeptide Y and CGRP, and increased anatomic interconnections between SP nerve fibers and MCs in the submucosa. It is hypothesized that damaged urothelial cells, as documented for epithelial cells, produce cytokines, such as stem cell factor and IL-3, and thus lead to MC proliferation [54].

Neurogenic Inflammation

Neurogenic inflammation is inflammation arising from the local release from afferent neurons of inflammatory mediators such as Substance P, VGRP Neurokinin A, neurokinin B, and CGRP. In a subgroup of patients with CPPS, chronic pain could be related to neurogenic inflammation [46]. Axon reflexes but also dorsal root reflexes may play a role [55]. While neurogenic inflammation is not by definition negative but more an adaptive response helping for local defense, it can in other instances be negative. Its role in several conditions as asthma, arthritis, migraine, and BPS has been highlighted [56, 57]. In visceral pain conditions neurogenic inflammation appears also to be important in referred pain [58] and one can thesize the role in BPS, vulvodynia, and prostatitis IIIb. It has been shown in an animal study on uterine pain in the rat [59]. It might be involved in the edema and trophic changes in the skin, subcutaneous tissue, and muscle reported in the referred zones in chronic visceral pain [60].

Pelvic Organs Cross Talk

The different pelvic functions are done in a coordinated way through complex integrative pathways that may converge peripherally and/or centrally. If pathology occurs, irritative, infectious, or traumatic, the shared afferent pathways may produce generalized pelvic sensitization or cross-sensitization to both chemical and mechanical stimuli, dependent on both intact bladder sensory innervation and neuropeptide content as shown bidirectionally for the bladder and bowel in animal models [61].

Pelvic pain associated with menstruation, i.e., dysmenorrhea, often co-occurs with other chronic painful conditions such as BPS and irritable bowel syndrome, demonstrating that pathophysiology in one organ can influence physiology and responses to pathophysiology in other organs: Bladder inflammation reduces the rate of uterine contractions and the effects of drugs on the uterus; colon inflammation produces signs of inflammation in the otherwise healthy bladder and uterus; a surgical model of endometriosis produces vaginal hyperalgesia, exacerbates pain behaviors induced by a ureteral stone, and reduces volume voiding thresholds in the bladder [62].

Conclusion

There are many aspects on nociceptive pain in BPS showing a wide involvement of neurophysiological mechanisms which also express a large plasticity and is associated with processes of sensitization. Further knowledge will show the way to better understand what goes on and will probably permit to gain improvement in diagnosis and treatment.

Neuropathic Pain with Special Attention to Pudendal Neuralgia

Pudendal neuralgia or Pudendal nerve entrapment is a painful neuropathic condition that involves the Pudendal nerve: for that reason it is classified among the peripheral neuropathy. The term Pudendal neuralgia has been used in the literature for a variety of neuropathic and non-neuropathic pelvic pain symptoms: burning, tingling, or heaviness in the perineum, rectum, or bladder, usually lasting for several years. Differential diagnosis requires a thorough investigation of urogynecological, andrological, colon-proctological, or neurological conditions due to the nonspecific clinical findings.

Peripheral neuropathy relates to a disorder of peripheral nerves: any part can be affected, but damage to axons is most common. It can be associated with poor nutrition, a number of diseases, and pressure or trauma. It can be caused by disease, nerve compression, entrapment, laceration, inflammation, or exposure to toxins. However a neuropathy can also be the result of radiculopathy, originating from nerve roots that exit the spinal canal through the neural foramen: degeneration of vertebral bone, herniation of the pulpy disc between vertebrae, narrowing of the spinal column (spinal stenosis), or trauma can compress or cut nerve roots and cause neuropathy.

Sign and symptoms of peripheral neuropathy depend on the type of nerve affected (e.g., motor, sensory, autonomic) and where the nerve is located in the body:

1. Motor nerve damage can produce muscle weakness, cramps, and spasms.
2. Sensory nerve damage can produce tingling, numbness, and pain.
3. Autonomic nerve damage can produce bladder, bowel, and sexual dysfunction, abnormal blood pressure and heart rate, and reduced ability to perspire.

Neuropathic pain associated with sensory nerve damage is variously described as burning, shooting, stabbing, freezing, or electric-like, extreme sensitivity to touch: the distribution of pain will be along the course of a particular peripheral nerve.

The hallmarks of neuropathic pain are the following:

1. Chronic allodynia: Pain resulting from a stimulus that ordinarily does not elicit a painful response (e.g., light touch).
2. Hyperalgesia: An increased sensitivity to a normally painful stimuli: Primary hyperalgesia, caused by sensitization of C-fibers, occurs immediately within the area of the injury; secondary hyperalgesia, caused by sensitization of dorsal horn neurons, occurs in the undamaged area surrounding the injury.

Anatomical-Physiologic Background

The Pudendal nerve innervates the pelvic floor muscles, the sphincter, and the pelvic organs; the nerve roots S2–S4 mainly supply it. The ventral and dorsal lumbar and sacral nerve roots exit laterally through the nerve root foramina to form the lumbar and sacral plexuses that provide motor and sensory innervations of the bladder, bowel, and sexual organs.

The efferent parasympathetic outflow (via the pelvic nerves S2–S4) synapses on postganglionic neurons in the pelvic plexus or in ganglia of the bladder wall provide the major input to the bladder and an inhibitory input to the urethra. The parasympathetic afferents have their cell bodies in the S2–S4 dorsal root ganglia before entering the dorsal horn. Sympathetic supply to the pelvic organs (T10–L1) provides excitatory input to the bladder neck and urethra and inhibitory input to the bladder smooth muscle. The sympathetic afferents are in the T11–L2 dorsal root ganglia. The Pudendal Nerve provides the efferent somatic pathways. The Pudendal nerve derives its fibers from the ventral branches of the second, third, and fourth sacral nerves. It passes between the Piriformis and Coccygeus muscles and leaves the pelvis through the lower part of the greater sciatic foramen. It then crosses the spine of the ischium, and reenters the pelvis through the lesser sciatic foramen. It accompanies the internal pudendal vessels upward and forward along the lateral wall of the ischiorectal fossa, being contained in a sheath of the obturator fascia, termed Alcock's canal, and divides into two terminal branches: the perineal nerve and the dorsal nerve of the penis or clitoris. Before its division, it gives off the inferior rectal nerve.

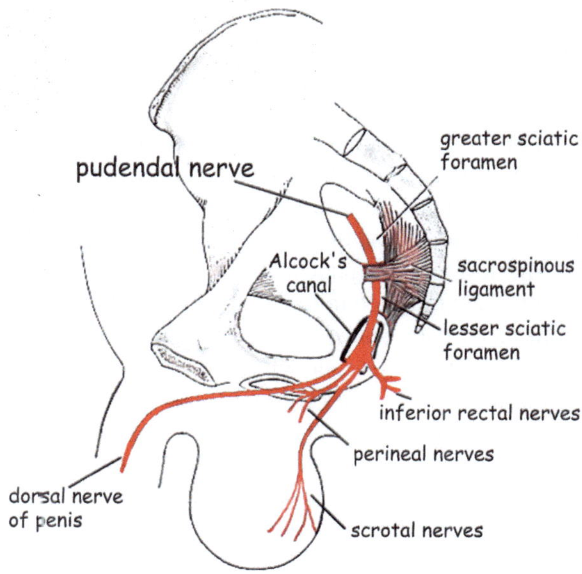

Fig. 6.1 Pudendal nerve anatomic schema. *Origin:* It is a major branch of the sacral plexus (S2S3S4). *Pathway:* It travels through the gluteal region, the Pudendal canal, and the perineum. *Fibers and function:* It is a mixed nerve with motor fibers (external anal and urethral sphincter, levator ani, bulbo and ischiocavernosus, deep and superficial perineal muscle), sensory fibers (perineal, genital area), and autonomic fibers (erection, bladder proprioception)

The pudendal nerve supplies the motor innervation to the urethral sphincter (rhabdosphincter) and pelvic floor muscle; the anterior horn cells lie in the ventral horn of sacral segments S2–S4 (Onuf's nucleus). It carries sensory fibers from the penis, urethra, anus, and pelvic floor muscles (Fig. 6.1).

Etiology and Pathophysiology of Pudendal Neuralgia

Direct trauma of the pudendal nerve is uncommon due to its deep position between muscles; however it can be damaged during urological, gynecological, colorectal surgery, or lumbosacral neurosurgery.

A recent case series was presented of 32 patients who underwent a Stapled Transanal Rectal Resection (STARR) for rectal prolapse, who developed chronic pelvic pain due to Pudendal neuropathy [63]. Sacral fractures and pelvic injuries can also result in a direct damage of the nerve [64].

The structural and biomechanical properties of pudendal nerve may be modified as the nerve responds to the physical stresses placed upon it through extrinsic movements and postures [65]: as in the case of abnormal contraction of pelvi-trochanter muscles, in particular when the external rotators such as the obturator internus, which forms the Pudendal canal, are over-recruited, causing a damage of the nerve [66]. Even repetitive micro-traumatisms [67] might cause compressions in the pudendal canal. This canal contains the pudendal nerve and vessels and can act as a "pulley" for the neurovascular bundle; in particular situations the pulley action may be disrupted by disorders or defection of the obturator internus muscle leading to an entrapment syndrome [68, 69].

Pudendal neuropathy due to compression within the Alcock's canal has been previously described in cyclists [70] with major complaint of transient paresthesia in the perineum and penis due to Pudendal nerve neuropraxia [71]. Few cases of entrapment syndrome, revealed by transient hypoestesia or impotence, following traction of the lower limb after orthopedic surgery have been reported [72–74]. Stretch mechanism on the pudendal nerve [75, 76] or on a sacral root (e.g., protrusion or herniated LS disc [77]) is advocated as mechanism of indirect damage that leads to compression of the nerve.

The level of the pudendal nerve damage, its severity, and the type of fibers involved are reflected in the symptoms experienced by the individuals, which range from rectal pain, anal "leakage," perineal pain/numbness, genital pain/numbness, frequency, urgency to incontinence, difficult voiding to urinary retention, erectile dysfunction, ejaculatory dysfunction, or even loss of orgasmic sensation. Pelvic–perineal entrapment syndromes are therefore even more disabling than other entrapment syndromes, since numbness and pain in the area of nerve distribution are associated to urological and/or sexual dysfunction. The pain tends to be positional, relieved by standing or lying down, and provoked by sitting.

Goodson [78] first described the compression of pudendal nerve within its canal as a cause of pudendal neuralgia; Amarenco [79] used the term "Alcock's canal syndrome" and described perineal palsy secondary to prolonged compression of the pudendal nerve and repeated micro-traumatisms.

Nerve damage secondary to entrapment mechanism leads to pathophysiological alteration in nerve function. The chronic alteration is responsible for a neuroma to form allowing for somatosensory afferents to generate signals initiating a sensation of neuralgia. Change in the efficient conduction of impulses and reduction in the stability of the nerve membrane, as consequences of abnormal generation of impulses, are responsible for abnormal sensation such as paresthesias, numbness, some neuropathic pains, and abnormal muscular contractions.

Electrodiagnosis of Pudendal Neuropathy

Neurophysiological tests, in accordance with the International Continence Society "uro-neurophysiological" standards, represent the required integration to morphological and functional assessment in chronic pelvic pain and other sacral area dysfunction, when a neuropathy is suspected. By means of application of neurophysiological tests identifying site, type, and degree of neurogenic lesion, the diagnosis of neurogenic alteration is allowed. A thorough evaluation of pelvic floor is normally performed in patients with complaint of sacral area: exploration of Motor Units via pelvic floor Electromyography, conduction study of terminal branches of Pudendal nerve by means of terminal motor latency, somatosensory evoked potentials of Pudendal nerve which explore afferent pathway, and motor evoked potential of External Anal Sphincter for efferent pathway, sacral reflexes, and sympathetic skin response complete the diagnostic protocol. The picture resulting from the diagnostic evaluation defines the functional residual potential, which constitutes the basis to address to a proper therapeutic-rehabilitative program.

Conclusion

Pudendal neuralgia can be suspected based on history and symptoms and needs to be confirmed by multidisciplinary assessment, but requires electrodiagnosis to clarify the pathophysiology of the neural lesion.

References

1. Uemura E, Fletcher TF, Bradley WE. Distribution of lumbar and sacral afferent axons in submucosa of cat urinary bladder. Anat Rec. 1975;183:579–88.
2. Gabella G, Davis C. Distribution of afferent axons in the bladder of rats. J Neurocytol. 1998;27:141–55.
3. Wiseman OJ, Brady CM, Hussain IF, Dasgupta P, Watt H, Fowler CJ, Landon DN. The ultrastructure of bladder lamina propria nerves in healthy subjects and patients with detrusor hyperreflexia. J Urol. 2002;168:2040–5.
4. Wiseman OJ, Fowler CJ, Landon DN. The role of the human bladder lamina propria myofibroblast. BJU Int. 2003;91:89–93.
5. Mukerji G, Yiangou Y, Grogono J, Underwood J, Agarwal SK, Khullar V, Anand P. Localization of M2 and M3 muscarinic receptors in human bladder disorders and their clinical correlations. J Urol. 2006;176:367–73.
6. Sui GP, Wu C, Fry CH. Characterization of the purinergic receptor subtype on guinea-pig suburothelial myofibroblasts. BJU Int. 2006;97:1327–31.
7. Andersson KE. LUTS treatment: future treatment options. Neurourol Urodyn. 2007;26(6 Suppl):934–47.
8. Yossepowitch O, Gillon G, Baniel J, Engelstein D, Livne PM. The effect of cholinergic enhancement during filling cystometry: can edrophonium chloride be used as a provocative test for overactive bladder? J Urol. 2001;165:1441–5.
9. Tyagi S, Tyagi P, Van-le S, Yoshimura N, Chancellor MB, de Miguel F. Qualitative and quantitative expression profile of muscarinic receptors in human urothelium and detrusor. J Urol. 2006;176:1673–8.
10. Andersson KE. Bladder activation: afferent mechanisms. Urology. 2002;59(5 Suppl 1):43–50.
11. Morrison J, Steers WD, Brading A, Blok B, Fry C, De Groat WC, Kakizaki H, Levin R, Thor K. Neurophysiology and neuropharmacology. In: Abrams P, Cardozo L, Khoury S, Wein A, editors. Incontinence: 2nd International Consultation on Incontinence. Plymouth: Health Publication Ltd; 2002. p. 83–163.
12. Cruz F. Vanilloid receptor and detrusor instability. Urology. 2002;59(5 Suppl 1):51–60.
13. Ferguson DR, Kennedy I, Burton TJ. ATP is released from rabbit urinary bladder epithelial cells by hydrostatic pressure changes – a possible sensory mechanism? J Physiol. 1997;505:503–11.
14. Aizawa N, Igawa Y, Andersson KE, Iijima K, Nishizawa O, Wyndaele JJ. Effects of intravesical instillation of ATP on rat bladder primary afferent activity and its relationship with capsaicin-sensitivity. Neurourol Urodyn. 2011;30:163–8.
15. White JP, Cibelli M, Fidalgo AR, Nagy I. Extracellular signal-regulated kinases in pain of peripheral origin. Eur J Pharmacol. 2011;650(1):8–17.

16. Mukerji G, Yiangou Y, Agarwal SK, Anand P. Increased cannabinoid receptor 1-immunoreactive nerve fibers in overactive and painful bladder disorders and their correlation with symptoms. Urology. 2010;75(1514):e15–20.
17. Birder LA, Wolf-Johnston AS, Chib MK, Buffington CA, Roppolo JR, Hanna-Mitchell AT. Beyond neurons: involvement of urothelial and glial cells in bladder function. Neurourol Urodyn. 2010;29:88–96.
18. Jacobs BL, Smaldone MC, Tyagi V, Philips BJ, Jackman SV, Leng WW, Tyagi P. Increased nerve growth factor in neurogenic overactive bladder and interstitial cystitis patients. Can J Urol. 2010;17:4989–94.
19. Liu HT, Tyagi P, Chancellor MB, Kuo HC. Urinary nerve growth factor level is increased in patients with interstitial cystitis/bladder pain syndrome and decreased in responders to treatment. BJU Int. 2009;104:1476–81.
20. Vizzard MA. Upregulation of pituary adenylate cyclase-activating polypeptide in urinary bladder pathways after chronic cystitis. J Comp Neurol. 2000;420:335–48.
21. Vizzard MA. Alterations in neuropeptide expression in lumbosacral bladder pathways following chronic cystitis. J Chem Neuroanat. 2001;21:125–38.
22. Qiao LY, Vizzard MA. Cystitis-induced upregulation of tyrosine kinase (TrkA, TrkB) receptor expression and phosphorylation in rat micturition pathways. J Comp Neurol. 2002;454:200–11.
23. Aizawa N, Igawa Y, Nishizawa O, Wyndaele JJ. Effects of nitric oxide on the primary bladder afferent activities of the rat with and without intravesical acrolein treatment. Eur Urol. 2011;59(2):264–71.
24. Birder LA, Ruan HZ, Chopra B, Xiang Z, Barrick S, Buffington CA, Roppolo JR, Ford AP, de Groat WC, Burnstock G. Alterations in P2X and P2Y purinergic receptor expression in urinary bladder from normal cats and cats with interstitial cystitis. Am J Physiol Renal Physiol. 2004;287:F1084–91.
25. Dang K, Lamb K, Cohen M, Bielefeldt K, Gebhart GF. Cyclophosphamide-induced bladder inflammation sensitizes and enhances P2X receptor function in rat bladder sensory neurons. J Neurophysiol. 2008;99:49–59.
26. Iggo A. Tension receptors in the stomach and the urinary bladder. J Physiol. 1955;128:593–607.
27. Floyd K, Hick VE, Morrison JFB. Mechanosensitive afferent units in the hypogastric nerve of the cat. J Physiol. 1976;259:457–71.
28. Xu L, Gebhart GF. Characterization of mouse lumbar splanchnic and pelvic nerve urinary bladder mechanosensory afferents. J Neurophysiol. 2008;99:244–53.
29. Habler HJ, Janig W, Koltzenburg M. Myelinated primary afferents of the sacral spinal cord responding to slow filling and distention of the cat urinary bladder. J Physiol. 1993;463:449–60.
30. Habler HJ, Janig W, Koltzenburg M. Activation of unmyelinated afferent fibers by mechanical stimuli and inflammation of the urinary bladder in the cat. J Physiol. 1990;425:545–62.
31. Janig W, Koltzenburg M. On the function of spinal primary afferent fibres supplying colon and urinary bladder. J Auton Nerv Syst. 1990;30:S89–96.
32. Moss NG, Harrington WW, Tucker S. Pressure, volume, and chemosensitivity in afferent innervation of urinary bladder in rats. Am J Physiol. 1997;272:R695–703.
33. Morrison JFB. Sensory processing in spinal afferent pathways from the bladder. In: Grastyan E, Molnar P, Grastyan E, Molnar P, editors. Advances in Physiological Science, vol. 16. Oxford: Pergamon; 1981. p. 325–33. Vol 16: Sensory functions.
34. Yoshimura N, Seki S, Chancellor MB, de Groat WC, Ueda T. Targeting afferent hyperexcitability for therapy of the painful bladder syndrome. Urology. 2002;59:61–7.
35. Mennini T, Testa R. Are descending control pathways of the lower urinary tract and pain overlapping systems? Cent Nerv Syst Agents Med Chem. 2010;10:113–47.
36. Robbins MT, Uzzell TW, Aly S, Ness TJ. Characterization of thalamic neuronal responses to urinary bladder distention, including the effect of acute spinal lesions in the rat. J Pain. 2006;7(3):218–24.

37. Goff JR, Burkey AR, Goff DJ, Jasmin L. Reorganization of the spinal dorsal horn in models of chronic pain: correlation with behaviour. Neuroscience. 1998;82:559–74.
38. Vizzard MA. Alterations in spinal cord Fos protein expression induced by bladder stimulation following cystitis. Am J Physiol Regul Integr Comp Physiol. 2000;278:R1027–39.
39. Kavia RB, Dasgupta R, Fowler CJ. Functional imaging and the central control of the bladder. J Comp Neurol. 2005;493:27–32.
40. Griffiths D. Imaging bladder sensations. Neurourol Urodyn. 2007;26:899–903.
41. Fenton BW. Limbic associated pelvic pain: a hypothesis to explain the diagnostic relationship and features of patients with chronic pelvic pain. Med Hypotheses. 2007;69:282–6.
42. Twiss C, Kilpatrick L, Craske M, Buffington CA, Ornitz E, Rodríguez LV, Mayer EA, Naliboff BD. Increased startle responses in interstitial cystitis: evidence for central hyperresponsiveness to visceral related threat. J Urol. 2009;181:2127–33.
43. Jarrell J. Demonstration of cutaneous allodynia in association with chronic pelvic pain. J Vis Exp. 2009;28: pii:1232. doi: 10.3791/1232
44. Cervero F, Laird JMA. Pain: visceral pain. Lancet. 1999;353:2145–8.
45. Ray BS, Neill CL. Abdominal visceral sensation in man. Ann Surg. 1947;126:709–24.
46. Wesselman U. Neurogenic inflammation and chronic pelvic pain. World J Urol. 2001;19:180–5.
47. Barbanti G, Maggi CA, Beneforti P, Baroldi P, Turini D. Relief of pain following intravesical capsaicin in patients with hypersensitive disorders of the lower urinary tract. Br J Urol. 1993;71:686–91.
48. Lazzeri M, Beneforti P, Spinelli M, Zanollo A, Barbagli G, Turini D. Intravesical resiniferatoxin for the treatment of hypersensitive disorder: a randomized placebo controlled study. J Urol. 2000;164:676–9
49. De Wachter S, Wyndaele JJ. Intravesical oxybutinin: a local anesthetic effect on bladder C afferents. J Urol. 2003;169:1892–5.
50. De Laet K, De Wachter S, Wyndaele JJ. Systemic oxybutinin decreases afferent activity of the pelvic nerve of the rat: new insights into the working mechanisms of antimuscarinics. Neurourol Urodyn. 2005;25:156–61.
51. Iijima K, De Wachter S, Wyndaele JJ. Effects of the m3 receptor selective muscarinic antagonist darifenacin on bladder afferent activity of the rat pelvic nerve. Eur Urol. 2007;52:842–7.
52. Nazif O, Teichman JM, Gebhart GF. Neural upregulation in interstitial cystitis. Urology. 2007;69:24–33.
53. Peeker R, Aldenborg F, Dahlström A, Johansson SL, Li JY, Fall M. Increased tyrosine hydroxylase immunoreactivity in bladder tissue from patients with classic and nonulcer interstitial cystitis. J Urol. 2000;163:1112–5.
54. Bauer O, Razin E. Mast cell-nerve interactions. News Physiol Sci. 2000;15:213–8.
55. Lin Q, Wu J, Willis WD. Dorsal root reflexes and cutaneous neurogenic inflammation after intradermal injection of capsaicin in rats. J Neurophysiol. 1999;82:2602–11.
56. Elbadawi A. Interstitial cystitis: a critique of current concepts with a new proposal for pathologic diagnosis and pathogenesis. Urology. 1997;49:14–40.
57. Steers WD, Tuttle JB. Neurogenic inflammation and nerve growth factor: possible roles in ijnterstitial cystitis. In: Sant GR, editor. Interstitail cystitis. Philadelphia: Lippincot-Raven; 1997. p. 67–75.
58. Procacci P, Maresca M. referred pain from somatic and visceral structures. Curr Rev Pain. 1999;3:96–9.
59. Wesselman U, Lai J. Mechanisms of referred veisceral pain: uterine inflammation in the adult virgin rat results in neurogenic plasma extravasation in the skin. Pain. 1997;73:309–17.
60. Jänig W, Koltzenburg M. Pain arising from the urogenita tract. In: Maggi CA, editor. Nervous control of the urogentital system. Chur: Harwood academic; 1993. p. 525–78.
61. Ustinova EE, Fraser MO, Pezzone MA Cross-talk and sensitization of bladder afferent nerves. Neurourol Urodyn. 2010;29 77–81.
62. Berkley KJ. A life of pelvic pain. Physiol Behav. 2005;86:272–80.

63. Malaguti S. Chronic pelvic pain caused by pudendal and pelvic plexus neuropathy as neurological sequelae of anorectal surgery. Int Urogynecol J. 2009;20:S233.
64. Tonetti J, Cazal C, Eid A, Badulescu A, Martinez T, Vouaillat H, Merloz P. Neurological damage in pelvic injuries: a continuous prospective series of 50 pelvic injuries treated with an iliosacral lag screw. Rev Chir Orthop Reparatrice Appar Mot. 2004;90:122–31.
65. Topp KS, Boyd BS. Structure and biomechanics of peripheral nerves: nerve responses to physical stresses and implications for physical therapist practice. Phys Ther. 2006;86:92–109.
66. Hunt GC, Fromherz WA, Danoff J, Waggoner T. Femoral transverse torque: an assessment method. J Orthop Sports Phys Ther. 1986;7:319–24.
67. Malaguti S, Capodaglio P. Quando il pudendo duole. Sport & Medicina. 2002;5:35–40.
68. Shafik A, El-Sherif M, Youssef A, Olfat ES. Surgical anatomy of the pudendal nerve and its clinical implications. Clin Anat. 1995;8:110–5.
69. Robert R, Prat-Pradal D, Labat JJ, Bensignor M, Raoul S, Rebai R, Leborgne J. Anatomic basis of chronic perineal pain: role of the pudendal nerve. Surg Radiol Anat. 1998;20:93–8.
70. Amarenco G, Kerdraon J, Bouju P, Le Budet C, Cocquen AL, Bosc S, Goldet R. Treatments of perineal neuralgia caused by involvement of the pudendal nerve. Rev Neurol (Paris). 1997;153:331–4.
71. York JP. Sports and the male genitourinary system. Phys Sportsmed. 1990;18:92.
72. Hofmann A, Jones RE, Schoenvogel R. Pudendal nerve neurapraxia as a result of traction on the fracture table. J Bone Joint Surg Am. 1982;64:136–8.
73. Schulak DJ, Bear TF, Summers JL. Transient impotence from positioning of the fracture table. J Trauma. 1980;20:420–1.
74. Goldet R, Kerdraon J, Amarenco G. Traction on the orthopedic table and pudendal nerve injury. Importance of electrophysiologic examination. Rev Chir Orthop Reparatrice Appar Mot. 1998;84:523–30.
75. Amarenco G, Kerdraon J, Albert T, Denys P. Stretch neuropathy of the internal pudendal nerve. Its relationship to urinary incontinence, anorectal, and genito-sexual disorders in women. Contracept Fertil Sex. 1994;22:235–8.
76. Engel AE, Kamm MA. The acute effect of straining on pelvic floor neurological function. Int J Colorectal Dis. 1994;9:8–12.
77. Garfin SR, Rydevik BL, Brown RA. Compressive neuropathy of spinal nerve roots. A mechanical or biological problem? Spine. 1991;16:162–6.
78. Goodson JD. Pudendal neuritis from biking. New Engl J Med. 1981;304:365. Letter to the Editor.
79. Amarenco G, Lanoe Y, Perrigot M, Goudal H. Un nouveau syndrome canalaire: la compression du nerf honteux interne dans le canal d'Alcock ou paralysie périnéale du cycliste. Presse Med. 1987;16:399.

Chapter 7
Syndromes Associated with Bladder Pain Syndrome as Clues to its Pathogenesis

John W. Warren, Joop P. van de Merwe, and J. Curtis Nickel

Early investigators of interstitial cystitis/painful bladder syndrome/bladder pain syndrome (which we will refer to as bladder pain syndrome or BPS in this chapter) rarely commented upon the presence of other syndromes or diseases in their patients. When they did, the significance of the report was unclear. For instance, in the first description of the characteristic ulcer that was to bear his name, Hunner in 1915 noted patients with "rheumatism" and headaches [1]. He presented no context in which to understand this observation, so it was unclear whether these disorders were more common in BPS patients than in those who did not have BPS. In other words, Hunner's study lacked proper controls, i.e., individuals who were otherwise similar but did not have BPS.

For most of the rest of the twentieth century, BPS was pursued as a disease of the urinary bladder and little substantive work was done in seeking associations with other diseases or syndromes (herein termed non-bladder syndromes, NBSs). However, the epochal definition of interstitial cystitis by the National Institute of Diabetes, Digestive and Kidney Diseases (NIDDK) in 1987 and 1988 [2] spurred research in BPS, increasingly including forays outside the bladder. Work seeking associations of BPS with NBSs occurred in the usual sequence seen in medical research, i.e., clinical observations followed by controlled studies. This chapter briefly surveys these investigations, critically evaluates selected reports, and discusses the implications of associations with other syndromes in revealing the pathogenesis of BPS.

J.W. Warren, M.D. (✉)
Medicine and Epidemiology and Public Health, University of Maryland School of Medicine, 10 South Pine St, Baltimore, MD 21201, USA
e-mail: Jwarren@medicine.umaryland.edu

J.P. van de Merwe, M.D., Ph.D.
Departments of Immunology and Internal Medicine, Erasmus MC, University Medical Center Rotterdam, Rotterdam, The Netherlands

J.C. Nickel, M.D., F.R.C.S.C.
Urology Department, Kingston General Hospital, Queen's University, Kingston, ON, Canada

J. Nordling et al. (eds.), *Bladder Pain Syndrome: A Guide for Clinicians*,
DOI 10.1007/978-1-4419-6929-3_7,

Clinical Observations

Studies of Patients with Other Syndromes

Some of the early reports actually came from investigations of patients who had other syndromes. In 1989, Maxton et al. reported that of 100 irritable bowel syndrome (IBS) patients queried for non-intestinal symptoms, 56% noted "urinary problems" [3]. Subsequently, other investigators reported what seemed to be high rates of BPS or relevant urinary symptoms in patients with fibromyalgia (FM) [4, 5], chronic fatigue syndrome (CFS) [5], temperomandibular disorder (TMD) [5], and chronic pelvic pain (CPP) [6].

Studies of BPS Patients

Not long after publication of the NIDDK definition, clinical investigators of BPS began reporting the presence in their patients of syndromes with symptoms outside the bladder. Van de Merwe in 1993 reported a case series of ten consecutive BPS patients from the Netherlands in which a careful search revealed what appeared to be a high prevalence of Sjögren's syndrome [7]. This study was eventually extended to 110 BPS patients: 7% met the criteria for Sjögren's syndrome and an additional 19% for Sjögren's-like syndrome [8].

The Interstitial Cystitis Data Base was an American multicenter study from which Simon et al. reported that 424 BPS patients had what seemed to be high prevalences of IBS, allergies, fibromyalgia, migraine, and systemic lupus erythematosus (SLE) [9]. A postal survey of 736 BPS patients who were members of a United Kingdom patient support group revealed apparently high rates of IBS, various allergies, arthritis, migraines, sinusitis, and vulvodynia [10]. Additionally, case series reported seemingly high prevalences in BPS patients of IBS, allergies, FM, vulvodynia, rheumatoid arthritis, and inflammatory bowel disease [11, 12].

In the preceding paragraphs, prevalence of NBSs has been modified by phrases like "seemed to be high" and "apparently high" because of the absence of controls in those studies. Researchers in two investigations in the early 1990s attempted to correct this problem. Koziol compared 565 BPS patients in California to 171 controls; the latter were described as either healthy volunteers or other types of urology patients [13]. Significantly more BPS patients than these controls reported the presence of IBS, various allergies, arthritis, and sinusitis. However, the controls were quite dissimilar from the cases in other ways: they were younger and, most significantly, only 60% were women compared to 88% of cases. Several of the putatively associated syndromes are known to be more common in women; thus, the relevance of the higher rates in BPS cases was uncertain.

A frequently cited study is a survey of 1,205 members of an American patient support group, the Interstitial Cystitis Association, in which Alagiri et al. compared self-report of 12 syndromes to prevalence reported in the general population [14]. Higher proportions of BPS patients claimed IBS, allergies, "sensitive skin," vulvodynia, FM, CFS, asthma, colitis/Crohn's disease, and SLE. The prevalences of migraine, endometriosis, and incontinence did not appear to differ from those in the general population. Problems with this type of comparison are many and include different population characteristics and investigators, and possibility different definitions of syndromes.

Indeed, each of these studies had a number of limitations, prominent ones being uncertain diagnostic criteria, lack of correction for age, sex, and other potentially confounding variables, and of course absent or inadequate controls. However, these studies were important because they generated the hypotheses that certain NBSs are associated with BPS.

Controlled Studies

These hypotheses were tested in two groups of controlled studies. Again, among the first were from the perspective of patients with other syndromes. Soon thereafter investigators compared the prevalence of NBSs in BPS patients and controls.

Studies of Patients with Other Syndromes

Investigators constructed controlled studies to assess the association of BPS (or of urinary symptoms) with syndromes not defined by bladder function. Several studies were of IBS patients. In 1986, Whorwell et al. compared 100 consecutive British IBS patients to controls matched on age, sex, and social class [15]. The IBS cases were significantly more likely to report each of urinary frequency, urgency, nocturia, hesitancy, and incomplete emptying of the bladder. Svedberg et al. later studied twins discordant for IBS and found "recurrent urinary tract problems" to be associated with IBS [16]. Whitehead et al. performed a retrospective comparison of non-gastrointestinal diagnoses in several thousand IBS patients and controls matched for age and sex: among the highest ORs for IBS were cystitis, urethritis, and prostatitis [17].

Twin studies of other NBSs have been informative. One demonstrated that CFS cases had a higher prevalence of physician-diagnosed BPS [18]. Another demonstrated that twins with FM ("chronic widespread pain") were more likely than those without to have "urinary tract problems" [19].

In two studies from Finland, Sjögren's patients and controls were compared for urinary symptoms or BPS. In a case series from a single hospital, more patients with Sjögren's (or SLE) reported "severe" urinary symptoms than did controls (14%, 9%, and 7%, respectively) [20]. Female members of a patient support group with self-reported physician-diagnosed Sjögren's syndrome ($N=870$) were compared to a population-based control group of women ($N = 1,304$) for BPS as diagnosed by the O'Leary–Sant scale. Adjusted for age, significantly more Sjögren's cases than controls had possible or probable BPS (14% vs. 2%) [21].

Studies of BPS Patients

Some of the first studies that compared BPS patients to controls examined the prevalence of single NBSs. The first was of FM by Clauw et al. in 1997 who reported that muscle pain, muscle spasms, morning stiffness, and swollen joints were significantly more common in 30 female BPS patients than 30 female controls [22]. Novi et al. [23] and Kennedy et al. [24] reported that gynecology patients with BPS were significantly more likely to have IBS than gynecology patients without BPS.

In the first decade of the twenty-first century, four investigations compared BPS patients to controls on *multiple* syndromes. Wu and colleagues in 2006 were the first to report their findings [25]. From a medical care database, they identified 749 cases with the International Classification of Disease (ICD) diagnosis of interstitial cystitis. They compared them to 1,498 controls, 2 for each case, randomly selected and matched on age, gender, residential region, and employee status. Significantly more cases than controls had each of IBS, FM, CPP, endometriosis, vulvodynia, depression, and anxiety (Table 7.1).

In a similar study in a health maintenance organization, Clemens et al. in 2008 identified 239 women with ICD-coded BPS and compared them to 717 women (1 case: 3 controls) matched on gender, age, and duration of membership [26]. Cases were compared to controls on apparently all ICD codes. Cases significantly exceeded controls in gastrointestinal symptoms, gynecologic pain and other symptoms, headache, myalgias, unspecified back disorders, depression, and anxiety. These authors specifically noted that they found no associations of BPS with inflammatory bowel disease, lupus, sinusitis, or rheumatoid arthritis. The authors of these two studies pointed out their limitations: dependence upon ICD coding, lack of confirmation of diagnoses, retrospective nature of the study, etc.

In a study more thoroughly discussed in the following section, Warren et al. in 2009 demonstrated that significantly more cases than matched controls had these 11 syndromes *before* BPS: FM, CFS, IBS, sicca syndrome (dry eyes and dry mouth in the absence of new medication), CPP, migraine, allergies, asthma, depression, panic disorder, and vulvodynia (see Table 7.1) [27].

In an international study from nine medical centers in the United States, Canada, Denmark, and India, Nickel et al. in 2010 compared 207 female BPS cases with 117 age- and gender-matched controls on the prevalence of IBS, FM, CFS, vulvodynia, migraine and tension headaches, TMD, and low back pain (see Table 7.1) [28]. There was a striking difference in the prevalence of IBS between cases and controls (38.6% vs. 5.2%, respectively) and FM (17.7% vs. 2.6%) with a less impressive but still statistically significant increased prevalence of CFS in cases compared to con-

Table 7.1 Proportions of BPS cases and controls with non-bladder syndromes (%)

Before/after BPS onset	Before			After			
Authors	Warren [27]			Wu [25]		Nickel [28]	
Publication date	2009			2008		2010	
Type participant	Case	Control	OR	Case	Control	Case	Control
Number	313	313		749	1,498	205	117
Non-bladder syndromes							
Chronic pelvic pain	36	11	4.5	22	4	ND	ND
Irritable bowel	27	11	2.9	7	1	39	5
Fibromyalgia	22	10	2.7	9	3	18	3
Chronic fatigue	20	9	2.5	ND	ND	10	2
Depression	42	24	2.3	7	2	ND[a]	ND[a]
Anxiety	29[b]	16[b]	2.2	5	1	ND[a]	ND[a]
Migraine	34	21	1.9	ND	ND	30	11
Sicca	19	10	2.2	ND	ND	ND	ND
Asthma	12	6	2.1	ND	ND	ND	ND
Allergies	77	68	1.6	ND	ND	ND	ND
Vulvodynia	2	0.3	NS[c]	18	3	17	1
Temperomandibular	ND	ND	–	ND	ND	12	5
Low back pain	ND	ND	–	ND	ND	47	19

The article by Clemens [26] is not included because we could not be sure that the ICD codes used in that study could be correlated with these non-bladder syndromes

OR odds ratio, *ND* not done

[a]Although mean scores on depression and anxiety scales were significantly greater in cases than controls [29]

[b]Panic disorder

[c]All case control comparisons within each study are significantly different ($p<0.05$) except for NS noted

trols (9.5% vs. 1.7%). Of the other conditions examined, the greatest difference between cases and controls was observed for vulvodynia (17% vs. 0.9%). All the other potentially associated medical conditions, including migraine and tension headaches, TMD, and low back pain, showed significantly higher prevalence in cases than controls. These associations were further verified using disease-specific questionnaires for IBS, FM, and CFS. Additionally, an earlier publication examining this database noted that BPS patients compared to controls reported significantly more depression and anxiety [29].

Summary

Controlled investigations of BPS cases have confirmed associations of certain NBSs and refuted others. The following syndromes have been shown by one or more controlled studies to be associated with BPS: FM, CFS, IBS, sicca syndrome, CPP, migraine, allergies, asthma, depression, anxiety, TMD, low back pain, and vulvodynia.

A recent systematic review of studies seeking associations of BPS with each of FM, CFS, TMD, and IBS was confirmatory [30].

In general, the conditions associated with BPS are not diseases with known pathogeneses and diagnostic findings. Rather, each is a collection of symptoms and signs, a syndrome. And these syndromes have many other similarities: symptom-based diagnoses, prominent pain in most, women overrepresented, normal or incidental local histopathology, non-diagnostic laboratory tests, fatigue, and exacerbation by stress, co-occurrence, chronicity, and unknown etiology. FM, CFS, IBS, and TMD are now commonly discussed together as functional somatic syndromes (FSSs). Others, i.e., CPP and migraine, are sometimes included as FSSs; and still others, i.e., depression and anxiety, are often associated with FSSs [31–35].

Associations with BPS of certain other syndromes hypothesized by the aforementioned clinical observations have not been confirmed. The study of antecedents to BPS by Warren et al. did not find cases to exceed controls in hypothyroidism, hyperthyroidism, mitral valve prolapse, shingles, cancer, Crohn's disease, ulcerative colitis, insulin-treated diabetes, diabetes treated with oral medication, Lyme disease, multiple chemical hypersensitivity, or SLE [27]. Although conceivable that associations with one or more of these conditions may appear during the course of BPS, a study of *prevalent* BPS cases that compared all ICD codes did not report any of these to be more common in BPS patients than in controls [26]. This study, however, only specifically noted that the following were not associated with BPS: inflammatory bowel disease, SLE, sinusitis, and rheumatoid arthritis.

Which Comes First?

So certain syndromes are epidemiologically associated with BPS. But association is not causation. One of the most important tenets of pathogenesis is that cause must precede effect [36]. Nickel et al. graphically illustrated this regarding BPS and associated NBSs [28].

Three studies have investigated the relative onsets of BPS and NBSs. Alagiri et al. apparently queried cases about onsets, for they note without presenting data that BPS "tended to precede FM, incontinence, and CFS, while it tended to follow allergies, migraine headaches, endometriosis, inflammatory bowel disease, asthma, and sensitive skin" [14]. Recall of such events may be inversely proportional to time elapsed since the events. Alagiri et al. do not note the interval between BPS onset and completion of their questionnaire but it must have been years: the mean interval between the onset of BPS symptoms and the *diagnosis* of BPS was a mean of 5.1 years.

The two other studies of relative onsets avoided this pitfall by using the onset date of BPS as a fulcrum. Wu et al., in an extension of the study above, defined the onset of BPS as the date when its ICD code first appeared, following a 6-month period of no such code [37]. They then looked at preceding syndromes in the large medical database population: individuals with antecedent CPP, vulvodynia, IBS, and FM were significantly more likely than those without to develop BPS.

Seeking risk factors for BPS, Warren et al. compared BPS cases to matched controls on antecedent NBSs [27]. Events Preceding Interstitial Cystitis (EPIC) nationally recruited incident female BPS cases (BPS symptoms of ≤12 months) through patient support and urology groups; the onset date (index date) was identified by a five-step iterative process including medical record review. Control patients were recruited by national random digit telephone dialing, matched by age, gender, and national region, and assigned an index date equivalent to the matched control. By telephone interview, 24 NBSs present before the index date were queried. For eight of these, i.e., CFS, FM, CPP, IBS, migraine, panic disorder, vulvodynia, and sicca syndrome, a series of questions addressed widely accepted expert consensus symptom-based diagnoses. For all but one of the other syndromes, diagnosis was by self-report of a physician diagnosis; the exception was allergies which were diagnosed solely by self-report.

Eleven syndromes, including all eight diagnosed by symptom-based expert consensus, were reported by more cases than controls (see Table 7.1). These findings were not confounded by demographic characteristics, prior surgeries [38], or reproductive health variables [39]. For most, there was little question of antecedence: in 71–95% of EPIC cases, these syndromes preceded IC by 12 months or more [27]. These syndromes were associated not only with BPS but also with each other. Indeed, factor analysis demonstrated that ten of these syndromes appeared in four clusters: (1) FM, CFS, IBS, sicca; (2) CPP, migraine; (3) allergy, asthma; and (4) depression, panic [27].

Further analysis showed that the odds ratios for BPS increased with increasing number of antecedent NBSs (Table 7.2) [40]. Types of NBSs were interchangeable in calculating these odds ratios [40]. The distribution of types of NBSs was skewed, allergy being overrepresented in those with few NBSs, and the classic functional somatic syndromes of FM, CFS, and IBS overrepresented in those with many NBSs [40].

Summary

Before the onset of BPS, 11 NBSs are present in significantly more BPS patients than controls. Most of the antecedent NBSs are associated with others; if a patient has one, she is likely to have others The odds of BPS increase with the number of antecedent NBSs.

Table 7.2 Prevalences and odds ratios, comparing cases to controls, for number of antecedent non-bladder syndromes [40]

No. of NBSs	No. of cases	No. of controls	Odds ratio (CI)
0	22	55	Reference
1	48	116	1.0 (0.6, 1.9)
2	70	68	2.6 (1.4, 4.7)
3	61	30	5.1 (2.6, 9.8)
4	41	21	4.9 (2.4, 10.0)
5	32	15	5.3 (2.4, 11.7)
6 or more	38	8	11.9 (4.8, 29.5)

CI 95% Confidence interval, *NBSs* non-bladder syndromes, *No.* number
From Warren JW, Wesselmann U, Morozov V, Langenberg PW. Numbers and types of non-bladder syndromes as risk factors for interstitial Cystitis/Painful bladder syndrome. Urology 2011;77:313–9. Reprinted with permission from Elsevier Ltd

Implications for BPS Pathogenesis

These three facts have emerged in the first decade of the twenty-first century: many NBSs are associated with BPS, the NBSs are associated with each other, and many NBSs antedate BPS. How do these facts help to reveal the pathogenesis of BPS?

Many NBSs are Associated with BPS

Baranowski et al. suggested a useful framework to conceptualize BPS [41]. They advised a distribution of BPS patients into three groups. One group would be those with only bladder symptoms. The second would be those with symptoms perceived in other pelvic organs. The authors suggested that this group might represent a phenomenon known as central sensitization: pain generated from one pelvic organ that is perceived in other pelvic sites because its second order neurons in the spinal cord also receive signals from those sites [42]. The third group would be BPS patients with systemic syndromes. The authors thought that this group would require mechanisms beyond referred pain at the level of the lower spinal cord to explain these associations. To our knowledge, to date only the studies by Warren et al. [27] and Nickel et al. [28] have published attempts to distribute BPS cases in such a way.

In EPIC, only 7% of the 312 cases had only BPS, i.e., with none of the 11 associated syndromes. Moreover, only 2% of the BPS cases had only pelvic syndromes (CPP, IBS, and/or vulvodynia) without accompanying systemic syndromes. The great majority of BPS cases, 91%, were in Baranowski's third category, i.e., with syndromes that manifested as symptoms beyond the pelvis [27].

These EPIC data suggest that very few BPS cases have only BPS, i.e., without one or more of the associated syndromes. Similarly, few BPS cases have additional pelvic syndromes without also having associated systemic syndromes. The implication is that central sensitization at the lower spinal cord level does not explain all the associations of NBSs in most BPS cases. Indeed, the overwhelming majority of BPS cases have one or more associated systemic syndromes. Therefore, to understand BPS, one must explain its association with this multitude of syndromes with symptoms well outside the pelvis.

The Nickel study [28] used three NBSs to assign BPS patients to three distinct clinical phenotypes which roughly correspond to the three groups proposed by Baranowski et al.: organ-centric (BPS only), regional pain syndrome (with IBS only), and systemic pain syndrome (with IBS plus FM and/or CFS). Of the 207 BPS cases, 176 were distributed into these phenotypes: organ-centric, $N=99$ (56%); regional, 48 (27%); and systemic, 29 (16%). There appeared to be a phenotypic progression, i.e., progression from organ to regional to systemic in terms of pain severity, stress, depression, sleep disturbance, sexual dysfunction, and diminished quality of life.

A comparison of these tripartite distributions by Warren et al. and Nickel et al. is instructive. An obvious distinction is that the more associated systemic NBSs used to define the groups, the fewer BPS cases that will remain in the BPS-only group or the pelvic group and the more that will be assigned to the systemic group.

The NBSs are Associated with Each Other

Not only are the NBSs associated with BPS, but many of them are also associated with each other [27]. As noted, many of the NBSs appear as clusters. For instance, if a woman had FM, she was more likely than if she did not have FM to have each of CFS, IBS, and sicca. And the boundaries of each cluster were indistinct; she might have NBSs outside the cluster as well [27]. Furthermore, the more NBSs, the more likely the case would have BPS, i.e., the higher the odds ratio. And this association of BPS with the number of NBSs was independent of the types of NBSs making up the number [40].

Many NBSs Antedate BPS

The association of certain NBSs with BPS and with each other generates three hypotheses: (1) that BPS initiates a pathophysiology that results in the NBSs, (2) that NBSs initiate a pathophysiology that results in other NBSs and in BPS, and (3) that a preceding pathophysiology results in the NBSs and BPS. There has not been a longitudinal study that has examined the temporal relationships among BPS and the NBSs. But data have been revealed that are consistent with each of these hypotheses.

Hypothesis: That BPS Initiates a Pathophysiology That Results in the NBSs

The study by Nickel et al. of prevalent BPS patients presented data that were consistent with the notion that in some patients BPS precedes certain NBSs. The pertinent observation was that the mean duration of BPS was in this pattern: BPS only < (BPS with IBS) < (BPS with IBS, and FM and/or CFS) ($p = 0.004$). The authors note the possibility of several explanations, including a temporal phenotypic progression from organ to regional to systemic pain syndrome.

Hypothesis: That NBSs Initiate a Pathophysiology That Results in BPS

On the other hand, two studies of incident BPS cases have shown that a number of NBSs precede BPS [27, 37]. One hypothesis to explain this is that syndrome A prompts a structural, physiological, environmental, or behavioral process that leads to syndrome B. An analogous situation may be diabetes mellitus as a risk factor for myocardial infarction. This reasoning becomes quite complicated when considering *multiple* NBSs. Is the process that leads to syndrome B the same that leads to syndrome C or is the latter a different one? Is that process also initiated by Syndrome A or is a separate one initiated by Syndrome B? Is a particular chronologic sequence important? Is a dominant NBS necessary for the appearance of others?

Hypothesis: That a Preceding Pathophysiology Results in the NBSs and BPS

An example would be atherosclerosis as the pathogenesis of each of myocardial infarction and ischemic stroke. That the NBSs—and BPS—are very similar in so many characteristics may be more consistent with this hypothesis. And of course this hypothesis would not require that any given syndrome precede any other syndrome.

Do Extant Data Allow a Distinction Among These Hypotheses?

Cross-sectional studies have provided provocative evidence of pathophysiologies *associated* with the NBSs and BPS: abnormalities in sensory processing, autonomic function, and the hypothalamus–pituitary–adrenal axis [43]; it is conceivable that other associated pathophysiologies will be found [44]. However, association is not causation and cross-sectional studies cannot distinguish among these three hypotheses.

This is because cross-sectional studies cannot answer the most basic question of pathogenesis: What comes first? In order to distinguish among these hypotheses, a prospective longitudinal study likely will be required. The ideal investigation would enroll young women without NBSs or BPSs, perform baseline testing of candidate pathophysiologies, and follow the participants for years with periodic reexamination for the onsets of the pathophysiologies, the NBSs, and BPS. Given the large number of patients and syndromes involved, perhaps all three hypotheses are correct.

Summary

Over the last decade, what were once distinct pathways to understanding the pathogenesis of BPS have become fainter. Fortunately, during this time several investigative groups intensively have been examining the association of NBSs with BPS and in so doing opened a new exploratory path. Three findings are pertinent to BPS pathogenesis: (1) many NBSs are associated with BPS; (2) many NBSs are associated with each other; and (3) many NBSs precede the onset of BPS. These findings have generated three hypotheses: (a) that BPS initiates a pathophysiology that results in NBSs, (b) that NBSs initiate a pathophysiology that results in BPS, and (c) that a preceding pathophysiology results in the NBSs and BPS. A well-designed longitudinal study likely will be necessary to distinguish among these three hypotheses.

References

1. Hunner GL. A rare type of bladder ulcer in women; report of cases. Boston Med Surg J. 1915;CLXXII(18):660–4.
2. Wein AJ, Hanno PM, Gillenwater JY. Interstitial cystitis: an introduction to the problem. In: Hanno PM, Staskin DR, Krane RJ, Wein AJ, editors. Interstitial cystitis. New York: Springer; 1990. p. 3–15.
3. Maxton DG, Morris JA, Whorwell PJ. Ranking of symptoms by patients with the irritable bowel syndrome. BMJ. 1989;299(6708):1138.
4. Stormorken H, Brosstad F. Fibromyalgia: Family clustering and sensory urgency with early onset indicate genetic predisposition and thus a "true" disease. Scand J Rheumatol. 1992;21(4):207.
5. Korszun A, Papadopoulos E, Demitrack M, Engleberg C, Crofford L. The relationship between temporomandibular disorders and stress-associated syndromes. Oral Surg Oral Med Oral Pathol Oral Radiol Endod. 1998;86(4):416–20.
6. Fenton BW, Durner C, Fanning J. Frequency and distribution of multiple diagnoses in chronic pelvic pain related to previous abuse or drug-seeking behavior. Gynecol Obstet Invest. 2008;65(4):247–51.
7. Van de Merwe J, Kamerling R, Arendsen E, Mulder D, Hooijkaas H. Sjogren's syndrome in patients with interstitial cystitis. J Rheumatol. 1993;20(6):962–6.
8. van de Merwe JP. Interstitial cystitis and systemic autoimmune diseases. Nat Clin Pract Urol. 2007;4(9):484–91.
9. Simon LJ, Landis JR, Erickson DR, Nyberg LM, the ICDB Study Group. The interstitial cystitis data base study: concepts and preliminary baseline descriptive statistics. Urology. 1997;49(Suppl 5A):64–75.

10. Tincello DG, Walker AC. Interstitial cystitis in the UK: results of a questionnaire survey of members of the interstitial cystitis support group. Eur J Obstet Gynecol Reprod Biol. 2005;118(1):91–5.
11. Peters KM, Carrico DJ, Diokno AC. Characterization of a clinical cohort of 87 women with interstitial cystitis/painful bladder syndrome. Urology. 2008;71(4):634–40.
12. Peeker R, Atanasiu L, Logadottir Y. Intercurrent autoimmune conditions in classic and non-ulcer interstitial cystitis. Scand J Urol Nephrol. 2003;37(1):60–3.
13. Koziol JA, Clark DC, Gittes RF, Tan EM. The natural history of interstitial cystitis: a survey of 374 patients. J Urol. 1993;149(3):465–9.
14. Alagiri M, Chottiner S, Ratner V, Slade D, Hanno PM. Interstitial cystitis: unexplained associations with other chronic disease and pain syndromes. Urology. 1997;49(5A Suppl):52–7.
15. Whorwell PJ, McCallum M, Creed FH, Roberts CT. Non-colonic features of irritable bowel syndrome. Gut. 1986;27(1):37–40.
16. Svedberg P, Johansson S, Wallander MA, Hamelin B, Pedersen NL. Extra-intestinal manifestations associated with irritable bowel syndrome: a twin study. Aliment Pharmacol Ther. 2002;16(5):975–83.
17. Whitehead WE, Palsson OS, Levy RR, Feld AD, Turner M, Von Korff M. Comorbidity in irritable bowel syndrome. Am J Gastroenterol. 2007;102(12):2767–76.
18. Aaron LA, Herrell R, Ashton S, Belcourt M, Schmaling K, Goldberg J, et al. Comorbid clinical conditions in chronic fatigue: a co-twin control study. J Gen Intern Med. 2001;16(1):24–31.
19. Kato K, Sullivan PF, Evengard B, Pedersen NL. Chronic widespread pain and its comorbidities: a population-based study. Arch Intern Med. 2006;166(15):1649–54.
20. Haarala M, Alanen A, Hietarinta M, Kiilholma P. Lower urinary tract symptoms in patients with sjogren's syndrome and systemic lupus erythematosus. Int Urogynecol J Pelvic Floor Dysfunct. 2000;11(2):84–6.
21. Leppilahti M, Tammela TL, Huhtala H, Kiilholma P, Leppilahti K, Auvinen A. Interstitial cystitis-like urinary symptoms among patients with sjogren's syndrome: a population-based study in finland. Am J Med. 2003;115(1):62–5.
22. Clauw DJ, Schmidt M, Radulovic D, Singer A, Katz P, Bresette J. The relationship between fibromyalgia and interstitial cystitis. J Psychiatr Res. 1997;31(1):125–31.
23. Novi JM, Jeronis S, Srinivas S, Srinivasan R, Morgan MA, Arya LA. Risk of irritable bowel syndrome and depression in women with interstitial cystitis: a case-control study. J Urol. 2005;174(3):937–40.
24. Kennedy CM, Bradley CS, Galask RP, Nygaard IE. Risk factors for painful bladder syndrome in women seeking gynecologic care. Int Urogynecol J Pelvic Floor Dysfunct. 2006;17(1):73–8.
25. Wu EQ, Birnbaum H, Mareva M, Parece A, Huang Z, Mallett D, et al. Interstitial cystitis: cost, treatment and co-morbidities in an employed population. Pharmacoeconomics. 2006;24(1):55–65.
26. Clemens JQ, Meenan RT, O'Keeffe Rosetti MC, Kimes TA, Calhoun EA. Case-control study of medical comorbidities in women with interstitial cystitis. J Urol. 2008;179(6):2222–5.
27. Warren JW, Howard FM, Cross RK, Good JL, Weissman MM, Wesselmann U, Langengerg P, Greenberg P, Clauw DJ. Antecedent nonbladder syndromes in case-control study of interstitial cystitis/painful bladder syndrome. Urology. 2009;73:52–7.
28. Nickel JC, Tripp DA, Pontari M, Moldwin R, Mayer R, Carr LK, et al. Interstitial cystitis/painful bladder syndrome and associated medical conditions with an emphasis on irritable bowel syndrome, fibromyalgia and chronic fatigue syndrome. J Urol. 2010;184:1358–63.
29. Nickel JC, Tripp DA, Pontari M, Moldwin R, Mayer R, Carr LK, et al. Psychosocial phenotyping in women with interstitial cystitis/painful bladder syndrome: a case control study. J Urol. 2010;183(1):167–72.
30. Rodriguez MA, Afari N, Buchwald DS, National Institute of Diabetes and Digestive and Kidney Diseases Working Group on Urological Chronic Pelvic Pain. Evidence for overlap

between urological and nonurological unexplained clinical conditions. J Urol. 2009;182(5):2123–31.
31. Aggarwal VR, McBeth J, Zakrzewska JM, Lunt M, Macfarlane GJ. The epidemiology of chronic syndromes that are frequently unexplained: do they have common associated factors? Int J Epidemiol. 2006;35(2):468–76.
32. Clauw DJ. The pathogenesis of chronic pain and fatigue syndromes, with special reference to fibromyalgia. Med Hypotheses. 1995;44(5):369–78.
33. Deary IJ. A taxonomy of medically unexplained symptoms. J Psychosom Res. 1999;47(1):51–9.
34. Kato K, Sullivan PF, Evengard B, Pedersen NL. A population-based twin study of functional somatic syndromes. Psychol Med. 2009;39(3):497–505.
35. Wessely S, Nimnuan C, Sharpe M. Functional somatic syndromes: one or many? Lancet. 1999;354(9182):936–9.
36. Hill AB. The environment and disease: association or causation? Proc R Soc Med. 1965;58:295–300.
37. Wu EQ, Birnbaum H, Kang YJ, Parece A, Mallett D, Taitel H, et al. A retrospective claims database analysis to assess patterns of interstitial cystitis diagnosis. Curr Med Res Opin. 2006;22(3):495–500.
38. Langenberg PW, Wallach EE, Clauw DJ, Howard FM, Diggs CM, Wesselmann U, et al. Pelvic pain and surgeries in women before interstitial cystitis/painful bladder syndrome. Am J Obstet Gynecol. 2010;202(3):286.e1–6.
39. Warren JW, Clauw DJ, Wesselmann U, Langenberg PW, Morozov V. Sexuality and reproductive health before interstitial cystitis/painful bladder syndrome. Urology. 2011;77:570–5.
40. Warren JW, Wesselmann U, Morozov V, Langenberg PW. Numbers and types of non-bladder syndromes as risk factors for interstitial cystitis/painful bladder syndrome. Urology. 2011;77:313–9.
41. Baranowski AP, Abrams P, Berger RE, Buffington CA, de C Williams AC, Hanno P, et al. Urogenital pain—time to accept a new approach to phenotyping and, as a consequence, management. Eur Urol. 2008;53(1):33–6.
42. Berkley KJ, Rapkin AJ, Papka RE. The pains of endometriosis. Science. 2005;308(5728):1587–9.
43. Williams DA, Clauw DJ. Understanding fibromyalgia: lessons from the broader pain research community. J Pain. 2009;10(8):777–91.
44. Buffington CA. Developmental influences on medically unexplained symptoms. Psychother Psychosom. 2009;78(3):139–44.

Part II
Clinical Presentations

Chapter 8
Bladder Pain Syndrome: Clinical Presentation

John Hughes and Mahindra Chincholkar

Definition

Bladder pain syndrome (BPS) encompasses a heterogeneous spectrum of poorly defined chronic disorders of unknown aetiology [1]. Although "Interstitial cystitis" originally represented a chronic inflammatory disease of the bladder, gradually the interpretation of this entity changed to describe a clinical diagnosis based on symptoms of pain related to the urinary bladder, following a considerable expansion of the understanding of the illness. Unfortunately though, following this transition, clinical research was severely hampered by lack of transparency of patient selection in the majority of clinical series, while terminology still suggested that inflammation is a decisive factor in all patients. The International Continence Society coined the term Painful Bladder syndrome (PBS) and reserved the term "Interstitial cystitis" for patients with typical cystoscopic and histological features, with the objective of improving precision of reporting in the literature [2]. Following this line of development, the ESSIC guidelines accepted that a clinical diagnosis can be made based on symptoms of pain that are perceived to be related to the urinary bladder, accompanied by at least one other symptom such as increased daytime or nighttime frequency. The guidelines also suggested standards for evaluation of patients and presentation of objective findings for clinical studies [3]. While the symptoms may resemble bacterial cystitis, there should be no proven urinary infection or other obvious pathology before making a diagnosis of BPS.

J. Hughes, M.B.B.S., F.R.C.A., F.F.P.M.R.C.A.
Pain Management Unit, The James Cook University Hospital, Marton Road,
Middlesbrough, TS4 3BW, UK

M. Chincholkar, M.D., F.R.C.A., F.F.P.M.R.C.A. (✉)
Department of Pain Management, Salford Royal Hospital,
Salford, UK
e-mail: mahindra.chincholkar@srft.nhs.uk

J. Nordling et al. (eds.), *Bladder Pain Syndrome: A Guide for Clinicians*,
DOI 10.1007/978-1-4419-6929-3_8,

There has been a large variation in the nomenclature used for this condition. The ESSIC guidelines proposed changing the original term "Interstitial Cystitis" to BPS, as inflammation is a feature in only a subset of patients. It proposed that the term BPS/Interstitial cystitis should be used in the interim. The Japanese Urological Association, on the other hand, felt that the term PBS was unacceptable, as a large proportion of patients with what they defined as interstitial cystitis do not express pain as the predominant symptom [4]. They proposed the term "hypersensitive bladder syndrome (HSB)" for the symptom syndrome associated with IC or IC-like conditions to avoid exclusion of patients without pain. The recent American Urology association guidelines have retained the use of Interstitial cystitis/Bladder pain syndrome (IC/BPS) and its definition as "an unpleasant sensation (pain, pressure, discomfort) perceived to be related to the urinary bladder, associated with lower urinary tract symptoms of more than 6 weeks duration, in the absence of infection or other identifiable causes" [5].

Clinical Presentation

The characteristic symptoms of this condition are pain, frequency and urgency. The presentation is quite variable. The onset is often insidious with only a single symptom of urgency/frequency, nocturia or pain [6]. The diagnosis is often delayed for years due to the failure of clinicians to appreciate the symptoms of this disease [7]. Over a period of time, other symptoms manifest. In a retrospective analysis of 45 patients, Driscoll and Teichman [6] found that 89% of patients presented with only one symptom. The median time to diagnosis was 2 years. Bacterial cystitis, prostatitis, endometriosis and chronic pelvic pain were the common initial misdiagnoses.

According to Parsons [8], patients often present with urgency/frequency in the early stages of the disease and the pain is only mild. As the disease progresses, pain becomes increasingly severe and becomes the dominant symptom. The symptoms can have a deleterious effect on patients' physical, professional and personal life.

The symptoms of urgency/frequency overlap with overactive bladder syndrome (OAB). However, patients with BPS void frequently to relieve pain whereas patients with OAB void to avoid leakage of urine, where urgency is the main symptom [9]. Abraham et al. [10] conducted qualitative interviews to identify key symptoms and the language used to identify them. They found that both OAB and BPS patients reported high day- and nighttime frequency. OAB patients did not experience pain associated with the urge.

In patients with BPS, urge had four components:

(1) Need to urinate driven by pain
(2) Need to urinate to avoid pain getting worse
(3) Constant need to urinate
(4) Sudden need to urinate

However Clemens et al. [11] found that 40% of patients with OAB also reported urgency due to pain, pressure and discomfort. They felt that urgency is not a clearly defined and commonly understood condition and cannot be used to differentiate between the two conditions. This emphasises the importance of language with individual patients using different words to describe similar sensations. When does pressure become pain and does discomfort mean pain or pressure? Taking a careful history helps elucidate what the patient actually perceives.

Pain can be felt to be in the bladder (or more accurately the area that the patient or the clinician perceives as from the bladder), abdomen or pelvis and the common descriptors used are "pressure", "burning", "sharp" and "discomfort". The pain is not limited to the suprapubic region but can be referred to locations throughout the pelvis, including the urethra, vagina, suprapubic area, lower abdomen, lower back, medial aspect of the thigh and inguinal area in any combination [8]. Consequently it is not always obvious that the pain is coming from the bladder due to this wide referral pattern. Intercourse and constrictive clothing can exacerbate the pain [12].

The natural history of the disease is characterized by exacerbations and remissions. Exacerbations can be triggered by stress, sexual activity, activation of allergies and premenstrual period [12, 13]. Most patients experience daily pain only during these exacerbations but some patients may always experience daily pain. In a national survey of 1,148 patients in the United Kingdom, 64% described daily pain during exacerbations and 37% described daily pain [14]. Longitudinal studies of long-term outcome are not available. Warren et al. [15] followed up 312 patients for a median duration of 33 months. In this study, 35% of patients reported improvement from baseline, including patients with moderate to severe disease. Although 9% of women reported temporary remission, complete disappearance of symptoms was very uncommon.

Irritable bowel syndrome, fibromyalgia and chronic fatigue syndrome are more common in patients with BPS/IC [16]. It has also been associated with immunological disorders such as Sjogrens syndrome, Systemic Lupus Erythematosus, thyroid disorders and presence of autoantibodies [17]. Increasing number of associated conditions (local, regional or systemic) has been shown to have a negative impact on quality of life including sexual function, increased pain, stress, sleep disturbances and depression [16]. It has been suggested that the disease progresses from an organ centric condition to a regional and eventually a systemic pain syndrome, leading to progression of symptoms and deterioration of cognitive and psychological parameters [16, 18].

This disease has a significant impact on patients' quality of life, both physical and psychological. The levels of pain and depression experienced by these patients are higher than those associated with other chronic pain populations [19]. Sleep disturbances, anxiety and depression are more common and are more difficult to treat [20]. The impact on the quality of life can be predicted by cognitive factors. Nickel et al. [21] used regression analysis to show that pain was associated with physical quality of life changes whereas depression, catastrophising and poor social support were associated with a reduction in mental quality of life. In particular, a maladaptive coping strategy such as catastrophising was strongly associated with greater pain, increased symptoms and poorer quality of life.

Heyhoe and Lawton [22] investigated the role of these illness perceptions in patients with BPS and their experience of psychological distress. They found that although illness perceptions differed between severely and non-severely distressed patients, there was no association with severity of symptoms. This suggests that psychological adaptation and outcomes can be at variance with measures of disease severity. Psychosocial interventions that target cognitive impairments may have a positive effect on patients' quality of life [23].

Patients with BPS may have a higher prevalence of sexual abuse and depression and all patients should be screened for sexual abuse [24]. Patients with a history of sexual abuse present with more pain and have fewer voiding problems, which may reflect increased central sensitization [25].

Conclusions

The diagnosis of BPS is often difficult due to the insidious onset of the condition, wide referral pattern and the inability to distinguish it from other diseases. A careful history with close attention to the terminology used by patients may allow the clinician to differentiate between BPS and other confusable diseases. Urgency/frequency may be the presenting symptoms with pain becoming the dominant feature as the disease progresses. The natural history of the disease is characterized by remissions and exacerbations, with some patients experiencing daily pain. It can be associated with other local, regional or systemic conditions, which suggests that the disease progresses from an organ centric to a systemic disease. The disease can have a significant impact on the physical and mental quality of life, particularly in patients who adopt maladaptive coping strategies. It is essential to screen all patients for sexual abuse, who may present with more pain and fewer voiding problems.

References

1. Fall M, Baranowski AP, Elneil S, et al. EAU guidelines on chronic pelvic pain. Eur Urol. 2010;57(1):35–48.
2. Abrams P, Cardozo L, Fall M, et al. The standardisation of terminology of lower urinary tract function: report from the standardisation sub-committee of the international continence society. Am J Obstet Gynecol. 2002;187(1):116–26.
3. van de Merwe JP, Nordling J, Bouchelouche P, et al. Diagnostic criteria, classification, and nomenclature for painful bladder syndrome/interstitial cystitis: an ESSIC proposal. Eur Urol. 2007;53(1):60–7.
4. Homma Y, Ueda T, Ito T, Takei M, Tomoe H. Japanese guideline for diagnosis and treatment of interstitial cystitis. Int J Urol. 2009;16(1):4–16.

5. International Painful Bladder Foundation. IPBF e-newsletter, Issue 2, June 2010. http://www.painful-bladder.org/Newsletters.html. Accessed 14 Jan 2010.
6. Driscoll A, Teichman J. How do patients with interstitial cystitis present? J Urol. 2001;166(6):2118–20.
7. Peeker R, Fall M. Toward a precise definition of interstitial cystitis: further evidence of differences in classic and nonulcer disease. J Urol. 2002;167(6):2470–2.
8. Parsons CL. Interstitial cystitis: epidemiology and clinical presentation. Clin Obstet Gynecol. 2002;45(1):242–9.
9. Moutzouris D-A, Falagas ME. Interstitial cystitis: an unsolved enigma. Clin J Am Soc Nephrol. 2009;4(11):1844–57.
10. Abraham L, Arbuckle R, Bonner N, et al. How do patients describe their symptoms of interstitial cystitis/painful bladder syndrome (IC/PBS)? Qualitative interviews with patients to support the development of a patient-reported symptom-based screener for IC/PBS. Value Health. 2009;12:A310.
11. Clemens JQ, Bogart LM, Liu K, Pham C, Suttorp M, Berry SH. Perceptions of "urgency" in women with interstitial cystitis/bladder pain syndrome or overactive bladder. Neurourol Urodyn. 2011;30(3):402–5.
12. Koziol J, Clark D, Gittes R, Tan E. The natural history of interstitial cystitis: a survey of 374 patients. J Urol. 1993;149(3):465–9.
13. Rosenberg M, Parsons CL, Page S. Interstitial cystitis: a primary care perspective. Cleve Clin J Med. 2005;72(8):698–704.
14. Tincello D, Walker A. Interstitial cystitis in the UK: results of a questionnaire survey of members of the Interstitial Cystitis Support Group. Eur J Obstet Gynecol Reprod Biol. 2005;118(1):5.
15. Warren JW, Greenberg P, Diggs C, Horne L, Langenberg P. A prospective early history of incident interstitial cystitis/painful bladder syndrome. J Urol. 2010;184(6):2333–8.
16. Nickel JC, Dean AT, Michel P, et al. Interstitial cystitis/painful bladder syndrome and associated medical conditions with an emphasis on irritable bowel syndrome, fibromyalgia and chronic fatigue syndrome. J Urol. 2010;184(4):1358–63.
17. Peeker R, Atanasiu L, Logadottir Y. Intercurrent autoimmune conditions in classic and non-ulcer interstitial cystitis. Scand J Urol Nephrol. 2003;37(1):60–3.
18. Labat JJ, Riant T, Delavierre D, Sibert L, Watier A, Rigaud J. Global approach to chronic pelvic and perineal pain: from the concept of organ pain to that of dysfunction of visceral pain regulation systems. Prog Urol. 2010;20(12):1027–34.
19. Rabin C, O'Leary A, Neighbors C, Whitmore K. Pain and depression experienced by women with interstitial cystitis. Women Health. 2000;31(4):67–81.
20. Clemens JQ, Brown SO, Calhoun EA. Mental health diagnoses in patients with interstitial cystitis/painful bladder syndrome and chronic prostatitis/chronic pelvic pain syndrome: a case control study. J Urol. 2008;180(4):1378–82.
21. Nickel JC, Tripp DA, Pontari M, et al. Psychosocial phenotyping in women with interstitial cystitis/painful bladder syndrome: a case control study. J Urol. 2010;183(1):167–72.
22. Heyhoe J, Lawton R. Distress in patients with interstitial cystitis: do illness representations have a role to play? Psychol Health Med. 2009;14(6):726–39.
23. Rothrock NE, Lutgendorf SK, Kreder KJ. Coping strategies in patients with interstitial cystitis: relationships with quality of life and depression. J Urol. 2003;169(1):233–6.
24. Goldstein H, Safaeian P, Garrod K, Finamore P, Kellogg-Spadt S, Whitmore K. Depression, abuse and its relationship to interstitial cystitis. Int Urogynecol J Pelvic Floor Dysfunct. 2008;19(12):1683–6.
25. Seth A, Teichman J. Differences in the clinical presentation of interstitial cystitis/painful bladder syndrome in patients with or without sexual abuse history. J Urol. 2008;180(5):2029–33.

Chapter 9
Pelvic Floor Dysfunction in Bladder Pain Syndrome

Mauro Cervigni and Franca Natale

Introduction

Pelvic floor dysfunction affects the anterior, apical or posterior vaginal compartment. There are two types: hypotonic or Low-tone pelvic floor dysfunction (LPFD), as occurs in urinary or faecal incontinence or in pelvic organ prolapse, and Hypertonic pelvic floor dysfunction (HPFD) (Table 9.1).

Many patients with Bladder pain syndrome (BPS) have concomitant HPFD, with muscle tenderness and spasm: they complain of voiding dysfunction and very high urethral pressure, which are both manifestations of the pelvic floor hypertonic component of their symptoms [1]. It has been estimated that the prevalence of HPFD in patients with BPS is 50–87% [2]. Pelvic floor dysfunction exacerbates BPS symptoms and has been reported to appear in response to events such as bladder inflammation, gait disturbance and trauma [3, 4].

Other pain disorders, such as Irritable bowel syndrome (IBS), Inflammatory bowel disease (IBD), Fibromyalgia, and Vulvodynia are all found to have a high prevalence in pelvic floor hypertonic dysfunction and myofascial pain [5–7]. All these disorders are frequently associated with BPS.

The term HPFD includes several conditions including:

- Non-neurogenic detrusor sphincter dyssynergia
- Spasm of the pelvic floor
- Tension myalgia of pelvic floor

M. Cervigni, M.D.
Department of Obstetrics and Gynecology, Catholic University, Rome, Italy

Department of Urogynecology, S. Carlo-IDI Hospital, via Ottorino Lazzarini, 5, Rome 00136, Italy

F. Natale, M.D. (✉)
Department of Urogynecology, S. Carlo-IDI Hospital,
via Ottorino Lazzarini, 5, Rome 00136, Italy
e-mail: f.natale@idi.it

J. Nordling et al. (eds.), *Bladder Pain Syndrome: A Guide for Clinicians*,
DOI 10.1007/978-1-4419-6929-3_9, © Springer Science+Business Media New York 2013

Table 9.1 Types of pelvic floor dysfunctions

Hypotonic disorders	Stress urinary incontinence
	Pelvic organ prolapse
	Faecal incontinence
Hypertonic disorders	Overactive bladder
	BPS
	Vulvodynia
	Chronic pelvic pain
	Overactive bowel
	Sexual dysfunction

- Proctalgia fugax
- Levator ani syndrome
- Coccygodynia
- Vaginismus
- Piriformis syndrome

These dysfunctions are generated by an antidromic reflex that is seen in an estimated 70% of women [8, 9]. In the colorectal literature it is defined also as tension myalgia and Levator ani syndrome [10–12] and can contribute to symptoms of frequency, urgency, dysuria, urinary and faecal retention, dyspareunia and/or vaginismus [8, 9, 13].

Pelvic Floor Anatomy

The pelvic floor consists of several components lying between the peritoneum and the vulvar skin. From above downwards, these are peritoneum, pelvic viscera and endopelvic fascia, deep genital muscles, perineal membrane and superficial genital muscles. The deeper layer, comprising the levator ani, is innervated by the levator ani nerve through S3–S5 sacral roots. The levator ani comprises the following: the pubococcygeus muscle anteriorly and the puborectalis muscle more posteriorly which are palpable during vaginal examination, and the ileococcygeus muscle, which extends from the symphysis to the obturator canal, and is anchored to the ischial spine posteriorly and to the obturator membrane or pubic bone anteriorly. The superficial layer includes the transversus perinei, ischiocavernous and bulbocavernous muscles, and also the distal urethral and anal sphincters innervated by the Pudendal nerve (PN) through S2–S4 sacral roots. The PN has three branches: the clitoral, perineal and inferior haemorrhoidal branches, which all innervate the clitoris, the perineal muscles, the inner perineal skin and the external anal sphincter [14].

As long as the muscles maintain their constant tone, they can keep the pelvic floor closed and give tonic support to the pelvic viscera via two types of fibres. Slow twitch fibres maintain urinary and faecal continence and fast twitch fibres perform active contraction. They are both activated by a sacro-spinal mechanism enhanced by mechanoreceptive parasympathetic impulses: the so-called guarding reflex.

A viscero-muscular reflex could cause a hypertonic contracted state of the pelvic floor muscles, resulting in decreased muscle function, increased myofascial pain and appearance of the myofascial trigger point [1].

In addition, the neural pathways that coordinate smooth and striated muscle activity of the pelvic organs may respond to ongoing long-term stimulation by distressing the nonirritated pelvic organs. This may lead to neurogenic inflammation and sensitization through the release of neurotrophic factors [15]. It has been proposed that a noxius stimulus may trigger the release of nerve growth factor and substance P in the periphery, causing the mast cells in the bladder to release proinflammatory substances leading to neurogenic inflammation. This can result in painful bladder symptoms, or vulvar and vaginal pain [1].

Literature Review

In 1937 Thiele created the term Coccygodynia to identify the spastic and painful pelvic floor musculature [11]. Paradis and Marganoff in 1969 proposed the term Coccygeus-Levator Spasm [16], Grant in 1975 Levator Syndrome [17] and Sinaki in 1977 Tension Myalgia of the Pelvic Floor [18]. Lilius et al. published a study on the prevalence of Levator Spasm in patients with BPS [19]. Twenty-five out of 31 patients (81%) were found to have spasm and tenderness of the levator ani, which they termed Levator Ani Spasm Syndrome.

Pathophysiology

In a normal bladder the peripheral way of transmission is mediated by Aδ(delta) fibres, myelinated, high-speed transmission nerves, that are associated with acute (sharp) pain, with sensation of temperature and pressure. Instead the unmyelinated C-fibres have a low-speed transmission and respond to stimuli which are stronger intensities and are the ones to account for the slow, dull, longer lasting, second pain (Fig. 9.1). They are normally silent, only becoming active in response to bladder inflammation or irritation. An inflammatory or pain disorder of the pelvic viscera, a trauma or exceptional behaviour may elicit noxious stimuli to sacral cord that set up a pelvic floor muscle dysfunction with sacral nerve hypersensitivity and a sacral cord wind-up (Fig. 9.2) [20].

The "Guarding Reflex" is a viscero-muscular reflex activated with the aim of increasing the tone of the pelvic floor during routine daytime activity [21]. In BPS patients there is an afferent autonomic bombardment that may enhance and maintain a guarding reflex that manifests itself as a hypertonus of the pelvic floor (Fig. 9.3).

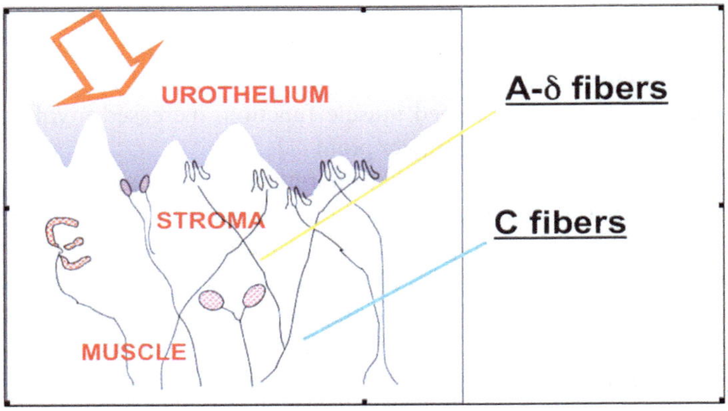

Fig. 9.1 Disposition of Aδ(delta)-fibres and C-fibres in the bladder

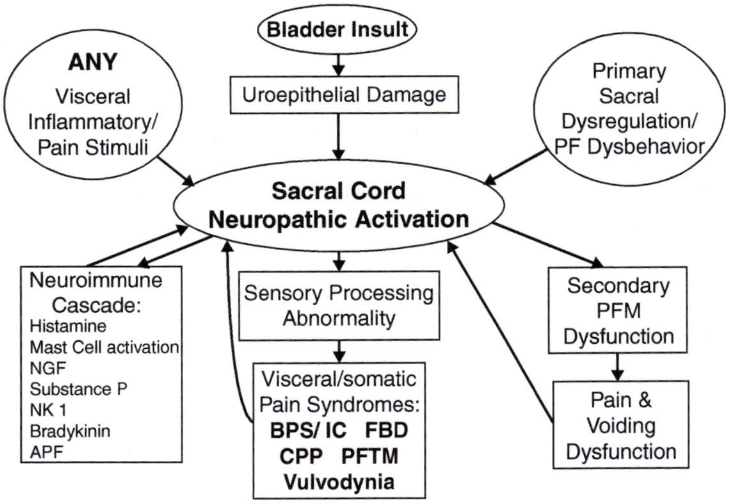

Fig. 9.2 Pathogenesis of pelvic neuropathic hypersensitivity. Modified from Butrick CW. Interstitial cystitis and chronic pelvic pain: new insights in neuropathology, diagnosis and treatment. Clin Obstet Gynecol. 2003;46(4):811–23

Vulvodynia

Vulvodynia, also known as Vulvar Vestibulitis or Vulvar Dysesthesia Syndrome, and more recently Vulvar Pain Syndrome, literally means pain, or an unpleasant altered sensation, in the vulva. It is characterized by itching, burning, stinging or stabbing in the area around the introitus of the vagina. Pain can be unprovoked, varying from constant to intermittent, or occurring only on provocation such as

Fig. 9.3 Role of guarding reflex in hypertonic pelvic floor disorders

HYPOTONIC DISORDERS	Voluntary guarding
HYPERTONIC DISORDERS	Guarding Reflex
	Antidromic reflex
	↓
	Pelvic floor dysfunction
	Voiding dysfunction
	Constipation

attempted vaginal penetration in sexual intercourse: a condition also known as Vestibulodynia. Symptoms may be highly localized or may be quite diffuse and may range from mildly irritating to completely disabling. Sometimes an area of redness may be visible, but more often the vagina and the vulva show no abnormalities on gynaecological or dermatological evaluation. This pain can affect women's sexual life and some women may become afraid to have sexual intercourse. This fear can lead to vaginismus, which is a spasm of the muscles around the vagina that makes sex painful and, in some cases, impossible. Moreover, dealing with pain for a long time causes mental health problems, such as low self-esteem, anxiety or depression. Vestibulodynia is diagnosed when there is no other obvious clinical pathology or infection present, and the vulvar pain has been present for at least 3 months [22]. Vestibulodynia has been reported in 11% of women with BPS [23] and was found to be the fourth most common IC-associated symptom (25%) [5].

The aetiology of vulvodynia is unknown, but it has been postulated that changes in the vulvar epithelium may lead to pelvic floor dysfunction and tightening, which stimulates the autonomic nervous system and increases pain. A history of pelvic surgery and abuse could play a role in BPS and its comorbidities. In a recent study more than one out of four BPS patients reported that they had suffered sexual, physical or emotional abuse at some time in their life [24].

Colorectal Pain Disorders

IBS is characterized by abdominal pain or discomfort, bloating and abnormal bowel habits (diarrhoea, constipation or both) in the absence of any structural or biochemical abnormalities. IBS is a classic example of a visceral pain syndrome and can induce central sensitization and secondary pelvic floor hypertonic disorders with dysfunctional defecation and colorectal pain [25]. It has a complex, multifactorial pathophysiology, involving biological and psychosocial elements resulting in dysregulation of the brain–gut axis. It is often associated with disorders of intestinal motility, hyperalgesia, immune disorders, disorders of the intestinal bacterial

Table 9.2 Prevalence of colorectal pain disorders in BPS patients

Colorectal pain disorders	BPS (%)	General population (%)
IBS	25–40	9
Constipation	68	3
IBD	7	0.07

microflora and autonomic and hormonal dysfunction. This syndrome is often associated with various types of chronic pelvic and perineal pain and is part of a global and integrated concept of pelviperineal dysfunction, without reference to a distinction between the posterior segment and the midline and anterior segments of the perineum [26]. Table 9.2 shows the association between BPS and colorectal pain disorders: this association is more frequent than in the general population.

Myofascial Pain Syndromes

Myofascial causes are involved in 12–87% of pelvic pain patients [27]. It is important to determine if it is a primary myofascial pain disorder or if it is secondary to another pain disorder such as BPS, Vulvodynia or IBS. If it is a secondary myofascial pain disorder, then the primary pain generator must be treated as well as the myofascial component.

Symptoms

Even though there are symptomatological similarities between BPS and PFD, there are also some differences related to pelvic floor non-relaxing behaviour (Table 9.3).

The pain symptoms are often vague and poorly localized, most commonly identified in the bladder followed by the pelvic floor, the vulvo-vaginal area and the bowel. Pain is described as achy, throbbing and as having a pressure or heaviness to it. Often this feeling is similar to the symptoms seen in patients with pelvic organ prolapse, yet on examination no significant prolapse is seen [7]. Pain often gets worse as the day progresses and is typically exacerbated by pelvic floor muscle activities, after sexual intercourse or after voiding. Factors such as job stress, constipation or menstrual cycle can trigger myofascial pain.

Patients with a significant myofascial component of their pain will often report leg or groin pain that occurs with bladder filling, and urinary frequency that is severe during the day but not at night. The pressure arising from hypertonicity of the pelvic floor is perceived as a need to void but during sleep the pelvic floor relaxes; therefore the need to void is generated only by bladder volume and not by the pelvic floor. As documented by many authors when pelvic floor therapy is used in patients with BPS the response to therapy is much better than bladder-directed therapy [28, 29].

Table 9.3 Symptomatological similarities and differences between BPS and PFD

BPS	PFD
Urgency	Urgency
Frequency	Frequency
Pelvic pain	Pelvic pain
Dyspareunia common	Dyspareunia common
Symptoms often worsened by stress	Symptoms often worsened by stress
Nocturia common	Nocturia uncommon
	Sensation of incomplete emptying
	Constipation
	Low back pain
	Straining with voiding

Table 9.4 Physical pelvic examination steps

1. Simple observation:	*Perineal strength*
	High tone
	Relaxation
2. Measure strength/high tone:	*Digital measurement*
	Perineometry
	EMG
3. Trigger point muscles	

Physical Examination

Table 9.4 shows the physical pelvic examination steps in BPS patients. Clinical evaluation of the pelvic floor begins with an observation of pelvic floor muscle activity during the process of squeezing and relaxation. It is often quite revealing to observe the perineum and introital area in the dorsal lithotomy position during the performance of a Kegel squeeze. Patients with HPFD are unable to produce more contractile strength and therefore cannot produce an effective squeeze. Spontaneous muscle fasciculation can be seen. A cotton swab (Q-tip) test for vulvodynia should be done. This involves touching the vestibule with the Q-tip at the 2, 4, 6, 8 and 10 o' clock positions (Fig. 9.4). Response to touch is rated on a VAS of 0–10 (no pain–worst pain event) [30].

At this point the doctor should place a generously lubricated single finger in the vagina to assess pelvic floor awareness (Fig. 9.5) and the ability to squeeze and relax the levator ani (Fig. 9.6). Many scales are available to document strength, tone and tenderness of each vaginal compartment (Oxford scale). Often patients with HPFD will have a "V" configuration and, as a finger is advanced, it will drop off the shelf caused by the contracted levator muscles and drop down onto the coccigeus muscle. Active trigger points are often identified by an exquisitely tender area palpable as a small 3–6 mm nodule within a taut band that reproduces the patient's pain as well as the referral pattern of her pain, on both the right and left side (Figs. 9.7 and 9.8).

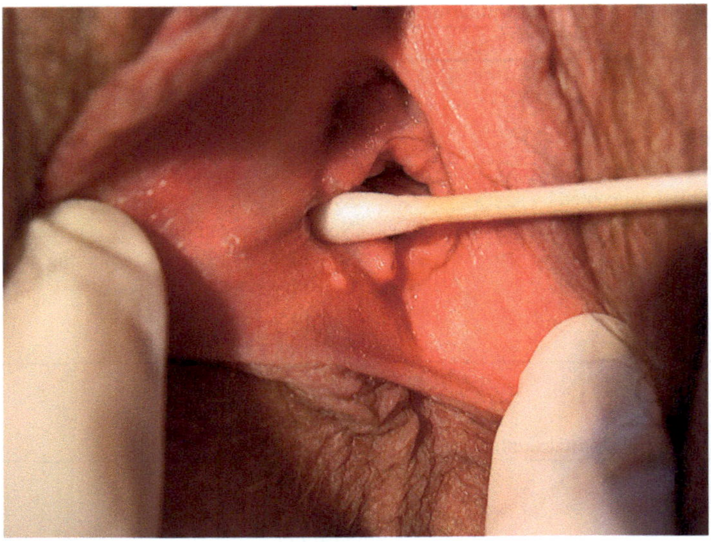

Fig. 9.4 Q-tip touch sensitivity test

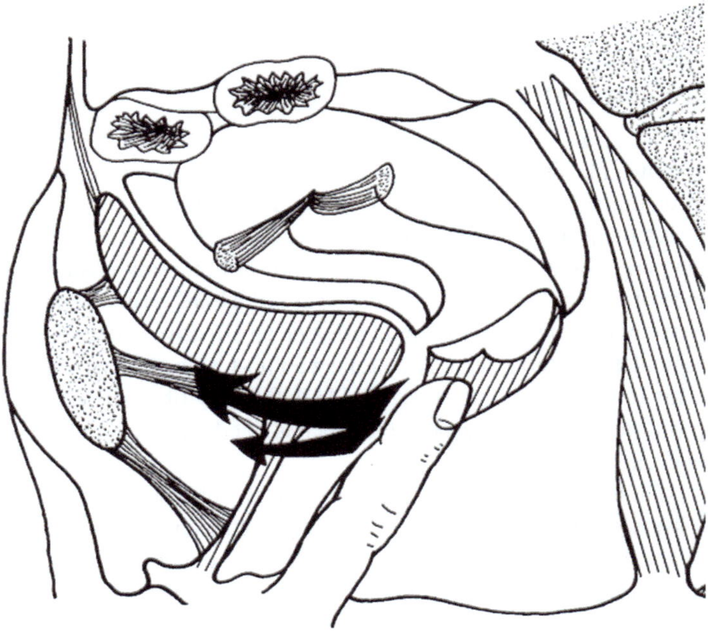

Fig. 9.5 Physical examination to assess pelvic floor awareness

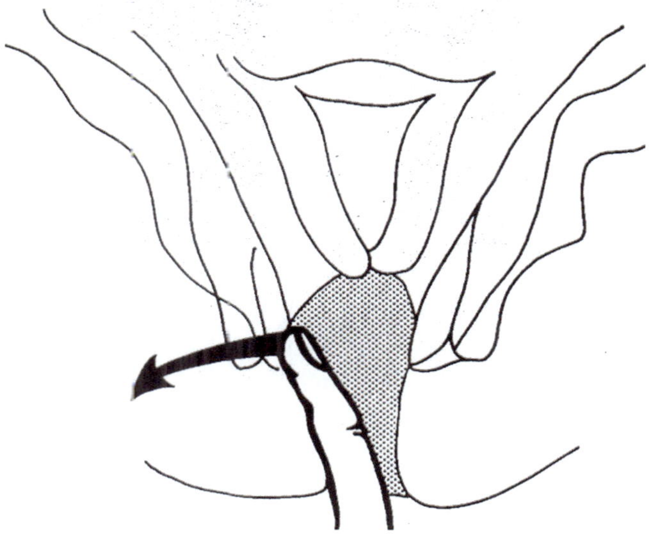

Fig. 9.6 Physical examination to assess levator ani tone

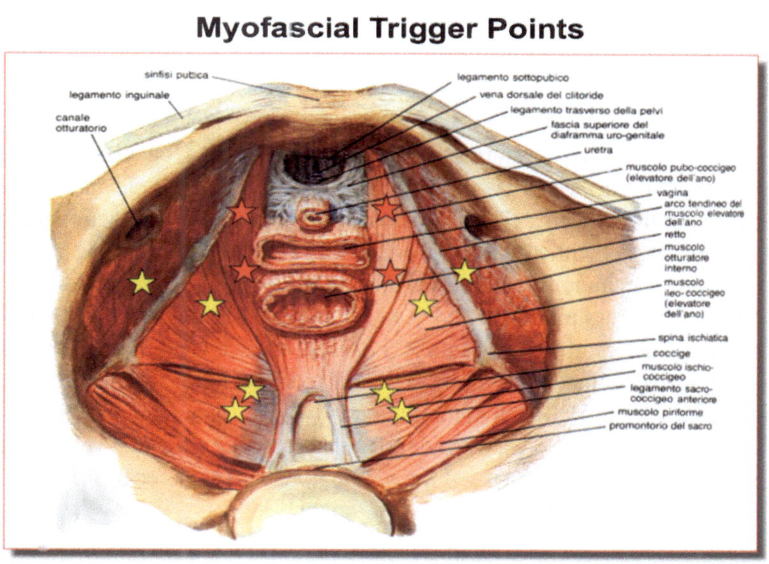

Fig. 9.7 Myofascial trigger point in female patients

Pressure is applied laterally at the ischial spines and anteriorly underneath the pubic rami. Often patients get referred pain to their low back, suprapubic area, groin or thighs.

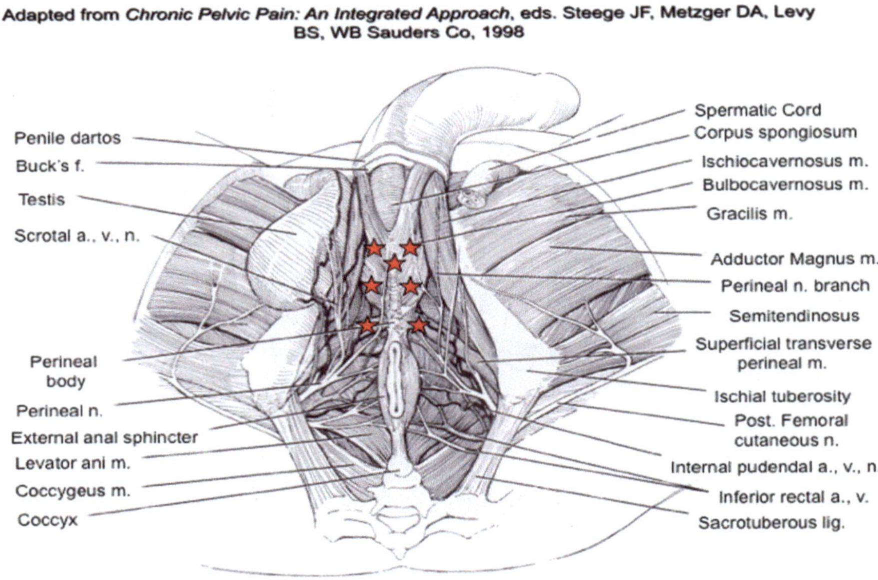

Fig. 9.8 Myofascial trigger point in male patients

Diagnostic Studies

Muscle activity can be measured using a perineometer or an electromyography probe [7, 13, 31]. Surface EMG readings can be as follows: (1) elevated and unstable resting baseline activity, (2) poor recovery, (3) poor post-contraction and relaxation and (4) spasms with sustained contractions and poor strength [32].

Urodynamics include fluctuating or interrupted flow, abnormal voiding studies, elevated urethral pressure at rest and urethral instability. Schmidt and Vapnek, performing urodynamics in patients with IC or severe urgency and frequency, observed that pain episodes coincided with behavioural increase in the sphincter tone, more than in the bladder [15]. When symptoms involve obstructed defecation and rectal pain, defecography can be used to identify the presence of a non-relaxing pelvic floor or even paradoxical activity of the pelvic floor during defecation.

Treatment Strategies

It is imperative, when approaching a patient with BPS, to focus not only on the bladder as a cause of the syndrome but also on the pelvic floor. If, in addition to the bladder, palpation of the levator muscles is painful, then pelvic floor therapy should be considered as a first-line treatment before any other systemic or intravesical medication. The goal of these stretching exercises is to lengthen the contracted muscles by decreasing tension, release trigger points in the levator muscles, re-educate the muscles to a normal range of motion and improve patient awareness.

Treatment of PFD in BPS

- Behaviour modification
- Muscle relaxants
- Local heat
- Physical therapy
- Pelvic floor manual therapy (Thiele's massage)
- Biofeedback and PFM
- Sacral neuromodulation (SNM)
- Posterior tibial nerve stimulation
- Trigger point injections
- Botulin toxin therapy

Behavioural Modification

Improvement in pelvic floor function begins with patient education on the normal function of the pelvic floor at rest and with bladder retraining including dietary modification, fluid schedules, bowel programmes and timed voiding. The application of heat using heating pads is also very helpful.

Pelvic Floor Rehabilitation

Physical therapy consists of teaching the patients how to contract or relax their pelvic floor. Manual therapy with the direct myofascial release, joint mobilization and strengthening and stretching of levator ani muscles all help the patient develop her awareness of the pelvic floor [33]. Surface electrodes applied to the perianal area or a vaginal probe can monitor the levator ani activity and teach the patient how to relax [34, 35]. The *Thiele massage* was first used for the management of coccydynia [36]. This technique encompasses a deep vaginal massage employing a back-and-forth motion over the pelvic floor musculature as well as a myofascial release manoeuvre for trigger points. Significant pain improvement can be obtained with biofeedback aimed to learn how to control voiding by relaxing pelvic floor spasm [37].

Sacral Neuromodulation

SNM is approved by the Food and Drug Administration for the treatment of idiopathic overactive bladder, urge urinary incontinence and chronic nonobstructive urinary retention. SNM is not yet an approved method for the treatment of other pelvic disorders, but data supporting its benefit are emerging. The major advantage of SNM lies in its potential to treat the bladder, urethral and anal sphincters and pelvic floor muscles simultaneously, which might result in better therapeutic effects [38, 39]. A significantly improved pain level and a reduction of opiate use were demonstrated in a paper that studied a group of long-term implanted SNM patients [40].

Posterior Tibial Nerve Stimulation

Posterior tibial nerve stimulation (PTNS) showed positive effect on pelvic pain management refractory to other previous treatments but the lack of a control study suggests that further studies are needed to confirm its real efficacy [41].

Trigger Point Injection

Trigger point injection (TPI) has the objective of deactivating the trigger point. TPI requires a series of 3–5 injections using the "wet" (with local anaesthetic) or dry with the advancement of 1–3 mm surrounding the trigger point and its associated taut band. The results show that at least 72% of patients report an improvement greater than 50% [42].

Botulin Toxin Therapy

The mechanism of pain relief with Botox involves muscle relaxation due to direct antinociceptive activity that causes a secondary decrease in central sensitization [43]. Botulin toxin A injected in the puborectalis and pubococcygeus muscles decreases pain scores, and improves quality of life and sexual function scores [44].

Conclusions

Chronic Pelvic Pain is a very common disorder affecting 16% of women. It could be related in more than 30% of cases to BPS that is frequently associated with pelvic floor dysfunction. Facing with such group of patients we need to observe not only the bladder but also "outside," considering the environment.

Therefore, it is of utmost importance to evaluate concomitant pelvic floor dysfunction that could cause associated conditions such as vulvodynia or IBS. In such cases, therapy should be oriented not only to treat bladder but also the myofascial component responsible for pain disorder.

Patients with bladder tenderness alone responded better than patients with multiple tender trigger points, possibly because in these cases the bladder is the only target organ and the patients are less severely affected than patients with multiple trigger points. Multimodal therapy remains the gold standard in the management of BPS patients.

References

1. Butrick C. Interstitial cystitis and chronic pelvic pain: new insights in neuropathology, diagnosis, and treatment. Clin Obstet Gynecol. 2003;46:811–23.
2. De Paepe H, Renson C, Van Laecke E, et al. Pelvic-floor therapy and toilet training in young children with dysfunctional voiding nad obstipation. BJU Int. 2000;85:889–93.
3. Travell JG, Simons DG. Myofascail pain and dysfunction: the triggerpoint manual. Baltimore: Williams and Wilkins; 1992.
4. Wallace K. Hypertonus dysfunction of the pelvic floor. In: Wilder E, editor. The gynecologic manual of the American Physical Therapy association. Saint Louis: University Press; 1997. p. 127–40.
5. Alagiri M, Chottiner S, Ratner V, Slade D, Hanno PM. Interstitial cystitis: unexplained associations with other chronic diseare and pain syndromes. Urology. 1997;49(5A Suppl):52–7.
6. van de Merwe JP, Yamada T, Sakamoto Y. Systemic aspects of interstitial cystitis, immunology and linkage with autoimmune disorders. Int J Urol. 2003;10(Suppl):S35–8.
7. Nickel JC, Tripp DA, Pontari M, et al. Interstitial custitis/painful bladder syndrome and associated medical conditions with an emphasis on irritable bowel syndrome, fibromyalgia and chronic fatigue syndrome. J Urol. 2010;184:1358–63.
8. Travell J, Simmons DG. Myofascial pain and dysfunction: the trigger point manual, vol. 2, the lower extremities. Baltimore, MD: Williams and Wilkins; 1998.
9. Moldwin RM. Similarities between interstitial cystitis and male chronic pelvic pain syndrome. Curr Urol Rep. 2002;3:313–8.
10. Thiele GH. Coccygodynia and pain in the superior gluteal region. JAMA. 1937;109:1271–5.
11. Fitzgerald MP, Kotarinos R. Rehabilitation of the short pelvic floor. II: treatment of the patients with the short pelvic floor. Int Urogynecol J Pelvic Floor Dysfunct. 2003;14:269–75.
12. Thiele GH. Coccygodynia: causes and treatment. Dis Colon Rectum. 1962;6:422–36.
13. Abrams P, Cardozo L, Fall M, et al. The standardization of terminology in lower urinary tract function. Report from the Standardization Sub-committee of the International Continence Society. Am J Obstet Gynecol. 2002;187:116–26.
14. Barber MD, Bremer RE, Thor KB, et al. Innervation of the female levator ani muscles. Am J Obstet Gynecol. 2002;187:64.
15. Pezzone MA, Liang R, Frazer MO. A model of neuronal cross-talk and irritation in the pelvis: implications for the overlap of chronic pelvic pain disorders. Gastroenterology. 2005;128:1953–64.
16. Paradis H, Marganoff H. Rectal pain of extrarectal origin. Dis Colon Rectum. 1969;12:306–12.

17. Grant SR, Salvati EP, Rubin RJ. Levator syndrome: an analysis of 316 cases. Dis Colon Rectum. 1975;18:161–3.
18. Sinaki M, Merritt JL, Stillwell GK. Tension myalgia of the pelvic floor. Mayo Clin Proc. 1977;52:717–22.
19. Lilius HG, Valtonen EJ. The levator ani spasm syndrome. A clinical analysis of 31 cases. Ann Chir Gynaecol Fenn. 1973;62:93–7.
20. Butrick CW. Pelvic floor hypertonic disorders: identification and management. Obstet Gynecol Clin North Am. 2009;36:707–22.
21. Chancellor MB, Perkin H, Yoshimura N. Recent advances in the neurophysiology of stress urinary incontinence. Scand J Urol Nephrol. 2005;39:21–4.
22. Reed BD. Vulvodynia; diagnosis and management. Am Fam Physician. 2006;73:1231–9.
23. Gordon AS, Panahian-Jand M, McComb F, Melegari C, Sharp S. Characteristics of women with vulvar pain disorders: responses to a Web-based survey. J Sex Marital Ther. 2003;19:45–58.
24. Carrico DJ, Sherer KL, Peters KM. The relationship of interstitial cystitis/painful bladder syndrome to vulvodynia. Urol Nurs. 2009;29:233–8.
25. Verne GN, Price DD. Irritable bowel syndrome as a common precipitant of central sensitization. Curr Rheumatol Rep. 2002;4:322–8.
26. Waltier A, Rigaud J, Labat JJ. Irritable bowel syndrome, levator ani syndrome, proctalgia fugax and chronic pelvic and perineal pain. Prog Urol. 2010;20:995–1002.
27. Peters KM, Carrico DJ, Kalinowski SE, et al. Prevalence of pelvic floor dysfunction in patients with interstitial cystitis. Urology. 2007;70:16–8.
28. Weiss JM. Pelvic floor myofascial trigger points: manual therapy for interstitial cystitis and the urgency-frequency syndrome. J Urol. 2001;166:2226–31.
29. Peters KM, Carrico DJ. Frequency, urgency and pelvic pain: treating the pelvic floor versus epithelium. Curr Urol Rep. 2006;7:450–5.
30. Haefner HK, Collins ME, Davis GD, et al. The vulvodynia guideline. J Low Genit Tract Dis. 2005;9:40–51.
31. Whitmore K, Kellogs-Spadt S, Fletcher E. Comprehensive assessment of the pelvic floor. Issues Incontinence. 1998;Fall:1–10.
32. White G, Jantos M, Glazer H. Establishing the diagnosis of vulvar vestibulitis. J Reprod Med. 1997;42:157–60.
33. Lukban JC, Whitmore KE, Kellogs-Spadt S, et al. The effect of manual physical therapy in patients with interstitial cystitis, high tone pelvic floor dysfunction, and sacroiliac dysfunction. In: NIDDK interstitial cystitis and bladder research symposium; 2000 Oct 19–20; Minneapolis: Minn; 2000
34. Rosenbaum TY, Owens A. The role of pelvic floor physical therapy in the treatment of pelvic and genital pain-related sexual dysfunction (CME). J Sex Med. 2008;5:513–23.
35. Clemens JQ, Nadler RB, Schaeffer AJ. Biofeedback, pelvic floor re-education, and bladder training for male chronic pelvic pain syndrome. Urology. 2000;56:951–5.
36. Holzberg A, Kellog-Spadt S, Lukban J, et al. Evaluation of transvaginal Thiele massage as a therapeutic intervention for women with interstitial cystitis. Urology. 2001;57((6 Suppl 1)):120.
37. Strohbehn K. Urogynecology and pelvic floor dysfunction. Obstet Gynecol Clin North Am. 1998;25:691–3.
38. Dudding TC. Future indications for sacral nerve stimulation. Colorectal Dis. 2011;13 Suppl 2:23–8.
39. Wehbe SA, Whitmore K, Ho MH. Sacral neuromodulation for female lower urinary tract, pelvic floor, and bowel disorders. Curr Opin Obstet Gynecol. 2010;22:414–9.
40. Peters KM, Konstandt D. Sacral neuromodulation decreases narcotic requirements in refractory interstitial cystitis. BJU Int. 2004;93:777–9.
41. Van Balken MR, Vandoninck V, Gisolf K, et al. Posterior tibial nerve stimulation as neuromodulative treatment of lower urinary tract dysfunction. J Urol. 2001;166:914–8.

42. Langford CF, Udvari Nagy S, Ghoniem GM. Levator ani trigger point injections: an underutilized treatment for chronic pelvic pain. Neurourol Urodyn. 2007;26:59–62.
43. Aoki KR. Evidence for antinociceptive activity of botulinum toxin type A in pain management. Headache. 2003;43 Suppl 1:S9–15.
44. Jarvis SK, Abbott JA, Lenart MB, et al. Pilot study of botulinum toxin type A in the treatment of chronic pelvic pain associated with spasm of the levator ani muscle. Aust N Z J Obstet Gynaecol. 2004;44:46–50.

Chapter 10
Psychosocial Risk Factors and Patient Outcomes for Bladder Pain Syndrome

Dean A. Tripp and J. Curtis Nickel

Abbreviations

BDI	Beck depression inventory
BPS	Bladder pain syndrome
CBT	Cognitive behavioral therapies
CFS	Chronic fatigue syndrome
CNS	Central nervous system
HPA	Hypothalamic pituitary adrenal
HRSD	Hamilton rating scale of depression
IBS	Irritable bowel syndrome
IC/PBS	Interstitial cystitis/painful bladder syndrome
LUTS	Lower urinary tract symptoms
NIH	National Institutes of Health
PCS	Pain catastrophizing scale
QoL	Quality of life
UCPPS	Urogenital chronic pelvic pain syndromes

Introduction

Bladder pain syndrome/interstitial cystitis (BPS/IC) was first clinically described as a painful female medical condition characterized by bladder ulceration approximately 100 years ago [1]. From this description, the lexicon of clinical terms associated with

D.A. Tripp, Ph.D. (✉)
Departments of Psychology, Anesthesia & Urology, Queen's University, Kingston, ON, Canada K7L 3N6
e-mail: dean.tripp@queensu.ca

J.C. Nickel, M.D., F.R.C.S.C.
Department of Urology, Kingston General Hospital, Queen's University, 76 Sturart Street, Kingston, ON, Canada K7L 2V7

J. Nordling et al. (eds.), *Bladder Pain Syndrome: A Guide for Clinicians*,
DOI 10.1007/978-1-4419-6929-3_10, © Springer Science+Business Media New York 2013

this painful disorder has grown, including Hunner's lesions and petechial hemorrhages seen under anesthetized bladder hydrodistension (classic interstitial cystitis) as well as those with symptoms, but no objective findings (painful bladder syndrome, PBS). For all BPS patients with symptoms of urinary urgency, frequency, and distressing pelvic pain other confusable diseases such as urinary tract infections, endometriosis, and cancer of the bladder are ruled out [2].

A progression from the original criteria was important because practitioners were missing more than 60% of patients using ulcer-based criteria [3]. Furthermore, prevalence rates indicate that IC/PBS is common in the United States [4]. A large European study estimated that over 16% of the sample reported moderate–high IC/PBS symptom and problem scores, with the highest prevalence reported by middle-aged women. Approximately 66% of the moderate–high-risk patients also reported diminished QoL, 35% reported an effect of IC/PBS on their sexual life, and stress was correlated with the report of IC/PBS. Although men are diagnosed with IC/PBS and some respond to therapy [5, 6], IC/PBS is diagnosed primarily in women. In fact, the only unambiguous risk factor for IC/PBS was being female (female/male ratio 9:1) [3]. Thus, in this chapter, the literature reviewed is female data.

Due to criticisms that "interstitial cystitis" was a terminology reflective of a specific, organ-based condition, PBS describes a disorder characterized by pain related to bladder filling, usually accompanied by urinary frequency and urgency in the absence of a proven urinary tract infection or other pathology [7]. The diagnostic term of IC/PBS was suggested in the past to limit communication of the clinical difficulties facing the patient, attending general practitioner, or urologist, because much of the comorbid presentation of IC/PBS may be centrally mediated as suggested for one of its primary symptoms: pain [8]. However, the nomenclature for this condition remains in flux and many are now advocating the more restrictive "BPS" as the appropriate diagnostic term [8, 9]. This chapter discusses the existing literature of patients reporting pelvic pain perceived to be related to the bladder associated with voiding symptoms, no matter whether it is called interstitial cystitis, PBS, or BPS, as it applies to psychosocial risk factors and patient outcomes associated with this medical syndrome. While much of the literature refers to IC or PBS, in this chapter we use the general term BPS to describe the patient populations discussed.

BPS is conceptualized as a visceral pain syndrome associated with heightened sensitivity to stimuli arising from changes in both the visceral and central nervous system (CNS), where previously insensible visceral inputs are now consciously apparent and often can be very painful [10–12]. As pain transitions from acute to chronic in state, it is suggested that afferent signaling from both primarily affected internal organs and the sensitized nociceptors associated with these viscera increase afferent pain signaling and CNS sensitization, thus facilitating the maintenance of chronic pain symptoms. Pain is a cardinal complex feature of BPS and its psychosocial comorbidity must be understood. Urologists must recognize the important psychosocial risk factors as they apply to BPS in order to optimize therapeutic strategies for this difficult-to-manage syndrome, which is especially true because no curative therapy has been established.

As a final introductory note, this chapter has a predominant focus on patient pain and quality of life (QoL) as outcomes. The study of patient pain and QoL is essential in medical syndromes where etiology is not understood and no cure exists. The deteriorative effect of pain on QoL runs across all ages. The pain literature suggests that persistent pain is associated with activity impairment, effects that persist after adjusting confounds such as age, gender, race, and cognitive status, and conditions as arthritis, stroke, congestive heart failure, or Parkinson's disease [13]. In BPS, patient management must reduce patient suffering and targets of psychosocial risk factors associated with diminished QoL are timely.

In this chapter, the urologist will learn about the pitfalls associated with conceptualizing BPS from a purely biomedical model. The next section briefly describes the literature associated with several psychosocial risk factors for BPS pain and/or QoL: stress, social support, catastrophizing, sexual functioning, depression, and abuse. A final section then focuses on management strategies for consideration.

Bladder Pain Syndrome as a Biomedical Problem

Surprisingly high prevalence rates exist for BPS in females. Some studies suggest that over 6% of American women exhibit symptoms of IC/BPS [14], suffering urinary urgency, frequency, pelvic pain, dysuria, and sexual pain, while others suggest that the overall prevalence of symptoms suggestive of BPS was 3% with twice the prevalence in women as men [15]. BPS pain may be constant and many characterize it as severe/excruciating [16] and progressive symptoms are common for 3–7 years before diagnosis [17]. BPS QoL is rated worse than persons receiving hemodialysis [18] and 50% of BPS patients report work disability [19].

The current clinically employed definition accepted by the NIH, ESSIC, and World Health Organization committees [8, 20] describes significant symptoms of chronic pelvic pain perceived to be related to the urinary bladder, usually accompanied by other urinary symptoms such as daytime and nighttime urinary frequency and/or urgency. As noted in the introduction, other conditions of chronic pelvic pain are ruled out before diagnosis of BPS is made. At best, traditional therapies for BPS provide some amelioration of symptoms that are said to wax and wane over time. These somewhat disappointing biomedical treatments are likely related to the fact that BPS etiology is poorly understood [21], but also that the whole syndrome is not being treated. Significant psychological comorbidities are unmistakable in BPS patients [22, 23]. The job of the treating physician is to recognize all outcome factors in BPS and strategize pertinent management options.

The Biomedical Model of Bladder Pain Syndrome

The current understanding of pain experience was formed by various theoretical, cultural, and scientific shifts [24]. Pain models predate Grecian medicine but many consider Descartes' dualistic pain concept a cornerstone [24]. Descartes assumed that pain was reported in equal amounts to the observable physical pathology: a one–one ratio of effect between tissue damage and perception. This mechanical model argued that the mind held little to no authority over nociceptive processes and that pain was experienced as a "straight-through" system [24]. Mid 1900s research provided impetus for a shift in pain understanding. Descartes' biomedical pain model could not explain why highly anxious individuals reported significantly greater pain than low-anxiety people [25]. Further, the model could not explain why soldiers in war hospitals for wound treatment used significantly less pain medication than did civilians having similar procedures, and soldiers' psychological disposition of relief from war was a suggested factor [26]. Biomedical pain models were pushed to evolve based on such findings and advances in pathophysiology.

The Gate Control Theory was a large advance in suggesting pathways to understand the impact of cognitive influences on pain experience and expression [27]. Physiological pain pathway activity was suggested to either augment or reduce subjective pain experiences. Afferent nervous system signaling travels the CNS from the extremities, and efferent pathways assist the neurophysiological influence of emotional and cognitive activity travel down the spinal cord, modulating incoming afferent signals at the dorsal horn. Thus, strong negative emotional states act to increase subjective reports of pain through facilitated sensory processing, while positive emotions may decrease subjective pain through decreased afferent processing, like the swinging gate analogy [28]. Pain is more than a sensory experience but varies based on subjective personal appraisals [29]. Cognitive factors can be either protective or inflammatory to pain experience (stress, catastrophizing versus optimistic). Anxious states are often associated with eventual appraisals of helplessness exacerbating pain experience further. Negative ruminatory or helpless pain appraisals (catastrophizing) are prominent in predicting poor experimental and clinical pain outcomes [29].

More recently, pain was suggested to occur in a neuromatrix pattern where individual genetic/characteristic patterns of nerve impulses are activated by sensory or central input often independent of peripheral activation [30]. Injury alters bodily homeostasis stressing the organism to initiate neural, hormonal, and behavioral activation to achieve normal baseline state. Whether physiological or psychological, stress activates the limbic system and emotional processing. In chronic activation, a predisposition for CNS sensitization to repeated stimulation patterns might act in developing chronic pain states. Thus, a neuromatrix model is a diathesis–stress process wherein physiological predispositions interact with the acute stressors manifesting in a person's experience [31]. Pain is "stress" that reduces bodily homeostasis. The presence of persistent pain creates a constant physiological activation and other physiological loads, helplessness or anxiety, can also reduce bodily homeostasis, further augmenting pain. Several underlying neuroanatomical pathways, neurophysiological mechanisms, and several well-known psychosocial factors can therefore be involved in pain experience [32].

Chronic pain is not simply a symptom but can be conceptualized as a disease process unto itself [33]. The International Association of the Study of Pain defines chronic pain as "an unpleasant sensory and emotional experience associated with actual or potential tissue damage, or described in terms of such damage." In the particular case of BPS, and as mirrored in the neuromatrix model of pain, chronic pelvic pain likely results from many changes in the pain signaling pathways associated within somatic and visceral structures and the excitatory processes in both the peripheral and CNS. Such changes can witness initial trauma in the viscera transformed into processes of peripheral sensitization, and with windup responses central sensitization may converge producing referred pain and referred pathophysiology [33]. There are no second-order neurons for the viscera and visceral and somatic afferents converge on the second-order neurons of the CNS, which can be associated with neuroexcitatory transmission and sensitization of the CNS. When neuroinflammatory response changes are noted referred pain or pathology can occur. For example, a neurotropic virus induces BPS but its neuroinflammatory responses can be halted by interrupting the neural connections [34]. This concept of convergence explains how neurogenic inflammation, its pain, and pathology can stretch between organ systems in chronic pain states [35]. Indeed, BPS is associated with distinct clinical phenotypes based on identification of overlapping syndrome patterns (BPS and no other symptoms; BPS and irritable bowel syndrome only; BPS and fibromyalgia only; BPS and chronic fatigue syndrome only; multiple associated conditions) [36]. Also, as associated conditions increased, the patient moved from a localized to more regional or even systemic presentation, with pain, stress, depression, and sleep disturbance increasing while social support, sexual functioning, and QoL deteriorated. Both anxiety and catastrophizing (negative appraisals of pain management ability) remained increased across phenotypes. Increased symptom duration was also associated with phenotypic progression (localized, regional, systemic) [23].

Biomedical approaches to BPS management may miss the complexity of pain and the "psychology" of the nervous system. The biopsychosocial model asserts that biological aspects of chronic illness (changes in muscles, joints, or nerves generating nociceptive input) affect psychological factors (anxiety, catastrophizing, helplessness) and the social context of the individual (social activity, activity of daily living, interpersonal relationships) in a recursive manner [37]. It is the general understanding that biomedical pain models focused on etiological and pathophysiological explanations for BPS are deficient.

Psychosocial Risk Factors for Bladder Pain Syndrome

There is increasing interest concerning BPS pain, QoL, and associated psychosocial risk factors across the urological, psychological, and pain literatures. Identifying risk factors assists clinicians in understanding the recursive dynamics between patients' physical, psychological and social experiences. Stress, depression, social support, pain catastrophizing, sexual dysfunction, and abuse have garnered research and clinical attention. Brief reviews of these risk factors and management suggestions are offered below.

Stress/Anxiety

Patients with BPS reporting greater medical comorbidity also reported high pain, poor physical QoL, depression, sexual dysfunction, and greater stress [23, 36]. BPS-associated stress and anxiety are important markers initiating and worsening functional urinary symptoms [38, 39]. The majority of BPS patients report symptom exacerbation under periods of stress [17], that acute stress increases bladder pain and urgency [40], and that associations between stress and pain increase when severity of other symptoms increases [41].

Another interesting finding comes from the large BACH study [15]. These authors produced a multivariate logistic model predicting symptoms suggestive of BPS between men, women, and overall effects. The results indicated that the primary predictive effects came from younger age, low physical activity, and greater reported stress ("worry about a sibling"; "trouble paying for life basics"). A potential genetic link between BPS and anxiety is suggested by a fourfold higher incidence of panic disorder to controls [42].

Hypothalamic pituitary adrenal (HPA) axis and sympathetic nervous system dysregulation by stress may be important mechanisms underlying BPS symptoms. Animal models can help us explain this stress–anxiety-symptom connection in BPS. Studies show that protracted psychological stress can boost bladder pain responses in high-anxiety rats [43]. Further, BPS patients exhibit increased activation of defensive emotional responses with threatened abdominal pain [44]. Finally, stress and pain may be exacerbated in BPS by dysfunctional cognitive filtering in the CNS. Hypersensitivity of interoceptive processing may be a general deficit in filtering interoceptive and exteroceptive stimuli due to altered pre-attentive processing augmented by emotional-cognitive factors [45] like catastrophizing.

In a recent BPS phenotyping study, patient questionnaires were contrasted with age, partner status, and education-matched controls. Patients reported greater pain, diminished physical QoL, greater dysfunctional sleep, more depression, catastrophizing, anxiety, and stress. Certain psychosocial risk factors (stress, anxiety, depression, catastrophizing) were also shown to further correlate with BPS-specific symptoms and strongly with decreased QoL. In particular, pain was strongly associated with physical QoL, while social support, depression, catastrophizing, and stress significantly predicted diminished mental QoL [23].

Social Support

Greater social support is associated with better patient outcomes. Lower levels of social support are associated with diminished QoL, greater depression, disability, pain severity, and pain behavior in patients with pain [46]. Indeed, persistent pain impairs daily functioning, influences marital discord, and negatively impacts both men and women but few BPS studies have examined social support or coping in the form of social engagement.

One previous study examined the association of the active seeking of social support or personal expression of distress to another as forms of social engagement in relation to depression and QoL in BPS [22]. In particular, venting (patients express themselves to another letting unpleasant feelings "escape") was found to be associated with greater depression and poorer mental health QoL. Although focused expressions of strong emotions are considered to be functionally beneficial in acute situations, protracted rumination or focus on anguish may maintain depression by reducing chances for interpersonal problem solving. This type of negative coping may be unpleasant interpersonally and may be associated with negative responses from the significant others, but this study did not assess such reactions. Additionally, seeking instrumental support (asking for assistance with activities or duties) was associated with less depression.

Recent research has examined responses of social support from the significant others. Such responses are operationalized into solicitous ("tries to get me to rest," "does some of my chores"), distracting ("tries to get me involved in some activity"), and negative or punishing ("gets angry with me"). In the chronic pain literature, negative responses to a partner's pain are associated with depression [47], pain catastrophizing [48], and greater pain [49]. Solicitous responses are related to greater pain [50], pain catastrophizing [48, 51], and depression [49]. Distracting responses from spouses are associated with greater pain [49, 50] and depression [52]. There has only been one study that examined the influence of spousal support and the association between pain and QoL, pain and depression, and pain and patient disability in BPS [53]. Results indicated that "distracting" behaviors from the patient spouses, in response to the patient's pain behavior, diminished the negative impact of patient pain on patient mental QoL. The effect of distracting spouses when in pain was also tested for the association between pain and physical QoL and depression and disability, but was not significant. This novel finding suggests that at higher levels of distracting responses, the correlation between pain and mental QoL was not significant. By contrast, the correlation between pain and mental QoL was significant at moderate and lower levels of distracting spousal responses. In essence, distracting spousal responses act to "buffer" the deleterious effects of pain on mental QoL in BPS. This study also tested the effects of "negative" spousal responses as well as "solicitous" spousal responses but no significant relationships were found.

Catastrophizing

Pain-related "catastrophizing" is broadly considered as a set of negative, exaggerated cognitive schema engaged when a patient is undergoing pain or is anticipating pain [54]. Catastrophizing is one of the most robust predictors of pain across clinical and nonclinical samples [29]. In initial BPS studies, patients reporting greater catastrophizing also reported greater depression, poorer mental health, social functioning, and greater pain [22]. In particular, this study used a series of regression models to test the independent contributions of catastrophizing and social coping variables to depression and QoL in BPS finding that greater catastrophizing predicted decreased social functioning. Further, catastrophizing, not age or symptom severity, was related to more severe symptoms for both depression and QoL. Finally, catastrophizing significantly predicted greater pain. These findings suggested that catastrophizing-exhibited impact in patients with BPS was similar to other pain samples [22].

Pain experience and catastrophizing in the lab were examined in generalized cutaneous hypersensitivity [55]. Patients with BPS were tested against controls for habituation to supra-threshold thermal stimuli applied at T12 and S3 dermatomes for 60 s while periodically rating the intensity of stimuli. They found that patients were less sensitive to warm stimuli in the T12 dermatome than asymptomatic controls but otherwise had similar thermal and vibratory thresholds and that habituation to supra-threshold stimuli at T12 and S3 dermatomes was more common in controls than BPS subjects. Catastrophizing was correlated with the duration of BPS symptoms and with thresholds to warm stimuli at T12 dermatome, suggesting that habituation to somatic stimuli is impaired in patients. Though cautionary, the authors suggested that the physical and psychological differences found in their study could potentially predispose patients suffering from BPS to chronic pain.

As suggested for stress above, BPS phenotyping research examined patient and controls on several important outcome risk factors [23]. Pain catastrophizing was shown to be strongly associated with pain and diminished QoL in patients with BPS. Catastrophizing had a significant association with decreased QOL (particularly poor mental QoL), greater pain, and a greater severity of BPS symptoms and bother. It was suggested that this was the first time any comparisons of BPS catastrophizing have been made with a control sample of healthy matched females. Importantly, this study cannot determine the cause and effect between catastrophizing and BPS outcomes.

The BPS catastrophizing findings have directed current efforts in the area of clinical assessment and management of psychosocial factors for improved patient adjustment. Using the clinically practical UPOINT phenotyping classification system for patients diagnosed with BPS [23, 56, 57], the psychosocial domain of the UPOINT system (i.e., catastrophizing, depression) identified patients with BPS that also reported greater pain, urinary urgency, and frequency [57]. Although cause and effect relations between pain, BPS symptoms, and psychosocial parameters were not feasible from this study design, psychosocial factors and catastrophizing in particular significantly impact BPS outcomes.

Sexual Functioning

Sexual functioning and its association to QoL has become a BPS research topic of interest. Pain and reduced sexual functioning are associated with poorer psychological functioning in other chronic pain conditions [58, 59]. Sexuality is significant to patients with BPS [60] and patients are intensely uneasy about the decreased sexual function [61]. Further, it is suggested that bladder pain and lower urinary tract symptoms (LUTS) related to BPS have a negative correlation with sexual function, prompting the opinion that physicians consider pain relief and control in LUTS but also sexual functioning when managing patients with BPS [62].

One of the initial evaluations of sexual functioning as a predictor of QoL was carried out in a large cohort of patients with refractory BPS [63]. These women were enrolled in a clinical trial of intravesical bacillus Calmette–Guerin, providing demographic data and responses to several questionnaires covering BPS symptoms and bother, sexual functioning, and QoL at baseline. The authors documented the severity, frequency, and bother of pain, urinary urgency, and frequency as well. They showed that physical and mental QoL were low. They found that employment, pain, and sexual functioning predicted physical QoL. Further, this study identified poorer sexual functioning as a primary predictor of diminished mental QoL in women with treatment refractory BPS suggesting that sexual functioning may be a salient therapeutic target.

A study of sexual functioning and QoL in patients with BPS enrolled in a 32-week treatment trial of pentosan polysulfate sodium showed that improvement in BPS symptoms was associated with significant improvement in sexual functioning [64]. In particular, patients showed statistically significant improvement in BPS symptoms and sexual functioning scores across treatment, and their reduction in symptom index score was moderately associated with improvement in their sexual functioning score at the end of the study. There was also a positive correlation noted between the mean change scores of sexual functioning score and improvements reported for physical and mental QoL leading authors to suggest that sexual dysfunction is moderate–severe in significantly decreased QoL, and treatment-associated reduction in BPS symptoms may improve sexual functioning, which may bolster patient QoL [64].

A cohort of urology clinic patients with BPS were examined for unique and shared associations between QoL, BPS symptoms, catastrophizing, depression, pain, and sexual functioning [65]. Women recruited from three North American centers completed measures and hierarchical regressions tested both unique and combined factor effects on QoL. They showed that diminished physical QoL scores were predicted by longer symptom duration and greater pain severity. However, poorer mental composite QoL scores were predicted by older age and greater pain catastrophizing (helplessness subscale). These data showed that longer symptoms, pain, older age, and anxious/helpless thinking about their pain (catastrophizing) were superior predictors of poorer QoL over sexual functioning when included in analyses.

BPS negatively impacts QoL suggesting that symptom duration, pain severity, depression, poor coping, stress, sleep disturbance, and sexual functioning have been identified as key predictors. However, much of this research did not examine all of these relevant psychosocial variables in a BPS cohort versus controls. Thus, extending the recent work [65], a phenotyping study examined prominent variables (symptom duration, pain severity, depression, poor coping, stress, sleep disturbance, sexual functioning) for impact on BPS QoL versus matched controls [23]. When compared to controls, patients reported significantly more sleep dysfunction, depression, anxiety, stress, catastrophizing, and moderately more sexual and social support dysfunction. Regression models within the BPS patient group showed that sexual dysfunction was not associated with either mental or physical QoL. Physical QoL was only predicted by increased pain and mental QoL was predicted by stress, lower social support, and catastrophizing.

Current research asserts that sexual dysfunction is high in women suffering from BPS [66]. In a large phone survey, 88% of women with a current sexual partner reported at least one or more general sexual dysfunction symptoms with 90% reporting at least one or more BPS-associated sexual dysfunction symptom in the past month. Further, they found that BPS-associated sexual dysfunction was significantly associated with more severe BPS symptoms, younger age, higher depression scores, and poorer perceptions of their general health. Their final regression analyses showed that general sexual dysfunction was predicted by ethnicity (non-Latino), being married, and having greater depressive symptoms [66]. It is clear that sexual dysfunction is a significant factor for patient QoL and that several biopsychosocial variables exert influence on this relationship.

Depression

Depression is a major healthcare issue affected up to 10% of primary care cases [67, 68]. Depression symptoms include sadness, helplessness, low energy, little interest in previously pleasurable activities, and negative thoughts about one's self and the future. Women suffering from BPS are at risk for depression but some qualify this in suggesting that not all women are suffering from severe levels [69]. Further, studies have shown that QoL assessment can be confounded with the measurement of depression [65]. Tripp et al. showed that a commonly used BPS QoL assessment (Medical Outcomes Survey short-form; SF-12) [70] may have a mental composite scale that can be redundant with depression scores ($r=0.77$) [71]. In such cases, mental QoL may be characterized as depression or depression as mental QoL.

In a study by Clemens and colleagues, urinary frequency and urgency, depression scores, and lower education level were independent predictors of worse symptom severity in both IC/BPS and CP/CPPS, and depression acted as one of the strongest predictors of symptom severity [72]. Women with BPS also reported greater depressive symptoms when they reported increased comorbid medical conditions [23]. The rate of mental health disorders in male and female patients with CP/CPPS and IC/BPS versus controls showed disorders reported in 13% of CP/CPPS versus 4% of controls with 23% of IC/BPS cases versus 3% of controls [72]. Further, this study reported that psychoactive medications were being consumed differentially by patient versus controls and suggested that the medication data imply that there may be a relationship between treatment efficacy for mental health disorders and the presence of urological pain symptoms. The authors suggested that there were an inordinate number of patients with BPS taking psychoactive medications for depression, anxiety, or stress (39%) versus controls that also had a mental health diagnosis (depression or anxiety) (14%) and postulated that whether the increased proportions of depressive symptoms among cases are a reaction to the experience of pelvic pain or predate the pelvic pain is of importance but has not yet been examined [73].

Other research has used multiple depression assessments to gauge the scope of symptoms across scales. Their research suggested that patients with BPS tend to present with averaged reports reaching only mild depressive symptoms, with approximately 10% of patients scoring in the moderate–severe range of depressive symptoms on one measure (Hamilton Rating Scale of Depression, HRSD) [69]. When using another measure (Beck Depression Inventory, BDI) that included somatic and the usual cognitive indicators, patient ratings again reflected mild depression with 17% falling into the moderate–severe depression range. What was interesting about this study was that greater BPS symptom severity did not correlate with increases in depressive symptoms, or general indices of QoL [69]. On the other hand, greater pain did significantly correlate with QoL and depression scores (BDI; HRSD). BPS frequency was only associated with physical functioning, and urgency and nocturia were also not associated with depression.

To summarize, those with greater pain were more likely to have poorer outcomes and pain was the most critical BPS symptom for predicting depression and diminished QoL. Whether depression precedes chronic pain or follows from it is still not well understood and must be considered through a careful history, but a direct relationship exists with pain and depression often promoting the other [74].

Abuse

Abuse history has been a hotly debated subject in urology for some time. Recent years have seen research suggesting prevalence, physical, and functional comorbidities and abuse's predictive impact on severity of BPS symptoms. Indeed, patients with chronic pelvic pain with abuse histories have been reported to suffer from diminished functional and health status, greater pain-associated dysfunction, more complaints of general medical symptoms, a greater lifetime propensity for surgeries, and greater overall disability compared to suffering chronic pelvic pain without an abuse history [75]. In reviews of the literature, some conclude that many women have been the victims of sexual assault and that sexual assault is a known risk factor for chronic pelvic pain [76].

The prevalence of BPS symptoms was more common in those abused, in those who were worried about someone close to them, and in those who were having trouble paying for basics, even when adjusting for subject depression [15]. They suggested that BPS might be associated with previous trauma and stress. In particular, their data showed that men and women who had reported abuse during adolescent years were more likely to have symptoms suggestive of BPS, with increasing prevalence of symptoms for those who experienced multiple types of abuse. This is interesting because although there was an indication of differences in physical or sexual abuse for men and women in the study, only the experience of multiple adult abuses was reported as significant in predicting BPS symptoms in final multivariable analysis. This study also found that abuse was associated with urinary frequency and urgency, and nocturia. These findings corroborate earlier questionnaire-based reports of abuse experienced during the lifetime of individuals with BPS suggesting that up to 18% reported sexual abuse, 17% reported physical abuse, and nearly 32% reported emotional abuse [77].

There is likely some association between depression and abuse history in BPS. Almost 70% of BPS patients reported mild depression but for those meeting the depression cutoff, the average score was of moderate depression [78]. Further, 36% of this BPS sample reported sexual abuse and 21% childhood sexual abuse. This study could not address causality in the relations between depression and abuse history in women and the authors suggest that it is too simplistic to suggest that sexual abuse causes BPS.

Other survey research suggests that BPS symptoms may not be associated with sexual abuse [79]. The authors sought to evaluate the relationship of childhood maltreatment on the prevalence of pain conditions comorbid with migraine in clinic population. They reported a diagnosis of BPS in 6.5% ($n=85$) of their sample, finding that patients reporting childhood physical abuse had a higher prevalence of arthritis; childhood emotional abuse had a higher prevalence of irritable bowel syndrome (IBS), fibromyalgia, chronic fatigue syndrome (CFS), and arthritis; and childhood physical neglect was associated with higher prevalence of IBS, CFS, arthritis, and BPS.

In another BPS abuse study, newly diagnosed women with BPS were stratified into those reporting a history of sexual abuse or no abuse and contrasted on demographics, frequency and urgency, nocturia, voided volumes, pelvic pain urgency frequency, BPS symptom and problem scores, and sexual functioning [80]. Up to 25% reported histories of sexual abuse including vaginal penetration, rape, and inappropriate touching of the genitals. Participants with sexual abuse histories showed larger voided volumes, less daytime frequency, and nocturia. Further, differences were also reported for palpation tenderness of the suprapubic area, vulva, posterior vaginal wall, cervical motion, and rectum, and perhaps accordingly lower sexual function scores. Interestingly, the BPS symptom and bother scores were similar between groups. These findings suggest that sexually abused patients with BPS present varied physical and functional problems. Further, abused patients may have inflamed pain responses due to central HPA dysregulation, as discussed earlier in this chapter.

Collectively, these studies show associations between histories of abuse, depression, physical and functional symptoms, and BPS diagnosis. As suggested in an abuse and BPS review [81], what cannot be causally determined from these reports is whether or not one factor leads to the development or maintenance of another. Further, the papers reviewed in this chapter have suggested that the negative psychological experience associated with the abuse may physically change the functional priorities of the CNS and/or peripheral visceral nerves in response to pain or somatic stimuli. This CNS windup may then set the stage for continued nerve sensitization caused by a cascading effect of localized inputs. Either way, the patient with BPS should be screened for depression and abuse impact amongst the other psychosocial risk factors pertinent to patient pain and QoL. Quantifying the severity of past abuse experiences presents with significant methodological challenges but it is necessary.

BPS Psychosocial Risk Factor Management

There has been increased desire to model Urogenital Chronic Pelvic Pain Syndrome (UCPPS) management into a multimodal therapy approach. UPOINT is a six-point clinical classification system categorizing phenotypes of UCPPS patients into six clinically identifiable domains including Urinary, Psychosocial (catastrophizing, depression), Organ Specific, Infection, Neurological/Systemic, and Tenderness (muscle) [23, 56, 57]. Of the psychosocial risk factors identified in this chapter, catastrophizing and depression have been provided particular attention within the UPOINT system [23, 57]. The reviewed studies suggest that cognitive and emotional factors are important to the creation, amplification, and perhaps maintenance of pain and diminished QoL in UCPPS, and suggest that standard patient care not addressing these domains may be ineffective [23, 56]. For example, there are at least three distinct BPS clinical phenotypes based on identification of overlapping syndrome patterns [36]. Here, 50.3% of the IC/BPS cohort reported no other associated medical conditions, 24.4% reported IC/BPS and IBS only, 2.5% reported IC/BPS and fibromyalgia only, and 1.5% reported IC/BPS and CFS only, while 20.2% reported multiple associated conditions. As the number of associated conditions increased and the patient moved from a localized to a more regional or even systemic presentation, pain, stress, depression, and sleep disturbance increased while social support, sexual functioning, and QoL deteriorated. Anxiety and catastrophizing remained increased in all groups. Interestingly, increased symptom duration was associated with this apparent phenotypic progression from localized, regional, to systemic [36].

The phenotyping research aids in understanding patient disease complexity [23, 36, 56, 57], but the cure of refractory urogenital conditions such as BPS remains elusive. BPS is not described as a standard disease or an inflammatory process and treatment must be individualized. Urologists are not expected to be psychologists, but are advocates for patient well-being. Patients with any type of chronic pain often report maladaptive coping (catastrophizing); may suffer from depression, relationship strain, and stress; and/or have a history of sexual or other physical abuse. Patients demonstrating these features can benefit from counseling, cognitive behavioral therapy (CBT), and/or antidepressant medications [82].

If we consider BPS to be as devastating to patient well-being as other chronic pain conditions, and to share some features in regard to psychosocial and physical predictors, models developed in CBT protocols to address anxiety, depression, and pain are relevant. Pain appraisals and catastrophizing have been of particular therapeutic interest in such treatment models. CBT is not a replacement for ongoing biomedical efforts to ease patient symptoms, but it must be considered as a serious adjunct in such treatment plans. CBT approaches help develop coping skills to manage their physical symptoms and the accompanying distress necessitated from persistent symptoms. Persistent pain and its associated comorbidities are a chronic disease; thus patients can improve QoL when engaged in symptom self-management. Treatment that has focused on decreasing negative thinking and emotional responses to pain, decreasing perceptions of disability, and increasing orientation toward self-management is predictive of favorable treatment outcomes [82–84].

CBT programs are problem oriented, use self-management skills in regard to monitoring and challenging dysfunctional and unsupported thinking, teach communication skills, use homework-based exercises, promote activity engagement, and prepare patients to anticipate setbacks in using these new skills [85–87]. These tasks help patients identify and modify significant problems in adjusting to persistent symptoms and the framework is malleable and can be used in settings of one-to-one engagement or group settings as is often found in multidisciplinary pain management programs.

Recent UCPPS treatment models optimized for a psychosocial Risk Factor Reduction Program (RFRP) have been proposed [88] and recently examined for feasibility in men suffering from CP/CPPS [89]. The goals of the RFRP are similar in nature to those of most CBT approaches and are designed to target stress, social support, catastrophizing, and mood. Issues of sexual functioning are usually drawn into sessions focused on partner support and couples issues, but the RFRP does not address histories of sexual abuse directly because the RFRP is a present focused intervention. It is recommended that adjunctive treatment should be pursued by referral in cases where previous abuse is a point of concern.

The four major goals of the RFRP are to: (1) Initiate a *sense of hope* by helping patients establish the belief that the self-management of their symptoms can shift from a state of being devastating to manageable. (2) Promote *self-efficacy* in symptoms management through the acquisition of new thinking- and new wellness-focused behavioral coping strategies. New strategies such as non-catastrophic thinking, positive self-coping statements, and mild–moderate exercise (i.e., walking program) are suggested to and evaluated by patients. The practice of new skills allows patients to stop being reactive in the face of their symptoms providing a sense of mastery. (3) Break established patterns of *schema-based automatic thinking*. In the RFRP, the practice of self-management skills takes direct aim at breaking patterns of negative or catastrophic thinking with the "Reaction Record" tool (see Fig. 10.1). The use of the Reaction Record allows patients to build confidence that they have the ability to evoke change in the management of their condition. (4) *Facilitate long-term adjustment* by helping patients anticipate problems with their attempts at self-management. The closing session of the RFRP provides explicit education and discussion about self-management into the future. Patients are encouraged to practice their new skills on a regular basis, not just in times of

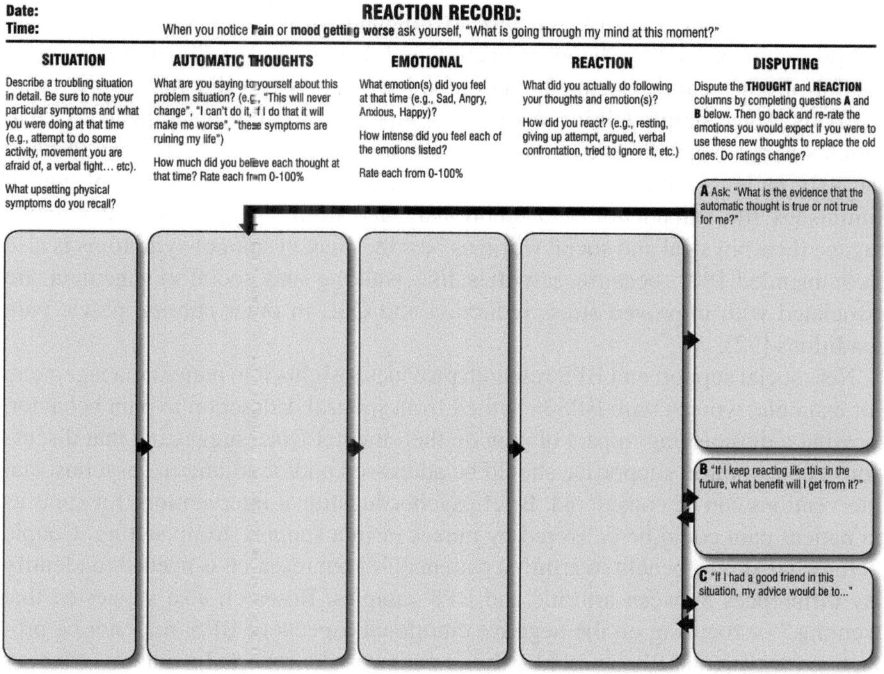

Fig. 10.1 Cognitive-behavioral thought analysis model used in psychosocial risk factor reduction program (© *D.A. Tripp 2010*)

perceived need. It is suggested that the RFRP can be adapted for use within group settings, which allows patients to share their experiences and in the process normalize their experiences when viewed in others.

Management Suggestions

Treatment models optimized for psychosocial risk factor reduction highlight the importance of rational wellness-focused thinking along with social and behavioral adaptation [88]. Urologists can have a significant impact on patient adjustment and the doctor–patient relationship is the key. Patient factors such as anger, noncompliance, and having an external locus of health control (needy, demanding) are associated with complex doctor–patient relationships. Physician factors predominantly include weight of workload (too rushed, not available) or physician communication skills or personality (low empathy) [90]. Of course, factors inherent to the health care system (financial pressure, availability of referral resources) are expected to hold some influence as well. How a physician is affected by his or her professional concerns and challenges of the health care system are primary factors in doctor–patient relationship quality [91].

Patient stress and negative self-talk are crucial to how patients feel and behave, and programs promoting the identification and disputing of such patterns are successful in other pain-associated conditions [88]. Stress is a disorder of the mind and body. Thus, simply talking, exhibiting empathy, and offering clinical advice to patients about their interpretations of stressful events and their reactions to them can help patients adjust. Patients can be "stressed" by their environment, which diminishes life satisfaction and emotional adaptation. Suggesting that patients engage their physical and social world as best they can in spite of symptoms is also recommended [88], because activities like walking and social engagement are associated with improved stress reduction and QoL in other chronic pelvic pain conditions [92].

New social support and BPS research provides insights into patient management. For example, women with BPS benefited from spousal distraction to pain behavior, showing a diminishing impact of pain on their mental QoL, suggesting that discussions about spousal supportive should be addressed and/or adjunctive psychosocial interventions can be considered. Brief psychoeducational interventions for spouses on patient pain could be delivered by nurses or in a support group setting. Couple therapy has shown benefit to arthritis patients [93] but research is needed to identify any differences between arthritis and BPS samples. Research also suggested that "venting," or focusing on the negative emotional aspects of BPS, may not be productive for patients. Rheumatoid arthritis patients who reported using this strategy in some social environments were more likely to show greater severe disease status with time as well as increased distress [94]. The pitfalls of such a strategy can be discussed with patients from within a supportive approach.

Helplessness catastrophizing is a predominant pain and QoL predictor in BPS and is often present in pain durations between 4 and 7 years [95]. Therefore, the present relation between helplessness and pain may not be specific to BPS but may be a manifestation of suffering from persistent pain. Developing from initial rumination and magnification of their pain and the threat it poses to their life, enduring pain symptoms in the context of ineffective medical therapy likely generates feelings of helplessness. Interventions targeting catastrophizing and helplessness have been shown to be feasible and to have particular value in reducing catastrophizing [89]. Programs such as RFRP are expandable and patient specific because the primary targets are developed from pertinent empirical literatures [88]. This type of treatment provides an optimistic speculation in BPS because behavioral therapy showed a reduction in disability and pain that was partially mediated by reducing catastrophizing [96]. In short, models for the amelioration of many psychosocial risk factors exist and need to be adapted for BPS.

Although sexual dysfunction is common in female BPS, there is little discussion about standardized treatment. Urologists should be aware of the types of treatments to reduce sexual dysfunctions associated with BPS. The first step to awareness is assessment; thus urologists should query women with BPS on sexual functioning because many may be reluctant to start such discussions due to embarrassment, gender differences between physician and patient, or stigma about discussing sexual behavior. Treating the medical aspects of sexual dysfunction is challenging and requires a team effort from urology, physical therapy, and perhaps sex therapy. Whenever possible, treatment and psychotherapy must involve the patient's sexual partner to increase social support. This engagement will aid in joint awareness and better communication in couples about sexual issues, concerns about intimacy, and patient pain. CBT approaches have been successfully used to teach patients pain self-management, which focuses on altering unwanted thoughts, feelings, and behaviors to gain control over their sexual experiences. For example, CBT has been used effectively to reduce vulvar pain among women with vulvodynia [97].

Medication use data suggest that anxiety and depression may be more difficult to treat in patients with urological pain syndromes than in controls [73]. Thus, a referral for talk therapy may be a useful form of treatment for more serious depression in UCPPS patients [36]. A model was proposed for UCPPS psychosocial risk factors (depressed mood, social support, catastrophizing) [88], and a recent feasibility study examined these specific factors [89]. Although depressive symptoms did decrease, they did not significantly change over the course of the feasibility trial. Caution is always to be exercised when managing depression and notable depression should be monitored appropriately by the clinic nurse or by a referred practitioner, particularly under suspicions of suicidal tendencies. Due to the strong comorbidity of depression and BPS it is suggested that routine screening be available for all incoming patients.

The management of previous sexual or physical abuse in patients may be one of the most challenging tasks of healthcare professionals but this is no reason to shy away from the issue. It is important for clinicians to empathically query in hopes of eliciting an abuse history and be prepared to provide support and appropriate referrals to mental health professionals or community agencies. BPS with abuse may present with a different pathophysiology, implying that abused patients may respond to therapy differently [80]. By its nature, abuse may lead patients with chronic pelvic pain to central sensitization and limbic dysfunction that might respond to pelvic floor physiotherapy and/or antidepressant pharmacotherapy [98] but such treatment approaches wait on satisfactory trials.

Concluding Comments

BPS is a chronic pain condition, to be examined in light of the theory and research related to the physiology of pain and the psychological suffering that such conditions manifest. In this sense, pain and other associated prominent BPS symptoms cannot be viewed from a biomedical model. By its nature, pain is more than a physical phenomenon but rather a complex physical, emotional, and interpersonal fusion associated with negative outcomes. The research and suggestions offered in this chapter help emphasize the role that psychosocial risk factors play in patients' responses to BPS symptoms. The urologist must consider the influences of an individual's prior history with pain, their cognitive pain appraisals (catastrophizing), and the social milieu in which the pain occurs. In cases of females with BPS, empathy and directive advice from physicians may be helpful when combined with appropriate referrals.

References

1. Hunner GL. A rare type of bladder ulcer in women: report of cases. Boston Med Surg J. 1915;172:660.
2. Peters K, Carrico D. Interstitial cystitis. In: Potts J, editor. Genitourinary pain syndromes: with and without inflammation. NJ: The Humana Press Inc.; 2008. p. 235–55.
3. Clemens JQ, Joyce GF, Wise M, et al. Interstitial cystitis and painful bladder syndrome. In: Litwin MS, Saigal CS, editors. Urologic diseases in America. Washington: Government Publishing Office; 2007. p. 124–54. NIH Publication No. 07-5512.
4. Clemens JQ, Meenan RT, O'Keeffe MC, et al. Prevalence of interstitial cystitis symptoms in a managed care population. J Urol. 2005;174:576.
5. Nickel JC, Johnston B, Downey J, et al. Pentosan polysulfate therapy for chronic nonbacterial prostatitis (chronic pelvic pain syndrome category IIIA): a prospective multicenter clinical trial. Urology. 2000;56:413.
6. Berger RE, Miller JE, Rothman J, et al. Bladder petechiae after cystoscopy and hydrodistension in men diagnosed with prostate pain. J Urol. 2001;159:83.
7. Abrams P, Cardozo L, Fall M, et al. The standardization of terminology of lower urinary tract function: report from the Standardization Subcommittee of the International Continence Society. Neurourol Urodyn. 2002;21:167.
8. van de Merwe J, Nordling J, Bouchelouche P, et al. Diagnostic criteria, classification, and nomenclature for painful bladder syndrome/interstitial cystitis: an ESSIC proposal. Eur Urol. 2008;53:60.
9. Hanno P, Lin A, Nordling J, et al. Bladder pain syndrome international consultation on incontinence. Neurourol Urodyn. 2010;29:191.
10. Coutinho SV, Meller ST, Gebhart GF. Intracolonic zymosan produces visceral hyperalgesia in the rat that is mediated by spinal NMDA and non-NMDA receptors. Brain Res. 1996;736:7.
11. Yoshimura N, de Groat WC. Increased excitability of afferent neurons innervating rat urinary bladder after chronic bladder inflammation. J Neurosci. 1999;19:4644.
12. Fitzgerald MP, Koch D, Senka J. Visceral and cutaneous sensory testing in patients with painful bladder syndrome. Neurourol Urodyn. 2005;24:627.
13. Katz N. The impact of pain management on quality of life. J Pain Symptom Manage. 2002;24:38.
14. Curhan GC, Speizer FE, Hunter DJ, et al. Epidemiology of interstitial cystitis: a population based study. J Urol. 1999;161:549.
15. Link C, Pulliam SJ, Hanno P, et al. Prevalence and psychosocial correlates of symptoms suggestive of painful bladder syndrome: results from the Boston area community health survey. J Urol. 2008;180:599.
16. Walker EA, Katon WJ, Hansom J. Psychosomatic diagnoses and sexual victimization in women with chronic pelvic pain. Psychosomatics. 1995;36:531.
17. Koziol JA, Clark DC, Gittes RF, et al. The natural history of interstitial cystitis: a survey of 374 patients. J Urol. 1993;149:465.
18. Held PJ, Hanno PM, Wein AJ, et al. Epidemiology of interstitial cystitis. In: Hanno PM, Staskin DR, Krane RJ, Wein AJ, editors. Interstitial cystitis. New York: Springer; 1990. p. 29.
19. Ratner V, Slade D, Green G. Interstitial cystitis: a patient's perspective. Urol Clin North Am. 1994;21:1.
20. Hanno PM. Re-imagining interstitial cystitis. In: Nickel JC, editor. New developments in infection and inflammation in urology, urologic clinics of North America. Philadelphia: Elsevier Science; 2008. p. 91–100.
21. Rosenberg M, Jackson MI, Page S. Interstitial cystitis/painful bladder syndrome: symptom recognition is key to early identification, treatment. Cleve Clin J Med. 2007;74:54.
22. Rothrock NE, Lutgendorf SK, Kreder K. Coping strategies in patients with interstitial cystitis: relationships with quality of life and depression. J Urol. 2003;169:233.

23. Nickel JC, Tripp DA, Pontari M, Moldwin R, Mayer R, Carr LK, Doggweiler R, Yang CC, Mishra N, Nordling J. Psychosocial phenotyping of women with IC/PBS: a case control study. J Urol. 2010;183:167.
24. Rey R. History of pain. Paris: La Decouverte; 1993.
25. Hill H, Kornetsky C, Flanary H, et al. Effects of anxiety and morphine on the discrimination of intensities of pain. J Clin Invest 1952;31:473.
26. Beecher HK. Relationship of significance of wound to the pain experienced. JAMA. 1956;16:1609.
27. Melzack R, Wall PD. Pain mechanisms: a new theory. Science. 1965;50:971.
28. Melzack R, Wall PD, Ty TC. Acute pain in an emergency clinic: latency of onset and descriptor patterns related to different injuries. Pain. 1982;14:33.
29. Sullivan MJL, Thorn E, Haythornthwaite J, et al. Theoretical perspectives on the relation between catastrophizing and pain. Clin J Pain. 2001;17:52.
30. Melzack R. From the gate to the neuromatrix. Pain Suppl. 1999;6:121.
31. Turk DC. A diathesis-stress model of chronic and disability following traumatic injury. Pain Res Manag. 2002;7:9.
32. Loeser JD, Butler SD, Chapman CR, et al. Bonica's management of pain. 3rd ed. Philadelphia: Lippincott Williams & Wilkins; 2001.
33. Gunter J. The neurobiology of chronic pelvic pain. In: Potts J, editor. Genitourinary pain syndromes: with and without inflammation. NJ: The Humana Press Inc.; 2008. p. 3–17.
34. Jasmin L, Janni G. Experimental neurogenic cystitis. Adv Exp Med Biol. 2003;539:319.
35. Fields HL, Basbaum AI, Heinrichier MM. Central nervous system mechanisms of pain modulation, Chapter 7. In: Wall P, Melzack R, editors. Textbook of pain. 5th ed. London: Elsevier; 2006. p. 125–42.
36. Nickel JC, Tripp DA, Pontari M, et al. Interstitial cystitis/painful bladder syndrome and associated medical conditions with an emphasis on irritable bowel syndrome, fibromyalgia and chronic fatigue syndrome. J Urol. 2010;184:1358.
37. Turk DC, Okifuji A. Psychological factors in chronic pain: evolution and revolution. J Consult Clin Psychol. 2002;70:678.
38. Macaulay AJ, Stern RS, Holmes DM, et al. Micturition and the mind: psychological factors in the etiology and treatment of urinary symptoms in women. Br Med J. 1987;294:540.
39. Baldoni F, Ercolani M, Baldaro B, et al. Stressful events and psychological symptoms in patients with functional urinary disorders. Percept Mot Skills. 1995;80:605.
40. Lutgendorf SK, Kreder KJ, Rothrock NE. Stress and symptomatology in patients with interstitial cystitis: a laboratory stress model. J Urol. 2000;164:1265.
41. Rothrock NE, Lutgendorf SK, Kreder KJ, et al. Daily stress and symptom exacerbation in interstitial cystitis patients. Urology. 2001;57:422.
42. Weissman MM, Gross R, Fryer A, et al. Interstitial cystitis and panic disorder: a potential genetic syndrome. Arch Gen Psychiatry. 2004;61:273.
43. Robbins MT, DeBerry J, Ness TJ. Chronic psychological stress enhances nociceptive processing in the urinary bladder in high-anxiety rats. Physiol Behav. 2007;91:544.
44. Twiss C, Kilpatrick L, Craske M, et al. Increased startle responses in interstitial cystitis: evidence for central hyperresponsiveness to visceral related threat. J Urol. 2009;181:2127.
45. Kilpatrick LA, Ornitz E, Ibrahimovic H, et al. Gating of sensory information differs in patients with interstitial cystitis/painful bladder syndrome. J Urol. 2010;184:958.
46. Leonard MT, Cano A, Johansen AB. Chronic pain in a couples context: a review and integration of theoretical models and empirical evidence. J Pain. 2006;7:377.
47. Cano A, Gillis M, Heinz W, et al. Marital functioning, chronic pain, and psychological distress. Pain. 2004;107:99.
48. Buenaver LF, Edwards RR, Haythornwaite JA. Pain-related catastrophizing and perceived social responses: inter-relationships in the context of chronic pain. Pain. 2007;127:234.
49. Cano A, Weisberg JN, Gallagher RM. Marital satisfaction and pain severity mediate the association between negative spouse responses to pain and depressive symptoms in a chronic pain patient sample. Pain Med. 2000;1:35.

50. Flor H, Turk DC, Rudy TE. Relationship of pain impact and significant other reinforcement of pain behaviors: the mediating role of gender, marital status and marital satisfaction. Pain. 1989;38:45.
51. Giardino ND, Jensen MP, Turner JA, et al. Social environment mediates the association between catastrophizing and pain among persons with a spinal cord injury. Pain. 2003;106:19.
52. Kerns RD, Haythornwaite J, Southwick S, et al. The role of marital interaction in chronic pain and depressive symptom severity. J Psychosom Res. 1990;34:472.
53. Ginting JV, Tripp DA, Nickel JC, et al. Spousal support decreases the negative impact of pain on mental quality of life in women with interstitial cystitis/painful bladder syndrome. BJU Int. 2010;107:1464-410.
54. Sullivan MJL, Bishop SR, Pivik J. The pain catastrophizing scale: development and validation. Psychol Assess. 1995;7:524.
55. Lowenstein L, Kenton K, Mueller ER, et al. Patients with painful bladder syndrome have altered response to thermal stimuli and catastrophic reaction to painful experiences. Neurourol Urodyn. 2009;28:400.
56. Shoskes DA, Nickel JC, Rackley RR, et al. Clinical phenotyping in chronic prostatitis/chronic pelvic pain syndrome and interstitial cystitis: a management strategy for urologic chronic pelvic pain syndromes. Prostate Cancer Prostatic Dis. 2009;12:177.
57. Nickel JC, Shoskes DA, Irvine-Bird K. Clinical phenotyping of women with interstitial cystitis/painful bladder syndrome: a key to classification and potentially improved management. J Urol. 2009;182:155.
58. Maruta T, Osborne D, Swanson DW, Halling JM. Chronic pain patients and spouses: marital and sexual adjustment. Mayo Clin Proc. 1981;56:307.
59. Flor H, Turk DC, Scholz OB. Impact of chronic pain on the spouse: marital, emotional and physical consequences. J Psychosom Res. 1987;31:63.
60. Webster DC. Recontextualizing sexuality in chronic illness: women and interstitial cystitis. Health Care Women Int. 1997;18:575.
61. Azevedo K, Nguyen A, Rowhani-Rahbar A, et al. Pain impacts sexual functioning among interstitial cystitis patients. Sex Disabil. 2005;23:189.
62. Yoon HS, Yoon H. Correlations of interstitial cystitis/painful bladder syndrome with female sexual activity. Korean J Urol. 2010;51:45.
63. Nickel JC, Tripp DA, Teal V, et al. Sexual function is a determinant of poor quality of life in women with treatment refractory interstitial cystitis. J Urol. 2007;177:1832.
64. Nickel JC, Parsons L, Forrest J, et al. Improvement in sexual functioning in patients with interstitial cystitis/painful bladder syndrome. J Sex Med. 2008;5:394.
65. Tripp DA, Nickel JC, Fitzgerald MP, et al. Sexual functioning, catastrophizing, depression and pain as predictors of quality of life in women suffering from interstitial cystitis/painful bladder syndrome. Urology. 2009;73:987.
66. Bogart LM, Suttorp MJ, Elliott MN, Clemens JQ, et al. Prevalence and correlates of sexual dysfunction among women with bladder pain syndrome/interstitial cystitis. Urology. 2011;77:576–80.
67. Simon G, Von Korff M. Recognition and management of depression in primary care. Arch Fam Med. 1995;4:99.
68. American Psychiatric Association. Diagnostic and statistical manual of mental disorders (text revision). 4th ed. Washington: American Psychiatric Association; 2000.
69. Rothrock N, Lutgendorf SK, Hoffman A, et al. Depressive symptoms and quality of life in patients with interstitial cystitis. J Urol. 2002;167:1763.
70. Gandek B, Ware JE, Aaronson NK, et al. Cross-validation of item selection and scoring for the SF-12 health survey in nine countries: results from the IQOLA project. International quality of life assessment. J Clin Epidemiol. 1998;51:1171.
71. Tabachnick BG, Fidell LS. Using multivariate statistics. 3rd ed. New York: Harper Collins; 1996. p. 100–85.

72. Clemens JQ, Brown SO, Kozloff L, et al. Predictors of symptom severity in patients with chronic prostatitis and interstitial cystitis. J Urol. 2006;175:963.
73. Clemens JQ, Brown SO, Calhoun EA. Mental health diagnoses in patients with interstitial cystitis/painful bladder syndrome and chronic prostatitis/chronic pelvic pain syndrome: a case/control study. J Urol. 2008;180:1378.
74. Fishbain DA, Cutler R, Rosomoff HL, et al. Chronic pain associated depression: antecedent or consequence of chronic pain: a review. Clin J Pain. 1997;13:116.
75. Leserman J. Sexual abuse history: prevalence, health effects, mediators, and psychological treatment. Psychosom Med. 2005;67:906.
76. Latthe P, Mignini L, Gray R, et al. Factors predisposing women to chronic pelvic pain: systematic review. BMJ. 2006;332:749.
77. Peters KM, Kalinowski SE, Carrico DJ, et al. Fact or fiction—is abuse prevalent in patients with interstitial cystitis? Results from a community survey and clinic population. J Urol. 2007;178:891.
78. Goldstein HB, Safaeian P, Garrod K, et al. Depression, abuse and its relationship to interstitial cystitis. Int Urogynecol J Pelvic Floor Dysfunct. 2008;19:1683.
79. Tietjen G, Brandes JL, Peterlin BL, et al. Childhood maltreatment and migraine (Part III). Association with comorbid pain conditions. Headache. 2010;50:42.
80. Seth A, Teichman JMH. Differences in the clinical presentation of interstitial cystitis/painful bladder syndrome in patients with or without sexual abuse history. J Urol. 2008;180:2029.
81. Mayson B, Teichman JMH. The relationship between sexual abuse and interstitial cystitis/painful bladder syndrome. Curr Urol Rep. 2009;10:441.
82. Shoskes DA, Nickel JC, Dolinga R, et al. Clinical phenotyping of patients with chronic prostatitis/chronic pelvic pain syndrome and correlation with symptom severity. Urology. 2009;73:538.
83. Morely S, Eccleston C, Williamson A. Systematic review and meta-analysis of randomized controlled trials of cognitive behaviour therapy and behaviour therapy for chronic pain in adults, excluding headaches. Pain. 1999;80:1.
84. McCracken L, Turk D. Behavioral and cognitive-behavioral treatment for chronic pain: outcome, predictors of outcome, and treatment process. Spine. 2002;27:2564.
85. Beck JS. Cognitive therapy: basics and beyond. New York: The Guildford Press; 1995.
86. Beck A, Rush AJ, Shaw B, Emery G. Cognitive therapy for depression. New York: The Guildford Press; 1979.
87. Persons J, Davidson J, Tompkins M. Essential components of cognitive-behaviour therapy for depression. Washington: American Psychological Association; 2001.
88. Nickel JC, Mullins C, Tripp DA. Development of an evidence-based cognitive behavioral treatment program for men with chronic prostatitis/chronic pelvic pain syndrome. World J Urol. 2008;26:167.
89. Tripp DA, Nickel JC, Katz L. A feasibility trial of a cognitive-behavioural symptom management program for chronic pelvic pain for men with refractory chronic prostatitis/chronic pelvic pain syndrome. Can Urol Assoc J. 2011;5:328–32.
90. Hahn SR, Kroenke K, Spitzer RL, et al. The difficult patient: prevalence, psychopathology, and functional impairment. J Gen Intern Med. 1996;11:1.
91. Vegni E, Visioli S, Moja EA. When talking to the patient is difficult: the physician's perspective. Commun Med. 2005;2:69.
92. Webster DC, Brennan T. Self-care effectiveness and health outcomes in women with interstitial cystitis: implications for mental health clinicians. Issues Ment Health Nurs. 1998;19:495.
93. Keefe FJ, Caldwell DS, Baucom D, et al. Spouse-assisted coping skills training in the management of osteoarthritic knee pain. Arthritis Care Res. 1996;9:279.
94. Griffin KW, Friend R, Kaell AT, et al. Distress and disease status among patients with rheumatoid arthritis: roles of coping styles and perceived responses from support providers. Ann Behav Med. 2001;23:133.
95. Sullivan MJL, Stanish W, Sullivan ME, et al. Differential predictors of pain and disability following whiplash injury. Pain Res Manag. 2002;7:68.

96. Smeets R, Vlaeyen JWS, Kester A, et al. Reduction of pain catastrophizing mediates the outcome of both physical and cognitive-behavioral treatment in chronic low back pain. J Pain. 2006;7:261.
97. Masheb RM, Kerns R, Lozano C. A randomized clinical trial for women with vulvodynia: cognitive-behavioral therapy vs. supportive psychotherapy. Pain. 2009;141:31.
98. Meltzer-Brody S, Leserman J, Zolnoun D, et al. Trauma and posttraumatic stress disorder in women with chronic pelvic pain. Obstet Gynecol. 2007;109:902.

Chapter 11
Bladder Pain Syndrome and Sexuality

Jennifer Yonaitis Fariello, Kristene E. Whitmore, and Robert M. Moldwin

Introduction

Sexual function is a primary predictor for mental quality of life (QOL) in the BPS patient, but is often overlooked by clinicians [1]. The presenting chronic symptoms of BPS, or those of comorbid conditions such as pelvic floor dysfunction, vulvodynia, fibromyalgia, or migraine headache, can negatively affect sexual intimacy resulting in depression and alterations in sexual functioning to the point of avoidance of sexual intimacy altogether [2, 3]. This chapter explores the relationship between interstitial cystitis, chronic pain, and sexual dysfunction, along with its physical and psychological impacts on patients and their partners.

Sexuality, Pain, and Sexual Dysfunction

Sexuality is a multi-faceted, physical, psychological, emotional, and spiritual experience incorporating intimacy, sensuality, and one's sexual identity. A delicate balance normally exists between these factors, which, in turn, is essential for a satisfactory sexual response. The sexual response has been redefined since Masters

J.Y. Fariello, M.S.N., C.R.N.P. (✉) • K.E. Whitmore, M.D.
Urology Division, Department of Obstetrics and Gynecology, FPMRS,
The Pelvic and Sexual Health Institute Drexel University College of Medicine,
207 N. Broad Street, 4th Floor, Philadelphia, PA, 19107, USA
e-mail: jfariello@gmail.com

R.M. Moldwin, M.D.
Urology Division, The Arthur Smith Institute for Urology, North Shore–Long Island Jewish Health System, New Hyde Park, NY, USA

Urology Department, The Hofstra University School of Medicine,
New Hyde Park, NY, USA
e-mail: rmoldwin@gmail.com

J. Nordling et al. (eds.), *Bladder Pain Syndrome: A Guide for Clinicians*,
DOI 10.1007/978-1-4419-6929-3_11, © Springer Science+Business Media New York 2013

Table 11.1 Effects of chronic pain on sexuality

Decreased libido
Alteration in sexual arousal
• Decreased transudation
• Erectile dysfunction
• Subjective lack of pleasure
Orgasmic dysfunction
• Anorgasmia
• Prolonged time to orgasm
• Decreased amplitude of orgasm
Dyspareunia (both men and women)
Avoidance of sexual activity/sexual intimacy

and Johnson's landmark work in 1966 as a fluid process of excitement, arousal, tension release, and reflection that is unique to each person.

Patients may have their own "typical" response pattern, but factors such as chronic pain may play a large role in altering that pattern with frequent patient complaints of decreased arousal, painful sexual activity, decreased libido, lowered self-confidence, and less frequent sexual encounters (Table 11.1) [4–6]. Diseases or syndromes intertwined with chronic pain that have a known effect on sexual function include fibromyalgia, ankylosing spondylitis, rheumatoid arthritis, osteoarthritis, depression, back pain, interstitial cystitis, and chronic prostatitis [7–14]. Ambler et al. surveyed 300 men with chronic back pain of whom 73 % reported some form of sexual difficulty [4]. Sexual dysfunction has been reported in 50–78 % of chronic pain patients [4–6, 15] with complete cessation of sexual activity identified in up to 40 % [5, 16, 17].

Sexual dysfunction can also have implications for the patient's partner including a decline in sexual activity and reduced relationship satisfaction [5, 16]. Desrosiers et al. surveyed 43 couples in which the woman suffered from vulvodynia. Frequency of intercourse per month, relationship characteristics, and psychosexual functioning of the couple were evaluated. The frequency of sexual intercourse reported by vulvodynia patients was found to be significantly lower than that of an age-matched cohort (4.52 times/month, 7.5 times/month, $P<0.01$, respectively) [18]. Martua et al. interviewed 66 chronic pain patients and their spouses independently to examine marital and sexual adjustment. They reported decreased frequency and quality of sexual activity in approximately two-thirds of the respondents; 68 % reported orgasmic dysfunction, and 58 % reported lack of interest or decreased libido [19].

The spouse's perception of the patient's disability often results in marital dissatisfaction and affective stress [20]. Fitchen et al. reported that male partners of women with orgasmic dysfunction were more likely to blame themselves for their partners' difficulty or inability to achieve orgasm which elicited stress in the relationship as indicated through questionnaires [21]. The frequent lack of physical findings in the setting of chronic pain may result in the partner's questioning the presence and severity of pain. Over time, many partners begin to believe that the patient does not have a physical problem, but rather is creating pain due to disinterest or lack of attraction. Jodoin et al. theorized that this is a salient factor promoting increased stress and can ultimately cause relational distress [22].

Indirect, but often profound, influences of pain upon sexual function include a negative self-image due to fatigue, pain, disfigurement, medication side effects, and dependency [23]. Partners also have a great influence in the modulation of pain, especially a man's intercourse-specific behavioral reactions [16, 18, 24–26]. Chronic pain patients report higher rates of depression, disability, and pain when their partners respond negatively or with hostility, solicitously, and/or they respond by trying to distract the patients from focusing on their pain [27–29].

With reference to vulvodynia, Desrosiers et al. postulated that solicitous reactions from the male partner could reinforce catastrophizing behaviors [18, 29–31]. Partner hostility, and their negative responses to the patient's pain, can increase depression and anxiety and impact pain and sexual functioning in women with chronic conditions such as BPS, pelvic floor dysfunction, vulvodynia, IBS, and endometriosis [9, 18, 31].

Bladder Pain Syndrome and Sexual Dysfunction

When compared with sexually active women without BPS, women with BPS who were sexually active were more likely to have alterations in sexual functioning domains including arousal, lubrication, desire, satisfaction, orgasm, and pain as evaluated on the Female Sexual Function Index (FSFI) [12]. Azevedo et al. conducted an ethno study that consisted of structured interviews of men and women diagnosed with BPS ($n=11$ and $n=38$, respectively). Narrative data were qualitatively analyzed and five domains relating to sexual dysfunction and BPS were identified: consequences of illness, kinds of loss, kinds of pain, steps in dealing with illness, and ways to feel. They concluded that the persistent pain associated with BPS impacts both the physical and emotional aspects of sexual intercourse [32]. Nickel et al. evaluated QOL and sexual functioning in women with BPS ($n=128$) for 32 weeks during treatment of pentosan polysulfate sodium (PPS). They reported significant improvement in symptom and sexual functioning scores: the mean change in sexual functioning score from baseline to week 32 was −2.97 ($P<0.00001$). Patients treated with PPS demonstrated an improved QOL, which positively correlated with improved sexual functioning [33]. This suggested that in patients with severe BPS, reduction of symptoms is associated with positive patient-reported outcomes, and sexual functioning is an important predictor of physical QOL in patients with and the only strong predictor of mental QOL [1, 33]. Contrary to previous findings, Tripp et al. found that sexual function was not a significant predictor of poorer physical or mental QOL in BPS patients [34].

Dyspareunia may be derived from BPS or common comorbid conditions such as endometriosis, irritable bowel syndrome, pelvic floor myalgia, or vulvodynia [11, 35]. Up to 87 % of women with chronic bladder conditions report dyspareunia [36]. In a survey of 565 women with BPS, more women reported pain localized to the

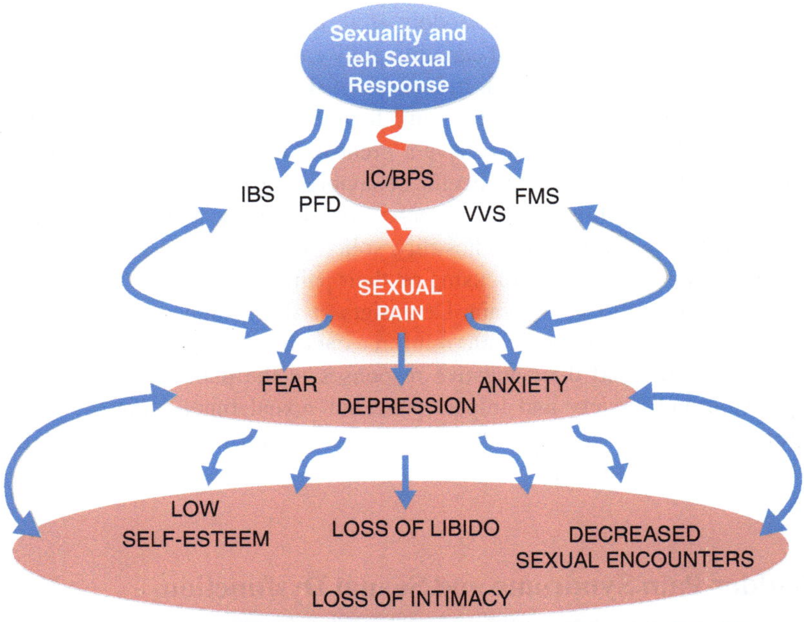

[redacted]

Fig. 11.1 The trickle down and cycling effects of chronic pain upon sexuality in IC/BPS. *IBS* irritable bowel syndrome, *PFD* pelvic floor dysfunction, *VVS* vulvodynia, *FMS* fibromyalgia

vaginal area than to either the lower abdominal or suprapubic areas (60.8 vs. 56.7 and 53.2 %, respectively) [37]. Gardella et al. compared women with BPS ($n=47$) to those without ($n=47$) for characteristics of vulvodynia. The prevalence of vulvodynia was 85.1 % in patients with BPS compared to 6.4 % in those without the disease ($p<0.0001$). Dyspareunia was described as "unbearable" in 31.9 % of the BPS group (15 of 47) and 4.3 % of the control group (2 of 47; $p=0.001$). Median total scores of the FSFI demonstrated significant sexual function impairment in women with BPS (13.8) compared to controls (28.7; $p<0.0001$) [35].

Sexual pain experienced with BPS may be exacerbated by psychological factors such as fear, anxiety, and depression [11, 38]. 54 % of BPS patients report avoidance of sexual intimacy due to pain resulting in negative outcomes for both the patient and her partner [39]. The result is often decreased sexual interest, feelings of inadequacy, isolation, and depression (Fig. 11.1).

Ginting et al. examined the impact of spousal response to BPS patient pain. Contrary to previous findings in the chronic pain literature, they concluded that in patients with BPS, distracting spousal responses from their pain may diminish psychological distress by preventing rumination [40].

Most of our understanding regarding sexual dysfunction in the male BPS patient originates from the clinically similar chronic prostatitis/chronic pelvic pain patient population [41]. The location of pain in the CP/CPPS patient is commonly described as perineal, testicular, or penile; and may radiate to other areas of the pelvis, lower abdomen, upper legs, and lower back [13]. A common feature of CP/CPPS is painful ejaculation. A prospective, longitudinal study sponsored by the NIDDK showed that close to 50 % of men with CP/CPPS reported intermittent ejaculatory pain, 24 % reported pain with every ejaculation, and 26 % reported no pain or post-ejaculatory pain ($n=486$) [42]. Fifty men with CP/CPPS were compared to a control group of 75 men comprising 25 with BPH and 50 with sexual dysfunction. Ejaculatory pain was more prevalent in men with chronic prostatitis than in men with BPH or sexual dysfunction ($P=0.07$ and $P<0.01$, respectively) [43, 44]. The effects of CP/CPPS on sexual function were evaluated through the use of the Pelvic Pain Symptom Survey (PPSS), an instrument with varied questions relating to sexual function. They found that 56 % of men (81/146) with refractory CP/CPPS had pain with ejaculation [45]. Forrest et al. reported that in men diagnosed with BPS ($n=92$), sexual dysfunction occurred in 60 % with the most common complaint being painful ejaculation [46].

There is a vast discrepancy in the reported prevalence of erectile dysfunction (ED) in men with CP/CPPS and BPS, ranging from 0.6 [47] to 48.3 % [14]. Factors that contribute to this variance may be poor research methods including lack of longitudinal studies, poor sampling methods, and the absence of detailed sexuality questions on the Chronic Prostatitis Symptom Index (CPSI) [13]. Decreasing male sexual function has been associated with increasing age; however, in the CP/CPPS population, ED may affect men indiscriminately [45, 48]. In general population surveys, ED is reported in approximately 1–3 % of men 40–54 years of age and 25 % of men 50–78 years of age [49, 50]. Comparatively, Anderson et al. report that of 146 men with a confirmed diagnosis of CP/CPPS, with a mean age of 42 years, 48 % report difficulty achieving erection ($n=70$) and 44 % difficulty maintaining erection ($n=64$) [45]. Only 10 % of the men were over the age of 60. Sexual dysfunction was highly prevalent among the CP/CPPS cohort. 92 % of the men reported one or more symptoms. In the absence of CP/CPPS, the authors concluded that the occurrence of sexual dysfunction in men in the early to mid fifth decade of life would be highly unexpected [45]. Davis et al. suggested ED in these patients, who are in their 30s and 40s, can have greater negative psychosocial effects due to the fact that these men are more likely to be in new relationships or in the process of forming them [13]. Self-reported prevalence of sexual dysfunction in men with CP/CPPS ($n=296$) was found to be 72 % ($n=214$). Men who reported both ED and ejaculatory difficulty reported worse CP/CPPS symptoms ($P=0.042$) and worse QOL ($P=0.006$) [14].

Psychological Effects of BPS on Sexual Function

Coping with chronic pain is life-long for some patients with BPS. They must continually assess stress, their cognitive, behavioral, and emotional responses, and subsequent reassessment of the situation [51]. Patients in chronic pain tend to cope in one of two ways, either through active or passive coping. Active coping is associated with less pain, depression, functional impairment, and a greater self-efficacy [51]. Active coping includes skills such as problem solving, collecting information and refocusing on the problem, and regulation of emotions. Conversely, maladaptive coping, such as avoidance and escape, results in greater depression, pain, episodes of disease "flare-ups," functional impairment, and lower self-efficacy [51].

Pain can disrupt the sexual response cycle. Patients who suffer from recurrent pain with sexual activity begin to associate pain with the activity. This anticipation of pain many times leads to decreased libido and arousal. The resultant lack of lubrication may then increase the pain further, making the experience overall unsatisfying and painful, perpetuating avoidance behavior. This can lead to a cycle of negative self-image, anxiety, loss of self-esteem, grief, and depression. In chronic pain syndromes, partner verbal and nonverbal reactions to the patient's pain response have been identified as pain intensity predictors [16, 24, 26].

Multidisciplinary therapy with referral to a certified sex therapist is often needed for BPS patients. Breton et al. evaluated 47 women with chronic pain with four 2-h cognitive behavioral therapy (CBT) sessions aimed at improving sexual function. They reported improved sexual function between pre-group and post-group scores on the Sexual Activity Questionnaire ($P < 0.05$) [52]. CBT has been shown to be efficacious in decreasing pain severity and affective distress and improving sexual function and self-efficacy in other chronic pain syndromes such as vulvodynia, chronic prostatitis, low back pain, rheumatoid arthritis, and fibromyalgia [53–55].

Managing BPS and Sexual Function

The symptoms of BPS and comorbid conditions must be controlled before any noteworthy improvement in sexual dysfunction can occur. An accurate and detailed history and physical examination are therefore of great importance to achieve an accurate assessment and treatment strategy. Q-tip testing for pain, identification of pelvic floor muscle tenderness, intravesical anesthetics, voiding diaries, and correlation of food, stress, or sexual activity triggers are various methods used to distinguish pain generators.

Initial treatment often includes behavior modification and dietary changes. Pharmacological treatment may include agents that improve pain and other urinary symptoms. While these medications can be efficacious in treating urinary and pain symptoms, they may have untoward effects on sexual function including decreased libido and arousal, erectile dysfunction, as well as orgasmic dysfunction (Table 11.2) [1, 23].

Although sexual dysfunction in the BPS population is common, assessment is often neglected. Zelman et al. conducted a survey of 281 pain clinicians to determine their awareness of sexual concerns among patients with pain, whether they typically ask the patient about their sexual problems, and their intervention strategies [15].

Table 11.2 Commonly used medications for BPS and sexual side effects

Drug class	Examples of medications	Possible sexual side effects
Anticholinergics	Oxybutynin, tolterodine, trospium, solifenacin, hyoscyamine	Vaginal dryness, fatigue, dry mouth, halitosis
Alpha-blockers	Tamsulosin, silodosin, alfuzosin, dutasteride	Retrograde ejaculation, ED, decreased libido, gynecomastia* (*found with the use of dutasteride)
SNRIs	Duloxetine, venlafaxine, desvenlafaxine, milnacipran	Weight changes, fatigue/somnolence, decreased libido, hyperhidrosis, nausea, headache, prolonged time to orgasm*, anorgasmia*, ED*, decreased libido* (*found to effect only men using duloxetine)
SSRIs	Escitalopram, fluoxetine, paroxetine, citalopram, sertraline	Decreased libido, prolonged latency to orgasm, anorgasmia, genital anesthesia, weight changes, ED, hyperhidrosis, nausea, fatigue/somnolence
Tricyclic antidepressants	Amitriptyline, nortriptyline, imipramine, doxepin	Fatigue, nausea, weight gain, decreased libido, prolonged latency to orgasm, anorgasmia, vaginal dryness, hyperhidrosis, (women: breast enlargement, galactorrhea; men: testicular swelling, gynecomastia)* (*with amitriptyline)
Antihistamines	Hydroxyzine	Fatigue, vaginal dryness
Neuroleptics	Gabapentin, pregabalin, topiramate	Fatigue, weight gain*, decreased libido, emotional labiality, hostility, thought disorder (*with gabapentin and pregabalin; weight loss/anorexia is associated with topiramate)
Skeletal muscle relaxants	Cyclobenzaprine, carisoprodol, metaxalone, tizanidine, diazepam	Fatigue, decreased libido, GI upset
Benzodiazepines	Diazepam, alprazolam	Fatigue, impaired coordination/attention, decreased libido, prolonged latency to orgasm, anorgasmia, vaginal dryness
Narcotics	Oxycodone, hydrocodone, morphine, hydromorphone, meperidine, fentanyl	Fatigue, headache, GI upset, mood changes, decreased libido, ED, vaginal dryness, prolonged latency to orgasm, anorgasmia
DMSO		Associated halitosis

The following medications are frequently used in the management of BPS and its associated comorbid conditions. While they may improve sexual function and QOL through management of the primary pain syndrome [33], the side effects of these medications that adversely impact patients' sexual functioning may outweigh the benefits. Physiological side effects of the medications listed below are not limited to the DSM-categories of sexual dysfunction. Included in this list are side effects that may impact patients' psychosexual response to the medication. For example, if weight gain is a side effect of a medication, it may have a negative effect on a patient's self-esteem subsequently altering his or her psychosexual response. Nausea and headache may cause decreased libido and/or arousal in some patients

Only 30 % of those surveyed regularly inquire about sexual function, 50 % believed sexual dysfunction was rare in the chronic pain population, and referrals to specialists such as sex therapists or urologists were scarce. 53 % of the respondents reported that the main barrier to discussing sexual function with patients was concern over embarrassment or offense to the patient [15].

Communication

Communication is fundamental to a healthy sexual relationship. Women in chronic pain reported that through communication with their partners about their sexual relationship, they went from feeling isolated and stigmatized to feeling connected and empowered [52]. BPS patients must communicate openly and honestly not only with their partners but also with their clinician. Discussing which activity or positions are painful, bringing the partner to an office visit, seeing a certified sex therapist, or going to support groups are all ways to enhance communication.

Self-Care

Self-care measures can help patients maintain sexual intimacy, thereby giving them a sense of control over their chronic illness [11]. If patients experience penetrative dyspareunia, they and their partners can explore alternatives such as "outercourse" and oral, anal, or manual sex play. They can also experiment with different positions for comfort, such as side-lying aka "spooning" or reverse missionary aka "woman-on-top," limit thrusting time or change thrusting motion to a "circular motion," use of a hypoallergenic lubricant to reduce urethral and vaginal irritation [56], and pre- and postcoital voiding to help alleviate bladder pressure during thrusting and orgasm [39]. Some BPS patients find it helpful to premedicate prior to sexual activity with analgesics, muscle relaxants, anticholinergenics, topical anesthetics, or intravaginal/intrarectal muscle relaxants. After intercourse, patients can use ice or topical anesthetics to ease pain and burning.

Changes in Sexual Scripts

Often, patients with BPS need to change their sexual scripts to maintain intimacy and sexual functioning in their relationship. What used to be arousing and satisfying for the couple may now be a source of pain. Patients and their partners need to explore new ways to become intimate, which at times may exclude penetrative intercourse altogether. Couples should be encouraged to negotiate sexual script changes prior to engaging in sexual activity. The bedroom is not the place for these discussions.

Couples oftentimes need to go "back to the basics" and reinstitute flirting, sex-texting (sexual flirting via text messaging), and touch into their repertoire. The focus should be on the experience, the intimacy, and the arousal. Orgasm is not the goal. The couple should discuss what was pleasurable and what was painful, what they liked and what they did not like. Keeping the lines of communication open will help facilitate a healthy relationship, promote intimacy, and foster positive sexual function.

Conclusion

Sexual dysfunction is common and often devastating to the QOL of the BPS patient. Pain associated with BPS and comorbid conditions appears to be the central underpinning of dysfunction Multifaceted secondary occurrences such as sexual fear, depression, loss of intimacy, and even the adverse effects of "therapeutic" medications may perpetuate or escalate the problem. Therapy lies in treating the patient on multiple fronts, with an emphasis on communication between the patient and his or her partner.

References

1. Nickel JC, Tripp D, Teal V, et al. Sexual function is a determinant of poor quality of life for women with treatment refractory interstitial cystitis. J Urol. 2007;177(5):1832–6.
2. Driscoll A, Teichman JM. How do patients with interstitial cystitis present? J Urol. 2001;166(6):2118–20.
3. Teichman JM, Parsons CL. Contemporary clinical presentation of interstitial cystitis. Urology. 2007;69(4 Suppl):41–7.
4. Ambler N, Williams AC, Hill P, Gunary R, Cratchley G. Sexual difficulties of chronic pain patients. Clin J Pain. 2001;17(2):138–45.
5. Maruta T, Osborne D, Swanson DW, Halling JM. Chronic pain patients and spouses: marital and sexual adjustment. Mayo Clin Proc. 1981;56(5):307–10.
6. Schlesinger L. Chronic pain, intimacy and sexuality: A qualitative study of women who live with pain. J Sex Res. 1996;33:249–56.
7. Tristano AG. The impact of rheumatic diseases on sexual function. Rheumatol Int. 2009;29(8):853–60.
8. Kalichman L. Association between fibromyalgia and sexual dysfunction in women. Clin Rheumatol. 2009;28(4):365–9.
9. Rosenbaum TY. Musculoskeletal pain and sexual function in women. J Sex Med. 2010;7(2 Pt 1):645–53.
10. Clayton A, Ramamurthy S. The impact of physical illness on sexual dysfunction. Adv Psychosom Med. 2008;29:70–88.
11. Whitmore K, Siegel JF, Kellogg-Spadt S. Interstitial cystitis/painful bladder syndrome as a cause of sexual pain in women: a diagnosis to consider. J Sex Med. 2007;4(3):720–7.
12. Ottem DP, Carr LK, Perks AE, Lee P, Teichman JM. Interstitial cystitis and female sexual dysfunction. Urology. 2007;69(4):608–10.

13. Davis SN, Binik YM, Carrier S. Sexual dysfunction and pelvic pain in men: a male sexual pain disorder? J Sex Marital Ther. 2009;35(3):182–205.
14. Lee SW, Liong ML, Yuen KH, et al. Adverse impact of sexual dysfunction in chronic prostatitis/chronic pelvic pain syndrome. Urology. 2008;71(1):79–84.
15. Zelman D, R J, Diller J. Addressing sexual impairment in chronic pain. Pain Medicine News. 2006;4:1–4.
16. Flor H, Turk D, Scholz OB. Impact of chronic pain on the spouse: Marital, emotional and physical consequences. J Psychosom Res. 1987;31:63–71.
17. Monga TN, T G, Ostermann HJ, et al. Sexuality and sexual adjustment of patients with chronic pain. Disabil Rehabil. 1998;20:317–29.
18. Desrosiers M, Bergeron S, Meana M, Leclerc B, Binik YM, Khalife S. Psychosexual characteristics of vestibulodynia couples: partner solicitousness and hostility are associated with pain. J Sex Med. 2008;5(2):418–27.
19. Maruta T, Osborne D. Sexual activity in chronic pain patients. Psychosomatics. 1978;19(9):531–7.
20. Geisser ME, Cano A, Leonard MT. Factors associated with marital satisfaction and mood among spouses of persons with chronic back pain. J Pain. 2005;6(8):518–25.
21. Fichten CS, Spector I, Libman E. Client attributions for sexual dysfunction. J Sex Marital Ther. 1988;14(3):208–24.
22. Jodoin M, Bergeron S, Khalife S, Dupuis MJ, Desrochers G, Leclerc B. Male partners of women with provoked vestibulodynia: attributions for pain and their implications for dyadic adjustment, sexual satisfaction, and psychological distress. J Sex Med. 2008;5(12):2862–70.
23. Basson R, Schultz WW. Sexual sequelae of general medical disorders. Lancet. 2007;369(9559):409–24.
24. Kerns RD, Haythornthwaite J, Southwick S, Giller Jr EL. The role of marital interaction in chronic pain and depressive symptom severity. J Psychosom Res. 1990;34(4):401–8.
25. Lousberg R, Schmidt AJ, Groenman NH. The relationship between spouse solicitousness and pain behavior: searching for more experimental evidence. Pain. 1992;51(1):75–9.
26. Boothby JL, Thorn BE, Overduin LY, Ward LC. Catastrophizing and perceived partner responses to pain. Pain. 2004;109(3):500–6.
27. Cano A, Gillis M, Heinz W, Geisser M, Foran H. Marital functioning, chronic pain, and psychological distress. Pain. 2004;107(1–2):99–106.
28. Cano A, Johansen AB, Franz A. Multilevel analysis of couple congruence on pain, interference, and disability. Pain. 2005;118(3):369–79.
29. Cano A, Weisberg JN, Gallagher RM. Marital satisfaction and pain severity mediate the association between negative spouse responses to pain and depressive symptoms in a chronic pain patient sample. Pain Med. 2000;1(1):35–43.
30. Schwartz L, Slater MA, Birchler GR. The role of pain behaviors in the modulation of marital conflict in chronic pain couples. Pain. 1996;65(2-3):227–33.
31. Payne KA, Binik YM, Amsel R, Khalife S. When sex hurts, anxiety and fear orient attention towards pain. Eur J Pain. 2005;9(4):427–36.
32. Azevedo K, Nguyen A, Rowhani-Rahbar A, et al. Pain impacts sexual functioning among interstitial cystitis patients. Sexuality and Disability. 2005;23(4):189–208.
33. Nickel JC, Parsons CL, Forrest J, et al. Improvement in sexual functioning in patients with interstitial cystitis/painful bladder syndrome. J Sex Med. 2008;5(2):394–9.
34. Tripp DA, Nickel JC, Fitzgerald MP, Mayer R, Stechyson N, Hsieh A. Sexual functioning, catastrophizing, depression, and pain, as predictors of quality of life in women with interstitial cystitis/painful bladder syndrome. Urology. 2009;73(5):987–92.
35. Gardella B, Porru D, Ferdeghini F, et al. Insight into urogynecologic features of women with interstitial cystitis/painful bladder syndrome. Eur Urol. 2008;54(5):1145–51.
36. Nickel JC. Interstitial cystitis: the paradigm shifts: international consultations on interstitial cystitis. Rev Urol. 2004;6(4):200–2.
37. Koziol JA. Epidemiology of interstitial cystitis. Urol Clin North Am. 1994;21(1):7–20.

38. Binik YM. Should dyspareunia be retained as a sexual dysfunction in DSM-V? A painful classification decision. Arch Sex Behav. 2005;34(1):11–21.
39. Webster DC, Brennan T. Use and effectiveness of sexual self-care strategies for interstitial cystitis. Urol Nurs. 1995;15(1):14–22.
40. Ginting JV, Tripp DA, Nickel JC, Fitzgerald MP, Mayer R. Spousal support decreases the negative impact of pain on mental quality of life in women with interstitial cystitis/painful bladder syndrome. BJU Int. 2010;108(5):713–7.
41. Eisenberg ER, Moldwin RM. Etiology: where does prostatitis stop and interstitial cystitis begin? World J Urol. 2003;21(2):64–9.
42. Shoskes DA, Landis JR, Wang Y, Nickel JC, Zeitlin SI, Nadler R. Impact of post-ejaculatory pain in men with category III chronic prostatitis/chronic pelvic pain syndrome. J Urol. 2004;172(2):542–7.
43. Krieger JN, Egan KJ, Ross SO, Jacobs R, Berger RE. Chronic pelvic pains represent the most prominent urogenital symptoms of "chronic prostatitis". Urology. 1996;48(5):715–21. discussion 721-712.
44. Lee SW, Cheah PY, Liong ML, et al. Demographic and clinical characteristics of chronic prostatitis: prospective comparison of the University of Sciences Malaysia Cohort with the United States National Institutes of Health Cohort. J Urol. 2007;177(1):153–7. discussion 158.
45. Anderson RU, Wise D, Sawyer T, Chan CA. Sexual dysfunction in men with chronic prostatitis/chronic pelvic pain syndrome: improvement after trigger point release and paradoxical relaxation training. J Urol. 2006;176(4 Pt 1):1534–8. discussion 1538–1539.
46. Forrest JB, Schmidt S. Interstitial cystitis, chronic nonbacterial prostatitis and chronic pelvic pain syndrome in men: a common and frequently identical clinical entity. J Urol. 2004;172(6 Pt 2):2561–2.
47. Collins MM, Stafford RS, O'Leary MP, Barry MJ. Distinguishing chronic prostatitis and benign prostatic hyperplasia symptoms: results of a national survey of physician visits. Urology. 1999;53(5):921–5.
48. Lutz MC, Roberts RO, Jacobson DJ, McGree ME, Lieber MM, Jacobsen SJ. Cross-sectional associations of urogenital pain and sexual function in a community based cohort of older men: Olmsted county, Minnesota. J Urol. 2005;174(2):624–8. discussion 628.
49. Blanker MH, Bosch JL, Groeneveld FP, et al. Erectile and ejaculatory dysfunction in a community-based sample of men 50 to 78 years old: prevalence, concern, and relation to sexual activity. Urology. 2001;57(4):763–8.
50. Panser LA, Rhodes T, Girman CJ, et al. Sexual function of men ages 40 to 79 years: the Olmsted County Study of urinary symptoms and health status among men. J Am Geriatr Soc. 1995;43(10):1107–11.
51. Bussing A, Ostermann T, Neugebauer EA, Heusser P. Adaptive coping strategies in patients with chronic pain conditions and their interpretation of disease. BMC Public Health. 2010;10:507.
52. Breton A, Miller CM, Fisher K. Enhancing the sexual function of women living with chronic pain: a cognitive-behavioural treatment group. Pain Res Manag. 2008;13(3):219–24.
53. Masheb RM, Kerns RD, Lozano C, Minkin MJ, Richman S. A randomized clinical trial for women with vulvodynia: cognitive-behavioral therapy vs. supportive psychotherapy. Pain. 2009;141(1-2):31–40.
54. McCracken LM, Turk DC. Behavioral and cognitive-behavioral treatment for chronic pain: outcome, predictors of outcome, and treatment process. Spine (Phila Pa 1976). 2002;27(22):2564–73.
55. Morley S, Eccleston C, Williams A. Systematic review and meta-analysis of randomized controlled trials of cognitive behaviour therapy and behaviour therapy for chronic pain in adults, excluding headache. Pain. 1999;80(1–2):1–13.
56. Kellogg-Spadt S, Albaugh JA. Intimacy and bladder pain: helping women reclaim sexuality. Urol Nurs. 2002;22(5):355–6.

Part III
Diagnosis

Chapter 12
Symptoms of Bladder Pain Syndrome

John W. Warren and Philip M. Hanno

Introduction

The cardinal symptoms of bladder pain syndrome (BPS) are four: pain perceived to be from the bladder, urinary urgency and frequency, and nocturia [1]. Over 200 BPS patients were asked which of these symptoms were "the worst part of IC": 87% said pain, 44% frequency, 43% urgency, and 34% nocturia (obviously, some said more than one was the "worst") (J.W. Warren, unpublished data).

This chapter discusses each of these four, briefly comments upon other symptoms experienced by BPS patients, critically reviews symptom questionnaires often used to diagnose BPS, and concludes with a discussion of the possible role of symptoms in helping to reveal the pathogenesis of BPS.

Pain

Several investigators have elicited detailed descriptions of the pain of BPS [2–4]. "Pain, pressure, or discomfort" appears to be appropriate phraseology to ask about this pain: 95% of female BPS patients endorsed this language as a good way to describe their sensations [4].

Some studies have used drawings of the anterior, posterior, and perineal views of the body upon which the patient shades in sites of pain. In one such study [4], 2/3 of

J.W. Warren, M.D. (✉)
Medicine and Epidemiology and Public Health, University of Maryland School of Medicine, 10 South Pine Street, Baltimore, MD 21201, USA
e-mail: Jwarren@medicine.umaryland.edu

P.M. Hanno, M.D., M.P.H.
Division of Urology, Department of Surgery, Hospital of the University of Pennsylvania, Philadelphia, PA, USA
e-mail: hannop@uphs.upenn.edu

J. Nordling et al. (eds.), *Bladder Pain Syndrome: A Guide for Clinicians*, DOI 10.1007/978-1-4419-6929-3_12, © Springer Science+Business Media New York 2013

226 BPS patients reported multiple pain sites. Adjectives from the McGill Pain Index [5] commonly used to describe all sites were "aching," "pressing," "throbbing," "tender," and "piercing." Almost all shaded areas could be consolidated into four sites: 83% of patients noted suprapubic pain, 36% urethral pain, 23% genital, and 29% reported non-genitourinary sites (mostly low back but also anterior thighs, buttocks, and posterior thighs). The pattern of suprapubic > urethral > genital > non-genitourinary also corresponded to the proportions of pain at each of these sites that changed with the urinary cycle. For instance, 76% of suprapubic pains worsened with bladder filling compared to 58% of urethral pains, 43% of genital pains, and 32% of non-genitourinary pains [4].

Other activities that were associated with change of BPS pains are noted in [4]. Of substantial interest is that 85% of BPS patients claimed that certain food or drink worsened their symptoms. This phenomenon has long been a known part of BPS and recently has been studied in detail by Shorter et al. [6]. They reported that 92/102 (90%) BPS cases noted that at least one food or drink worsened their BPS symptoms. Of 175 comestibles queried, 35 substantially worsened symptoms; prominent among them were coffee, tea, sodas, alcoholic beverages, some fruits and fruit juices, tomatoes, hot peppers, spicy foods, and certain artificial sweeteners. The authors concluded that BPS patients should experiment with avoiding capsaicin, citrus fruits, caffeine, and alcoholic and carbonated drinks. Interestingly, 75% of BPS cases also noted that large meals worsened their BPS symptoms.

Pain perceived to be from the bladder has become the sole necessary criterion of BPS [7–9]. Recently investigators asked patients why they perceived the pain of BPS to be from the bladder and recorded their responses [10]. Of 179 cases, 41% noted the location of pain; 34% pain increasing with bladder filling and/or decreasing with bladder emptying; 31% claimed the association of urgency and/or frequency; 23% described pain worsening during and/or after urination; and 17% mentioned the concurrence of other urinary symptoms. We note that these were verbatim answers to a specific question and that patients could have experienced other sensations [4] but not reported them in answer to this particular query.

In a discussion of BPS pain, a special mention should be made of urethral or genital pain sites. In addition to the McGill Pain Index adjectives above, urethral and genital pain sites were more likely than other sites to be described as "burning," "stinging," and "sharp" [4]. Moreover, urethral pain worsened with voiding, and genital pain worsened with touch, tampon insertion, and vaginal intercourse. Patients with such pains might be diagnosed with chronic urethral syndrome and vulvodynia, respectively. However, BPS cases with urethral or genital sites of pain did not differ from those without such sites in numerous patient characteristics [4, 11]. Peters et al. similarly noted that of 70 BPS patients, those with and without vulvar tenderness did not differ in important patient variables [11]. This type of comparison, known as identity of patient characteristics, has been used in other explorations to distinguish or consolidate diseases [12–14]. These data suggest that when urethral or genital pain is present in BPS patients, it usually is part of BPS and not a separate disease.

In the general population, the proportion of chronic urethral syndrome and vulvodynia patients who actually have BPS is unknown. However, we find it interesting that many patients who have been diagnosed with "chronic urethral syndrome" have frequency, urgency, and suprapubic pain [15] and that large minorities of vulvodynia patients have urgency and frequency [16]. A reasonable hypothesis would be that many such patients actually have BPS.

Urgency

The Standardization Subcommittee of the International Continence Society in 2002 defined urgency as "a sudden compelling desire to pass urine, which is difficult to defer" [17]. Three years later two of the experts in this group were among the authors of an opinion piece suggesting that this description applied more to overactive bladder (OAB) than to BPS [18].

Two studies have used questions to explore the nature of urgency in BPS. Greenberg et al. found that 65% of BPS patients reported that the urge to void was to relieve pain and 21% to prevent incontinence [19]. Clemens et al. compared BPS to OAB patients [20]. Among BPS patients, they found results similar to Greenberg et al.: 87% reported that the urge to urinate was "mainly because of pain, pressure, or discomfort" and 11% to avoid incontinence. Interestingly, they found that 42% of the OAB patients reported that their urgency was "because of pain, pressure, or discomfort" and only 49% that it was because of fear of incontinence. About 60% of each of the BPS and OAB groups reported that urgency started "suddenly," as opposed to over minutes or hours.

The definition and characterization of urgency are controversial at this point. Although many BPS patients complain of urgency, it is not a requirement for diagnosis of BPS.

We believe that the substantial overlap in descriptions of urgency by BPS and OAB patients precludes the use of urgency by itself to discriminate between these two syndromes.

Frequency

Reaching consensus on the definition of abnormal urinary frequency has been deceptively difficult. Increased daytime frequency has been defined by the International Continence Society as "the complaint by the patient who considers that he/she voids too often by day" [17]. However, large variation in the bother of urinary frequency [21] makes this approach subject to question.

Data suggest that urinary frequency in women can be defined as regularly having to void at intervals of less than 3 h [22, 23]. Based on a ninetieth percentile cutoff to determine the ranges of normality, in the fourth decade of life, for instance, "normal" frequency is up to six times for men and nine times for women [24]. But frequency is obviously dependent upon fluid ingestion and the number of voids per volume of intake may be more accurate than an absolute number.

However abnormal frequency is defined, many patients with BPS have it. The Interstitial Cystitis Data Base used 3-day voiding logs and reported this distribution of urinary frequency: <10 times/day, 33%, 11–14 times/day, 28%; and ≥15 times/day, 40% of BPS patients [3]. Anecdotal information indicates that some BPS patients have ≥50 urinations per day, an experience that much limits their activities. The reason for the urinary frequency of BPS is considered but not proven to be a result of the abnormal urge to void.

Nocturia

The International Continence Society first defined nocturia in 2002: "The number of voids recorded during a night's sleep: each void is preceded and followed by sleep" [25]. Of women older than 40 years, 25% have nocturia at least once [22, 23]. Because nocturia once a night is common and additionally is associated with minimal bother or change in quality of life [26], many investigators have considered clinically important nocturia to be two or more episodes/night.

Although it is one of the four main symptoms of BPS, nocturia in such patients has rarely been investigated. A recent study simply asked BPS patients which of these reasons caused them to awaken at night: urgency, pain, noise, or shortness of breath [27]. Of 257 BPS cases, 194 (76%) agreed with urgency, 110 (43%) with pain, 88 (34%) with noise, and 9 (4%) with shortness of breath. An examination of the interaction of urgency and pain revealed that the largest group, 39% of the total, reported both urgency and pain as reasons for awakening. A group of comparable size, 37%, reported urgency but not pain. Four percent reported that pain without urgency was the reason. Fifty three cases (21%) did not report either urgency or pain as reasons for awakening. Considering these data with those exploring urgency above, they suggest that pain may play a twofold role in the nocturia of IC/PBS: directly in awakening the patient and indirectly in generating the sensation of urgency.

The 21% of BPS cases who did not agree with either urgency or pain as reasons for awakening at night may constitute an interesting group. They were more likely than the other groups to be awakened by noise and had the fewest nocturnal urinations. These cases may wake up and urinate as opposed to wake up to urinate [25, 28].

Other Symptoms

Other genitourinary symptoms have been reported by BPS patients [2, 29] but comparisons to adequate controls generally have been lacking. These symptoms include difficulty starting urine flow (reported by 47% of BPS patients), burning with voiding (42%), difficulty emptying the bladder (51%), retention of urine (42%), and blood in the urine (22%). Some of these may constitute symptoms of pelvic floor dysfunction. Sensations perceived to be bladder spasms have been reported by 61% of PBS patients. Additionally, dyspareunia in the form of pain during intercourse was reported by 55% of BPS patients, and as pain for days after intercourse by 37%.

Using Symptoms to Diagnose BPS

Pain perceived to be from the bladder as well as urgency, frequency, and nocturia are symptoms characteristic of BPS. In the absence of signs, laboratory tests, or pathologic abnormalities sensitive and specific for BPS, questionnaires comprising these and other symptoms have been proposed as diagnostic tools for BPS.

There are three published BPS symptom questionnaires: (1) the University of Wisconsin IC Scale, (2) the O'Leary–Sant IC Symptom Index and IC Problem Index, and (3) the Pelvic Pain and Urgency/Frequency (PUF) Scale.

The University of Wisconsin IC Scale includes seven BPS symptoms [30]. It has not been validated for identification or diagnosis of BPS. It captures severity of symptoms [31]. BPS patients do not appear to indiscriminately report higher scores than controls for different somatic and general complaints [32]. Unlike the other two instruments, it addresses some quality-of-life issues, and this is an advantage when such issues are the subject of investigation. Its most attractive aspects are its face validity and its ease of implementation.

The O'Leary–Sant indices [33] comprise a questionnaire that was originally developed with the use of focus groups, subjected to test–retest reliability analysis, and validated by administration to IC patients and asymptomatic controls [33, 34]. Each of the symptom and problem indices has four questions, one on each of the four characteristic symptoms of BPS: bladder-associated pain, urgency, frequency, and nocturia. The questionnaire does not address generalized pelvic pain or symptomatology associated with sexual activity but not because these items were not initially considered. Indeed, the preliminary instrument comprised 73 questions including ones in those domains. However, only the four questions now in each instrument were needed to reliably and validly distinguish BPS patients from asymptomatic controls [35].

Another instrument is the PUF questionnaire (Fig. 12.1) [36]. It includes questions that reflect a variety of symptoms experienced by BPS patients. One-third of the questions address pelvic pain, including pain perceived in the vagina, labia, lower abdomen, urethra, perineum, testes, penis, or scrotum. A large study utilizing the PUF questionnaire has concluded that up to 23% of American females have BPS [36]. A total score of 10–14 = 74% likelihood of a positive potassium test (PST); 15–19 = 76%; and 20+ = 91%. To the extent that the PST is suspect, the reliability of PUF data comes into question. Question No. 4 of the PUF, on sexual activity, is

Patient's Name: ______________________ Today's Date______________

PELVIC PAIN and URGENCY/FREQUENCY
PATIENT SYMPTOM SCALE

Please circle the answer that best describes how you feel for each question.

		0	1	2	3	4	SYMPTOM SCORE	BOTHER SCORE
1	How many times do you go to the bathroom during the day?	3-6	7-10	11-14	15-19	20+		
2	a. How many times do you go to the bathroom at night?	0	1	2	3	4+		
	b. If you get up at night to go to the bathroom, does it bother you?	Never Bothers	Occasionally	Usually	Always			
3	a. Do you now or have you ever had pain or symptoms during or after sexual intercourse?	Never	Occasionally	Usually	Always			
	b. Has pain or urgency ever made you avoid sexual intercourse?	Never	Occasionally	Usually	Always			
4	Do you have pain associated with your bladder or in your pelvis (vagina, labia, lower abdomen, urethra, perineum, testes, or scrotum)?	Never	Occasionally	Usually	Always			
5	a. If you have pain, is it usually		Mild	Moderate	Severe			
	b. Does your pain bother you?	Never	Occasionally	Usually	Always			
6	Do you still have urgency after going to the bathroom?	Never	Occasionally	Usually	Always			
7	a. If you have urgency, is it usually		Mild	Moderate	Severe			
	b. Does your urgency bother you?	Never	Occasionally	Usually	Always			
8	Are you sexually active? Yes No							

SYMPTOM SCORE = (1, 2a, 3a, 4, 5a, 6, 7a)		
BOTHER SCORE = (2b, 3b, 5b, 7b)		
TOTAL SCORE (Symptom Score + Bother Score) =		

Fig. 12.1 Pelvic pain and urgency/frequency patient symptom scale (PUF). From Keller ML, McCarthy DO, Neider RS. Measurement of symptoms of interstitial cystitis. A pilot study. Urol Clin North Am. 1994;21(1):67–71. Reprinted with permission from Elsevier

problematic. Patients with identical BPS pain, urgency, frequency, and nocturia who are sexually active can gain up to six more points than those who are not. Moreover, the latter patients who over time begin sexual activities because they are feeling better would at that time receive a worse PUF score.

None of the questionnaires has been shown to be of value in diagnosis [37], though they may suggest those who should be screened further for the syndrome [38]. The O'Leary–Sant and University of Wisconsin instruments correlated strongly in a large population of patients with BPS [39]. Both the O'Leary–Sant and University of Wisconsin questionnaires are responsive to change over time and thus good for following the natural history of the disorder and the results of treatment.

A one-category change in a global response assessment, a balanced patient self-report on overall response to therapy, correlated with a 1.2 point change in the O'Leary–Sant and a 3.1 point change in the University of Wisconsin instruments [40].

A "Genitourinary Pain Index" adapted from the National Institutes of Health Chronic Prostatitis Symptom Index has recently been published and may prove to be a useful addition to the questionnaire battery used to follow patients in the future [41].

Preliminary work for a RAND prevalence study of BPS revealed a problem that may be generic to symptom-based diagnostic instruments for BPS and indeed may indicate more fundamental issues. These investigators reported difficulty in finding a single symptom-based definition for BPS that had sufficient sensitivity and specificity to separate BPS patients from those with physician-diagnosed OAB, vulvodynia, or endometriosis [42]. The authors noted three possible reasons for the difficulty in disentangling these syndromes: "the true overlap of symptoms across these conditions, and ... the accuracy of measurement and clinical diagnoses of these conditions."

Indeed, symptoms of other syndromes overlap those of BPS. These include not only the pelvic conditions studied by RAND but others such as irritable bowel syndrome (IBS) and even systemic syndromes such as fibromyalgia. To compound this confusion, many of these syndromes with overlapping symptoms are diagnosed in the same patient: vulvodynia, chronic pelvic pain, IBS, and fibromyalgia are epidemiologically associated with BPS [43–45].

And how good is the accuracy of measurement of these conditions? For instance, as noted, the characteristics of urgency of OAB overlap considerably with those of BPS. But it may be possible that other overlapping symptoms might be sufficiently different so as to distinguish between syndromes. Is the pain associated with endometriosis distinctive from that of BPS? What does the patient perceive that convinces her that a particular pain is not her IBS or fibromyalgia but rather "involves" her bladder? In other words, nuances of symptoms might allow discrimination of syndromes. This "splitting" would go against the trend of recent years of "lumping" symptoms [46]. Such work has begun on several of these symptoms [4, 19, 20, 47].

But what if adequate symptom description still were not able to yield accurate clinical diagnoses? A similarity of symptoms, particularly when coupled with the comorbidity of these syndromes, may have nosological implications: If boundaries cannot be identified between syndromes, are they different diseases? Almost 1,500 men and women with urinary symptoms were asked commonly used questions about symptoms thought to be characteristic of each of BPS, OAB, benign prostatic hyperplasia, and chronic prostatitis/chronic pelvic pain syndrome [48]. Two important findings emerged. The distributions of symptoms were similar between men and women. And within individuals, there was an overlap of the symptoms used to classify the different syndromes. These studies again suggest that work should be directed at nuances of pain, urgency, and other symptoms that might distinguish these pelvic syndromes. More importantly, these findings raise a provocative question which the authors of this comparison phrased as a statement: "If symptoms overlap to a large degree, it would imply that the distinction among these various syndromes is rather arbitrary" [48].

Do the Symptoms of BPS Provide Clues to Its Pathogenesis?

To answer this question, a scrutiny of the pain of BPS appears to be critical. Pain defines BPS [7–9] and in most patients drives urgency [19, 20], nocturia [27], and presumably urinary frequency.

Pain worsening with distention of a hollow organ is an important characteristic of visceral pain [49]. Clinical evidence of this phenomenon supports the involvement of bladder sensation in BPS patients. Eighty-four percent of BPS patients claimed that bladder filling worsened their pain; indeed, 94% reported this and/or that urination relieved BPS pain [50]. Additionally, the Interstitial Cystitis Data Base generated important but unpublished data of urodynamic studies during which conscious BPS patients were asked: "Does this feeling or sensation feel like your syndrome?" At the first sensation to void 224/269 (83%) and at maximal cystometric capacity 250/268 (93%) answered yes [50]. These findings imply that the bladder is a viscus involved in BPS [50].

But these observations do not confirm the bladder to be the root cause of BPS. This uncertainty in part comes from the concept of central sensitization [49, 51, 52]. The lower spinal cord receives sensory input from pelvic viscera such as the bladder, uterus, colon, and rectum as well as somatic structures such as the lumbar back, anterior abdominal wall, suprapubic region, anterior thighs, buttocks, and perineum. Convergence of afferent nerves at the same second order spinal neuron means that noxious stimuli from one pelvic organ can result in perception of pain from these other pelvic or somatic sites. And, importantly, the sites of these referred pains can themselves manifest allodynia [49, 51, 52]. Hence, that bladder filling evokes pain in BPS does not in and of itself distinguish between the bladder as the pain generator and the bladder as a referral site of pain that originated from another site.

The fact that some foods and drinks worsen the symptoms of BPS does not necessarily solve this conundrum. At least two hypotheses can be generated. The first is that these foods cause physiologic changes in the bowel that through central sensitization are perceived to be from the bladder. The comorbidity of IBS and BPS makes this an attractive possibility. Another hypothesis is that compounds in certain foods are released in the gut, absorbed into the bloodstream, carried to the kidney, and excreted in the urine, and in some way irritate the bladder of BPS patients. Consistent with this is the finding that denuded bladder epithelium in BPS patients is significantly associated with the pain of BPS [53].

And what is more troublesome in comprehending BPS pathogenesis is that more patients with BPS than controls have symptoms well outside the pelvis. Many such symptoms can be aggregated into syndromes like fibromyalgia, chronic fatigue syndrome, and migraine. These non-pelvic syndromes are not only associated with BPS but also with each other; additionally, many of these syndromes precede the onset of BPS. As described in the chapter, Syndromes associated with Bladder Pain Syndrome as clues to its Pathogenesis, these symptoms distant to the pelvis suggest in some patients that systemic pathophysiologies may be implicated in the pathogenesis of BPS.

Summary

Symptoms are the heralds of disease that prompt a patient to seek medical care. It then is the task of the patient and the clinician to reveal sufficient description of the symptoms so as to make an accurate diagnosis and thus initiate appropriate management of the disease. Hence, it is important to understand what sensory sensations BPS patients are experiencing. Open-ended descriptions followed, as necessary, by specific questions should be helpful. Graphic drawings of anterior, posterior, and perineal views of the human body may assist the patient in identifying sites of pain [4]. Asking whether the pain "gets worse, gets better, or stays the same" before, during, and after urination and other activities offers non-leading options to the patient about features that may improve or exacerbate the pain [4].

Inquiries about the symptoms of BPS may allow the clinician to accurately distinguish BPS cases from normal individuals. But present information indicates difficulty in constructing an instrument with adequate sensitivity and specificity to distinguish BPS from vulvodynia and endometriosis in women, BPH and CP/CPPS in men, and OAB and IBS in both sexes. Whether more detailed descriptions would be more discriminatory is unclear. Also unclear is the etiologic relationship of BPS to these pelvic syndromes and to systemic symptom-based syndromes such as fibromyalgia, chronic fatigue syndrome, and migraine.

References

1. Hanno P, Lin A, Nordling J, Nyberg L, van Ophoven A, Ueda T, et al. Bladder pain syndrome committee of the international consultation on incontinence. Neurourol Urodyn. 2010;29(1):191–8.
2. Koziol JA. Epidemiology of interstitial cystitis. Urological Clinics of North America. 1994;21(1):7–20.
3. Simon LJ, Landis JR, Erickson DR, Nyberg LM, The ICDB Study Group. The interstitial cystitis data base study: concepts and preliminary baseline descriptive statistics. Urology. 1997;49(Suppl 5A):64–75.
4. Warren JW, Langenberg P, Greenberg P, Diggs C, Jacobs S, Wesselmann U. Sites of pain from interstitial cystitis/painful bladder syndrome. J Urol. 2008;180(4):1373–7.
5. Melzack R. The McGill pain questionnaire: major properties and scoring methods. Pain. 1975;1(3):277–99.
6. Shorter B, Lesser M, Moldwin RM, Kushner L. Effect of comestibles on symptoms of interstitial cystitis. J Urol. 2007;178(1):145–52.
7. Abrams P, Andersson KE, Birder L Brubaker L, Cardozo L, Chapple C, et al. Fourth international consultation on incontinence recommendations of the international scientific committee: evaluation and treatment of urinary incontinence, pelvic organ prolapse, and fecal incontinence. Neurourol Urodyn. 2010;29(1):213–40.
8. van de Merwe JP, Nordling J, Bouchelouche P, Bouchelouche K, Cervigni M, Daha LK, et al. Diagnostic criteria, classification, and nomenclature for painful bladder syndrome/interstitial cystitis: an ESSIC proposal. Eur Urol. 2008;53(1):60–7.
9. Hanno et al. Diagnosis and treatment of interstitial cystitis/bladder pain syndrome: AUA guideline. Annual meeting of the American Urological Association; May 2010 San Francisci, CA

10. Warren JW, Diggs C, Horne L, Greenberg P. Interstitial cystitis/painful bladder syndrome: what do patients mean by "perceived" bladder pain? Urology. 2011;77(2):309–12.
11. Peters K, Girdler B, Carrico D, Ibrahim I, Diokno A. Painful bladder syndrome/interstitial cystitis and vulvodynia: a clinical correlation. Int Urogynecol J Pelvic Floor Dysfunct. 2008;19(5):665–9.
12. Coggon D, Martyn C, Palmer KT, Evanoff B. Assessing case definitions in the absence of a diagnostic gold standard. Int J Epidemiol. 2005;34(4):949–52.
13. Reading I, Walker-Bone K, Palmer KT, Cooper C, Coggon D. Anatomic distribution of sensory symptoms in the hand and their relation to neck pain, psychosocial variables, and occupational activities. Am J Epidemiol. 2003;157(6):524–30.
14. Kendell R, Jablensky A. Distinguishing between the validity and utility of psychiatric diagnoses. Am J Psychiatry. 2003;160(1):4–12.
15. Gormley EA. Irritative voiding symptoms: identifying the cause. Hosp Pract (Minneap). 1999;34(13):91–6. quiz 108.
16. Smith EM, Ritchie JM, Galask R, Pugh EE, Jia J, Ricks-McGillan J. Case-control study of vulvar vestibulitis risk associated with genital infections. Infect Dis Obstet Gynecol. 2002;10(4):193–202.
17. Abrams P, Cardozo L, Fall M, Griffiths D, Rosier P, Ulmsten U, et al. The standardisation of terminology of lower urinary tract function: report from the standardisation sub-committee of the international continence society. Neurourol Urodyn. 2002;21(2):167–78.
18. Abrams P, Hanno P, Wein A. Overactive bladder and painful bladder syndrome: there need not be confusion. Neurourol Urodyn. 2005;24(2):149–50.
19. Greenberg P, Brown J, Yates T, Brown V, Langenberg P, Warren JW. Voiding urges perceived by patients with interstitial cystitis/painful bladder syndrome. Neurourol Urodyn. 2008;27(4):287–90.
20. Clemens JQ, Bogart LM, Liu K, Pham C, Suttorp M, Berry SH. Perceptions of "urgency" in women with interstitial cystitis/bladder pain syndrome or overactive bladder. Neurourol Urodyn. 2010;30(3):402–5.
21. FitzGerald MP, Butler N, Shott S, Brubaker L. Bother arising from urinary frequency in women. Neurourol Urodyn. 2002;21(1):36–40. discussion 41.
22. Glenning PP. Urinary voiding patterns of apparently normal women. Aust N Z J Obstet Gynaecol. 1985;25(1):62–5.
23. Fitzgerald MP, Brubaker L. Variability of 24-hour voiding diary variables among asymptomatic women. J Urol. 2003;169(1):207–9.
24. Burgio KL, Engel BT, Locher JL. Normative patterns of diurnal urination across 6 age decades. J Urol. 1991;145(4):728–31.
25. van Kerrebroeck P, Abrams P, Chaikin D, Donovan J, Fonda D, Jackson S, et al. The standardisation of terminology in nocturia: report from the standardisation sub-committee of the international continence society. Neurourol Urodyn. 2002;21(2):179–83.
26. Tikkinen KA, Johnson 2nd TM, Tammela TL, Sintonen H, Haukka J, Huhtala H, et al. Nocturia frequency, bother, and quality of life: how often is too often? A population-based study in finland. Eur Urol. 2010;57(3):488–96.
27. Warren JW, Horne L, Diggs C, Greenberg P. Nocturia in interstitial cystitis/painful bladder syndrome. Urology. 2011;77(6):1308–12.
28. Weiss JP, Weinberg AC, Blaivas JG. New aspects of the classification of nocturia. Curr Urol Rep. 2008;9(5):362–7.
29. Held PJ, Hanno PM, Wein AJ, Pauly MV, Cahn MA. Epidemiology of interstitial cystitis: 2. In: Hanno PM, Staskin DR, Krane RF, Wein AJ, editors. Interstitial Cystitis. London: Springer; 1990. p. 29–48.
30. Keller ML, McCarthy DO, Neider RS. Measurement of symptoms of interstitial cystitis. A pilot study. Urol Clin North Am. 1994;21(1):67–71.
31. Goin JE, Olaleye D, Peters KM, Steinert B, Habicht K, Wynant G. Psychometric analysis of the University of Wisconsin interstitial cystitis scale: implications for use in randomized clinical trials. J Urol. 1998;159(3):1085–90.

32. Porru D, Tinelli C, Gerardini M, Giliberto GL, Stancati S, Rovereto B. Evaluation of urinary and general symptoms and correlation with other clinical parameters in interstitial cystitis patients. Neurourol Urodyn. 2005;24(1):69–73.
33. O'Leary MP, Sant GR, Fowler Jr FJ, Whitmore KE, Spolarich-Kroll J. The interstitial cystitis symptom index and problem index. Urology. 1997;49(5A Suppl):58–63.
34. Lubeck DP, Whitmore K, Sant GR, Alvarez-Horine S, Lai C. Psychometric validation of the O'leary-sant interstitial cystitis symptom index in a clinical trial of pentosan polysulfate sodium. Urology. 2001;57(6 Suppl 1):62–6.
35. O'Leary MP, Sant G. The interstitial cystitis symptom and problem indices: rationale, development, and application. In: Sant G, editor. Interstitial Cystitis. Philadelphia: Lippincott-Raven; 1997. p. 271–6.
36. Parsons CL, Dell J, Stanford EJ, Bullen M, Kahn BS, Waxell T, et al. Increased prevalence of interstitial cystitis: previously unrecognized urologic and gynecologic cases identified using a new symptom questionnaire and intravesical potassium sensitivity. Urology. 2002;60(4):573–8.
37. Moldwin R, K L. The diagnostic value of interstitial cystitis questionnaires. Meeting of the American Urological Association; 2004 May 9; San Francisco, CA. p. 96
38. Kushner L, Moldwin RM. Efficiency of questionnaires used to screen for interstitial cystitis. J Urol. 2006;176(2):587–92.
39. Sirinian E, Payne CK. Correlation of symptoms between 2 instruments among interstitial cystitis patients. Urology. 2001;57(6 Suppl 1):124–5.
40. Propert KJ, Mayer RD, Wang Y, Sant GR, Hanno PM, Peters KM, et al. Responsiveness of symptom scales for interstitial cystitis. Urology. 2006;67(1):55–9.
41. Clemens JQ, Calhoun EA, Litwin MS, McNaughton-Collins M, Kusek JW, Crowley EM, et al. Validation of a modified national institutes of health chronic prostatitis symptom index to assess genitourinary pain in both men and women. Urology. 2009;74(5):983–7. quiz 987. e1–3.
42. Berry SH, Bogart LM, Pham C, Liu K, Nyberg L, Stoto M, et al. Development, validation and testing of an epidemiological case definition of interstitial cystitis/painful bladder syndrome. J Urol. 2010;183(5):1848–52.
43. Alagiri M, Chottiner S, Ratner V, Slade D, Hanno PM. Interstitial cystitis: unexplained associations with other chronic disease and pain syndromes. Urology. 1997;49(5A Suppl):52–7.
44. Nickel JC, Tripp DA, Pontari M, Moldwin R, Mayer R, Carr LK, et al. Interstitial cystitis/painful bladder syndrome and associated medical conditions with an emphasis on irritable bowel syndrome, fibromyalgia and chronic fatigue syndrome. J Urol. 2010;184(4):1358–63.
45. Warren JW, Howard FM, Cross RK, Good JL, Weissman MM, Wesselmann U, Langengerg P, Greenberg P, Clauw DJ. Antecedent nonbladder syndromes in case-control study of interstitial cystitis/painful bladder syndrome. Urology. 2009;73:52–7.
46. Barry MJ, Fowler Jr FJ, O'Leary MP, Bruskewitz RC, Holtgrewe HL, Mebust WK, et al. The American Urological Association symptom index for benign prostatic hyperplasia. The measurement committee of the American Urological Association. J Urol. 1992;148(5):1549–57. discussion 1564.
47. FitzGerald MP, Kenton KS, Brubaker L. Localization of the urge to void in patients with painful bladder syndrome. Neurourol Urodyn. 2005;24(7):633–7.
48. Clemens JQ, Markossian TW, Meenan RT, O'Keeffe Rosetti MC, Calhoun EA. Overlap of voiding symptoms, storage symptoms and pain in men and women. J Urol. 2007;178(4 Pt 1):1354–8. discussion 1358.
49. McMahon SB, Dmitrieva N, Koltzenburg M. Visceral pain. Br J Anaesth. 1995;75(2):132–44.
50. Warren JW, Brown J, Tracy JK, Langenberg P, Wesselmann U, Greenberg P. Evidence-based criteria for pain of interstitial cystitis/painful bladder syndrome in women. Urology. 2008;71(3):444–8.
51. Malykhina AP. Neural mechanisms of pelvic organ cross-sensitization. Neuroscience. 2007;149(3):660–72.

52. Pezzone MA, Liang R, Fraser MO. A model of neural cross-talk and irritation in the pelvis: implications for the overlap of chronic pelvic pain disorders. Gastroenterology. 2005;128(7):1953–64.
53. Tomaszewski JE, Landis JR, Russack V, Williams TM, Wang LP, Hardy C, et al. Biopsy features are associated with primary symptoms in interstitial cystitis: results from the interstitial cystitis database study. Urology. 2001;57(6 Suppl 1):67–81.

Chapter 13
Clinical Evaluation and Diagnosis of Bladder Pain Syndrome

Jennifer Yonaitis Fariello and Kristene E. Whitmore

Introduction

Bladder pain syndrome (BPS) is a chronic condition of the bladder with symptoms of urinary frequency, urgency, and pelvic pain/pressure in the absence of infection, carcinoma, or other pathology [1]. Although the exact etiology of BPS is still an enigma, many experts theorize that it is multifactorial and therefore should be considered part of a visceral pain syndrome [2].

Adding to the difficulty in the diagnostic evaluation of a patient with BPS is the overlap of its symptoms with a wide range of other disorders including endometriosis, vulvodynia, pelvic floor muscle (PFM) dysfunction, overactive bladder, urinary tract infection, irritable bowel syndrome, chronic prostatitis, and chronic pelvic pain syndrome [3]. Due to pain generators originating in the pelvis other than the bladder, the diagnosis of BPS becomes even more confounding. On average, approximately eight healthcare providers evaluate a patient with BPS symptoms over 5–7 years prior to receiving a correct diagnosis [4].

Recent studies suggest that initiation of therapy early in the disease process leads to decreased symptomatology and better overall quality of life for the BPS patient [5, 6]. The caveat is that the diagnostic criteria established by the National Institutes of Arthritis Diabetes Digestive and Kidney Disease (NIDDK) in 1987 misses about

J.Y. Fariello, M.S.N., C.R.N.P. (✉)
The Pelvic and Sexual Health Institute, Drexel University College of Medicine,
207 N. Broad Street, 4th Floor, Philadelphia, PA 19107, USA

Urology Division, Department of Obstetrics and Gynecology, FPMRS,
Drexel University College of Medicine, Philadelphia, PA, USA
e-mail: jfariello@gmail.com

K.E. Whitmore, M.D.
Urology Division, Department of Obstetrics and Gynecology, FPMRS,
Drexel University College of Medicine, Philadelphia, PA, USA

J. Nordling et al. (eds.), *Bladder Pain Syndrome: A Guide for Clinicians*,
DOI 10.1007/978-1-4419-6929-3_13, © Springer Science+Business Media New York 2013

Table 13.1 Common patient symptoms, prevalence (%)

Urinary urgency, 57–98
Daytime frequency, 84–97
Pain with voiding or dysuria, 71–98
Nocturia, 44–90
Dyspareunia (women), 46–80
Subjective sensation of bladder spasms, 50–74
Pubic pressure, 60–71
Suprapubic pain, 39–71
Pubic pressure, 60–71
Depression, 55–67
Perineal pain, 25–56
Genital pain (men), 40–50
Rectal pain (men), 30–32

From Seth A, Teichman JM. Differences in the clinical presentation of interstitial cystitis/painful bladder syndrome in patients with or without sexual abuse history. J Urol. Nov 2008;180(5):2029–2033. Reprinted with permission from Springer

60% of patients with BPS [7]. These diagnostic criteria were developed for patient recruitment into research trials, not clinical practice. Currently there is no "definitive diagnostic test" for BPS and to date there are no biological markers to aid in the diagnostic process. Because of this, many clinicians regard BPS as a "diagnosis of exclusion" and make empirical diagnoses based on patient symptomatology [1]. Therefore, it is imperative that clinicians be able to identify symptoms associated with BPS in order to make a timely and accurate diagnosis. The most common symptoms patients present with are frequency, urgency, nocturia, and suprapubic pain or pressure/discomfort [8]. Suprapubic pain, pressure, or discomfort, hallmark symptoms of BPS, may not be early symptoms, may not be constant, may be flared by "triggers," or may be present from the very beginning [9–12]. The symptoms of BPS can be as enigmatic as the disease itself (Table 13.1).

Evaluation

Fundamental to the clinical diagnosis of BPS is a thorough history that includes voiding symptoms, pain characteristics, and triggers (Table 13.2) [13]. A complete medical and surgical history helps to establish a potential initiating event, a triggering event, as well as comorbid conditions associated with BPS and/or conditions whose symptoms imitate those of BPS (Table 13.3).

Diaries

The most common diary clinicians recommend to patients is the voiding diary. This is a self-recorded log of intake and output typically over a 3-day time span [14].

Table 13.2 Bladder symptom history taking

Ask questions about:
• Urinary urgency
• Urinary frequency
• Hematuria
• Incontinence
• Nocturia
• Pain/pressure in suprapubic region
• Length of symptoms
• Sentinel event
• Precipitating or alleviating factors
Is pain/pressure:
• Worse with bladder filling?
• Worse in the am?
• Triggered by any specific food?
• Worse with sexual activity?

Table 13.3 Differential diagnoses to BPS

Urological
• Urinary tract infection
• Overactive bladder
• Bladder carcinoma
• Urethritis
• Prostatits
Gynecological
• Endometriosis
• Pelvic inflammatory disease
• Vaginitis
• Vulvodynia (provoked and/or generalized)
Gastrointestinal
• Irritable bowel syndrome
Musculoskeletal
• Pelvic floor dysfunction

When evaluating the BPS patient, the clinician should remember to tell the patient to record episodes of nocturia, as well as pain upon bladder filling compared to bladder emptying. Mazurick and Landis et al. analyzed voiding diaries of 305 women enrolled in the National Interstitial Cystitis Data Base Study and concluded that voiding diaries can be reduced to a single day, as day 2 and 3 measures were not statistically significantly different from day 1 (1% level) [15]. They also found that there was no difference between weekend versus weekday measurements [15].

Along with the number of micturations, it may be helpful for both clinicians and patients to document on the voiding diary any "triggers" that may increase number of voids or pressure/pain. This is a good opportunity for the patient to attempt to correlate exacerbators of bladder symptoms such as food, sexual activity, or menstrual cycle-associated "flares."

Another type of diary is a pain diary. This can be used independent of, or in conjunction with, a voiding diary. A pain diary is used as a log of daily pain experienced by the patient, and its inciting events. Patients rate their symptoms on a scale of 0–10 (0 = no pain; 10 = severe pain) for an "overall" generalized pain assessment, and then into more specific categories. Patients can also determine precipitating factors that exacerbated pain and any measures that helped to alleviate pain.

Questionnaires

Questionnaires, or symptom impact severity indices, are tools utilized by clinicians to aid in diagnosis, assessing severity of disease, and evaluation of treatment response [13]. The most frequently used questionnaires for bladder symptoms are the O'Leary–Sant Interstitial Cystitis Symptom Index and Problem Index (ICSI) and (ICPI) and the Pain Urgency and Frequency score (PUF). The ICSI and ICPI were the first to be validated and were originally designed to be used to evaluate outcome measures [16, 17]; however they have since been shown to demonstrate therapeutic response to treatment [18, 19]. Lubeck et al. analyzed the use of this questionnaire in 376 female patients receiving pentosan polysulfate sodium of varying doses [19]. The ICSI was shown to be a valid, reliable, and responsive measure of change in BPS symptoms [19].

The PUF score is another questionnaire used as a screening tool for BPS. In addition to urinary questions, the PUF questionnaire also includes questions related to pelvic pain and pain related to sexual intercourse [13]. Validation of the PUF questionnaire was done through studies of both male and female patients utilizing the potassium sensitivity test (PST) as a correlate [20, 21]. Parsons et al. found that 74% of female patients with a PUF score of 10–14 had a positive PST; 76% of patients with a score of 15–19 had a positive PST; and 91% of those with a score of ≥20 had a positive PST [20]. Likewise, Parsons et al. also reported that 77% of men diagnosed with chronic prostatitis (CP) had a positive PST and a PUF score ≥7 [21].

Kushner and Moldwin assessed the validity of the ICSI/ICPI and the PUF questionnaires in screening for BPS and distinguishing it from other disease processes, finding the PUF questionnaire (with a score of ≥13) the more efficient of the two [22]. They concluded that while both questionnaires are unable to serve as a sole diagnostic indicator, they are helpful screening tools to distinguish patients who require further evaluation, as well as useful instruments to follow those who have been previously diagnosed [22].

An important aspect that should not be overlooked when evaluating the BPS patient is pain. A visual analogue scale (VAS) is a tool that assists both the patient and clinician quantify pain over the past 24 h. The VAS has been shown to be a valid and reliable assessment of both acute and chronic pain [23–27]. The patient is asked to indicate his or her average pain by placing a vertical line on a horizontal line that represents a continuum of no pain to worst pain from left to right, respectively.

The clinician is able to obtain a "final" score by measuring where along the horizontal line the patient marks using a 10 cm ruler (0 = no pain; 10 = worst pain). The two most common categories evaluated on the VAS are pain with daily activity and pain with sexual activity; however these are not exclusive and there are many variations available.

Physical Exam

A detailed physical exam is the hallmark component in the diagnosis of BPS. The exam for both men and women should begin with an external musculoskeletal examination in the standing and bending positions assessing for symmetry of the pelvic girdle, gait, kyphosis, lorcosis, or scoliosis. While supine and side lying, the patient should then be assessed for sacroiliac joint tenderness, symphysis pubis tenderness, bladder distention, hernias, and abdominal trigger points.

A pelvic exam is an integral part of the physical exam for the female BPS patient. The pelvic exam begins with inspection of the skin and vulvar structures. Pigmentation and structural changes associated with vulvar dermatoses or vulvar neoplasia should be noted. The clinician should then proceed with a Kauffman Q-tip touch sensitivity test (Fig. 13.1) in which a saline-moistened cotton swab applicator is lightly applied to each of the vestibular glands in a clockwise manner. There is a significant comorbidity rate of BPS and vulvodynia [28, 29]. During embryologic development, the reproductive and urinary systems initially develop from the intermediate mesoderm of the embryo. In the female embryo, the urogenital sinus develops into the bladder, urethra, vagina, vestibule, and vestibular glands. In the end, the endoderm that forms the urothelium of the bladder, trigone, and urethra is the same that forms the lower third of the vagina and vestibule [30, 31].

Assessment of the PFMs is done during the bimanual exam in women and the digital rectal exam (DRE) in men. Pelvic floor dysfunction (PFD) can be a comorbid condition with BPS or its own disorder. During palpation of the levator ani muscle groups, trigger points may be noted. Resting tone and the ability of the patient to contract and relax the muscles are graded by using the modified Oxford Scale (Table 13.4) [32]. A bimanual exam in women may also elicit posterior bladder wall or urethral tenderness while a digital rectal exam (DRE) in men may elicit tenderness of the prostate.

A more objective assessment of the pelvic floor can be obtained through perineometry. A pressure-sensitive intravaginal or intrarectal probe is zeroed and then inserted to measure the resting tone of the PFMs [32]. The patient is then asked to contract their PFMs, the maximum force of contraction recorded, and then the patient is asked to relax their PFMs. The final reading, the return to the flaccid state, enables the practitioner to evaluate if the patient is able to consciously bring his or her PFMs out of a contraction, back to his or her resting tone. Isherwood and Rane evaluated 263 women with both perineometry and digital exam using the Oxford scale [33]. Results showed concordance between the two methods of evaluation as highly significant ($P < 0.0001$) [33].

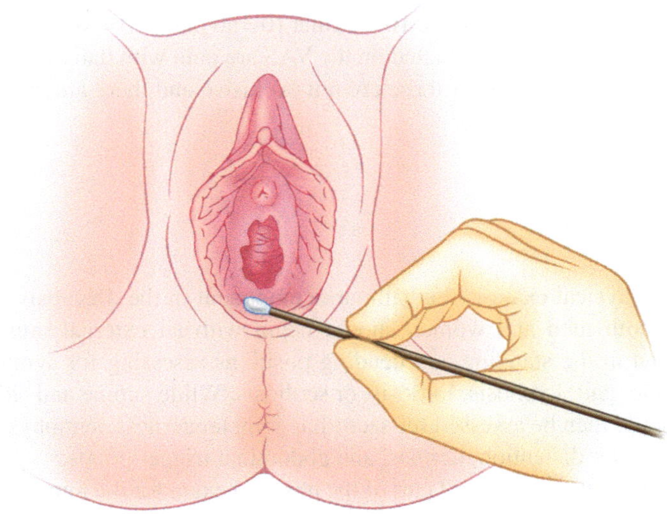

Fig. 13.1 Kaufmann Q-tip touch test

Table 13.4 Modified oxford scale: Pelvic floor muscle tenderness

0 = No pressure or pain associated with exam
1 = Comfortable pressure associated with exam
2 = Uncomfortable pressure associated with exam
3 = Moderate pain associated with exam, intensifies with contraction
4 = Severe pain associated with exam; patient is unable to perform contraction maneuver due to pain

From Lukban JC, Whitmore KE. Pelvic floor muscle re-education treatment of the overactive bladder and painful bladder syndrome. Clin Obstet Gynecol. Mar 2002;45(1):273–285. Reprinted with permission from Wolters Kluwer Health

Laboratory Testing

A urine dipstick should be done in the office as a preliminary screening tool; however a laboratory urinalysis and urine culture should be done to rule out microhematuria and infection. Additionally, urine cytology is warranted if microhematuria is identified or if any other risk factors for bladder carcinoma are present (Table 13.5). Studies have shown that 20–30% of patients with BPS have hematuria; however, despite the lack of clinical significance it is regarded as an incidental finding in this patient population [7, 34, 35]. Gomes et al. [36] did a retrospective chart review on 148 BPS patients with gross or microscopic hematuria that evaluated urine culture and cytology, cystoscopy, and intravenous urography or retrograde pyelography with renal ultrasound. They found that 41% (60/148) of patients had at least one episode of hematuria, which is higher than previously reported. Of the 56 patients

Table 13.5 Risk factors for bladder carcinoma

Smoking
Workplace exposure to certain chemicals
Caucasian
Over 50
Family history
History of chemotherapy or radiation therapy

who agreed to further evaluation, no malignancy was found [36]. Stanford et al. [37] prospectively evaluated 100 women with BPS for microscopic hematuria with post-void sterile catheterization along with urine culture, PST, cystoscopy with hydrodistention, and PUF questionnaire. Results showed a 24% prevalence of microhematuria in this patient cohort, thus leading the authors to conclude that microhematuria should be considered an incidental finding in the majority of BPS patients [37].

Urinary Markers

Recently, the potential use of urine tests that look for markers associated with BPS, specifically antiproliferative factor (APF) and Tamm–Horsfall protein (THP), has been reported. APF is thought to inhibit normal bladder urothelial cell proliferation and may induce reversible inhibition of heparin-binding epidermal growth factor-like growth factor (HG-EGF) and increase levels of epidermal growth factor (EGF) [38]. Keay et al. [39] evaluated the urine of women meeting the NIDDK criteria for BPS for elevated APF. In the cohort studied, they found that the test is 94% sensitive and 95% specific [39]. Keay et al. [40] compared the urine of three groups of men for the biomarkers APF, HG-EGF, and EGF: symptomatic CP/CPPS ($n=41$), BPS ($n=24$), and asymptomatic or no bladder disease, the control group ($n=36$). Their findings showed that the CP/CPPS group did not differ significantly from the control group for any of the markers ($P>0.49$) [40]; however the BPS group had significantly higher levels of APF and lower levels of HG-EGF than both the CP/CPPS and control groups ($P<0.00001$ for all markers tested) as well as higher EGF levels, though this did not reach significance ($P=0.06$) [40]. Studies on APF and its associated markers have yet to be reproduced. These studies included only BPS patients meeting the NIDDK criteria; therefore it remains to be seen if APF levels are abnormal in the early stages of the disease.

Tamm-Horsfall protein (THP) is a glycoprotein that contains sialic acid that is thought to protect the bladder urothelium from bacteria and other irritants [41]. Parsons et al. [42] compared patients with BPS ($n=22$) to controls ($n=20$) and found that although the mean concentration of THP was not significantly different ($P=0.6$), the mean sialic acid content was almost twofold lower ($P<0.0001$) [42]. Agarde et al. [43] also compared the THP concentration and the sialic acid content from urine samples of patients with BPS ($n=23$) to a control group ($n=24$). The findings were similar to the previous study as they found half the concentration of sialic acid in the BPS group [43]. Albeit this marker appears to be sensitive and specific, there are only a limited number of studies done due to its complexity, cost, and unavailability.

Potassium Sensitivity Test

The PST was first described by Parsons et al. as a diagnostic tool for BPS [44]. This test is based on the theory that there is a defect in the bladder epithelium or glycoaminoglycan (GAG) layer of BPS patients, thereby making it permeable to irritative substances. Forty ml of sterile water is instilled intravesically followed by 0.4 M potassium chloride (KCL). The patient's subjective responses to pain and urgency after each infusion are compared. It is thought that patients with normal bladder epithelium should not respond to either instillation; however, patients with a defective GAG layer will report pain, urgency, or both with the KCL instillation. The initial study reported that 75% of patients with IC have a positive KCL test compared with 4% of the control group [44]. All patients had a negative response to the water instillation. Follow-up studies report that in patients with a clinical diagnosis of IC, the PST has a sensitivity of approximately 80% [45, 46]. However, it should be noted that other inflammatory conditions that increase bladder epithelium permeability may produce false-positive results [47]. False-negative results can occur if the patient has been recently treated with intravesical therapy or has had a recent bladder hydrodistention [48].

Chambers et al. [49] compared the PST to history and cystoscopy with hydrodistention in a population with symptoms suggestive of BPS and found the PST to have a poor sensitivity and specificity (69.5 and 50%, respectively). The authors concluded that the PST has no added value over cystoscopy with hydrodistention [49].

There are advantages to the PST such as identification of BPS early in the disease process, localization of the origin of the pain to the bladder, and simplicity of the test [47]. A major disadvantage of the PST is the potential to cause intense pain to the patient [47]. In order to avoid elucidating additional pain in these patients, many clinicians are opting to use novel intravesical procedures, such as the intravesical anesthetic challenge (IAC), to aid in the diagnosis of BPS.

Anesthetic Challenge

The current diagnostic aid BPS experts are using more frequently is the intravesical anesthetic challenge (IAC). Though still an investigational procedure, the theory is that the reduction or elimination of pain with intravesical anesthetic is evidence of bladder origin of pain [9]. This procedure emphasizes symptom reduction rather than exacerbation, and therefore should only be used in patients in pain [50, 51].

Moldwin et al. [50] evaluated improvement in pain scores of BPS patients with Hunner's lesions versus those without Hunner's lesions after administration of an IAC. A 1:1 mixture of 0.5% bupivacaine and 2% lidocaine was instilled intravesically, remaining for 30 min. Patients were asked to score their BPS pain symptoms on a 0–10 VAS. A positive response to the IAC is a 50% reduction in the VAS score [50]. This innovative study showed that 89% ($n=28$) of Hunner's lesion-positive patients and 71% ($n=52$) of lesion-negative patients had a positive response to the IAC [50]. Additionally, the mean duration of relief in Hunner's lesion-positive patients was 11 days, and in Hunner's lesion-negative patients was 4 days, thus making the IAC a potential therapeutic option as well [50].

There are a variety of "cocktails" used in clinical practice for this procedure. Parsons reported statistically significant improvement in symptoms ($P<0.01$) and sustained symptom relief with the combination of heparin and alkalinized lidocaine [51].

Urodynamics

The use of urodynamics in the diagnosis of BPS is controversial. When compared to the findings of voiding diaries, urodynamic findings closely correlated, leading some experts to suggest that noninvasive voiding diaries capture adequate information [52]. However, when patients with BPS present with concomitant incontinence and/or retention, urodynamics can be a helpful diagnostic tool to rule out other disorders such as detrusor-sphincter dyssynergia, bladder outlet obstruction, and PFD (although PFD may be secondary to BPS) [17, 53].

Typically, patients with BPS will have sensory urgency, a low functional capacity, and an early first sensation. Sastry et al. [54] suggest that the severity of symptoms (PUF as assessed by validated questionnaires and VAS scales) was significantly associated with urodynamic parameters seen in earlier first sensation, first urge, strong desire, and a lower maximum cystometric capacity (MCC). They purport their findings illustrate that urodynamics is an objective measure of pain as well as confirmation of symptom severity in the BPS patient [54]. It has also been recognized that 15–25% of BPS patients demonstrate detrusor overactivity during the test [52, 55]. Kim et al. [56] performed a retrospective chart review of women with BPS ($n=40$) and compared their fluoroscopic urodynamic study results to women with idiopathic overactive bladder ($n=78$). This small study showed that the urodynamics results were significantly different between the two groups [56].

Cystoscopy with Hydrodistention

Cystoscopy with hydrodistention under anesthesia was established as the diagnostic tool for Interstitial Cystitis by the NIDDK. The criteria established by the NIDDK were glomerulations, and/or Hunner's ulcers [57]. Cystoscopy with hydrodistention is done with the patient under general or regional anesthesia or intravenous sedation.

A cystoscope is introduced into the bladder and a full evaluation is preformed. Lesions, tumors, masses, and ulcerations are ruled out as causes of hematuria and/or bladder symptoms [58]. The bladder is then filled by gravity with sterile water or saline at 70–100 cm H_2O pressure. Once capacity is achieved, bladder distention is maintained for a minimum of 2 min, drained, and a second cystoscopic examination is performed. Terminal bloody effluent when the bladder is drained, glomerulations (petechiae), and/or Hunner's lesions (fissures or cracks in the urothelium that are not ulcers) are findings consistent with BPS [57, 58]. It is imperative that the clinician remembers that a negative cystoscopy with hydrodistention does not rule out BPS.

Recent studies have called into question the sensitivity and specificity of this procedure for the diagnosis of BPS [58–60]. Braunstein et al. compared a cohort of patients meeting the NIDDK criteria for BPS with Hunner's lesion disease ($n=86$) to those with non-Hunner's lesion disease ($n=137$) [61]. They found no statistical significance in the parameters measured (symptom duration, history of gross hematuria, history of comorbid disease, or VAS pain scores) [61]. It was concluded that cystoscopy is needed to accurately identify Hunner's lesions in patients with BPS [61]. Conversely, Chai [62] states that in some BPS patients, the urothelium is very friable after hydrodistention, making identification and analysis of Hunner's lesions versus tears in the urothelium difficult.

Cystoscopy is necessary to rule out bladder cancer in patients with an abnormal cytology, or who present with hematuria and are in a high-risk category. It may also be used as an aid in the treatment of refractory cases of BPS. Anecdotal reports show that approximately half of the patients experience reduction in pain and urinary frequency and urgency for a mean duration of 2 months following hydrodistention [63]. Aihara et al. reported BPS patients (71%, 21/30) experienced continued therapeutic benefit one month post cystoscopy with hydrodistention [64]. Cystoscopy with hydrodistention may also play a role in assisting to stage BPS.

Bladder Biopsy

The International Society for the Study of BPS (ESSIC) states, as part of their guidelines for the evaluation of patients with BPS, that bladder biopsies with subsequent staining for mast cells be done on all patients undergoing a cystoscopy with hydrodistention [14]. According to these guidelines, three biopsies should be obtained and should include detrusor muscle for the purpose of eliciting mast cell counts [14]. Of the three biopsies, only the one with the greatest number of mast cells per mm^2 should be reported. If detrusor muscle is not present in the specimen, they must be disregarded and new ones obtained [14].

Currently in the United States, bladder biopsy is not recommended for the diagnosis of BPS, as there are no features specific to the disease to use as a confirmatory test [13]. No histological changes specific to BPS have yet been identified and

Table 13.6 Summary of AUA guidelines for IC/BPS (2011) [70]

Diagnosis
Guideline #1
• Careful history, physical examinations, and laboratory testing to document signs and symptoms characteristic of IC/BPS, excluding other disorders that could be the cause of the patient's symptoms.
Guideline #2
• Obtain baseline voiding symptoms and pain levels in order to evaluate subsequent treatment effects.
Guideline #3
• Cystoscopy and/or urodynamics should be considered when the diagnosis of IC/BPS is questionable or the patient is refractory to treatment; these tests are not necessary for making a diagnosis in uncomplicated presentations.
Treatment
Guideline #6
• Multiple, concurrent treatments may be considered if it is in the patient's best interest; baseline and regular symptom assessment are essential to evaluate efficacy or single and combined treatments. *Clinical principle*
Guideline #7
• Ineffective treatments should be discontinued after a clinically meaningful interval. *Clinical principle*
Guideline #9
• Reconsider the IC/BPS diagnosis if no improvement occurs after multiple treatment approaches. *Clinical principle*
First-line treatment
• Education and expectations. *Clinical principle*
• Self-care practices and behavioral modifications. *Clinical principle*
• Stress management practices. *Clinical principle*
• Coping techniques for management of stress-induced symptom exacerbations. *Clinical principle*
Second-line treatment
• Physical therapy (including manual therapy). ***Pelvic floor strengthening exercises (e.g., Kegel exercises) should be avoided.*** *Clinical principle*
• Multimodal pain management approaches should be initiated (e.g., pharmacological, stress management, manual therapy if available). *Expert Opinion*
• Amitriptyline, cimetidine, hydroxyzine, or pentosan polysulfate may be administered orally (listed in alphabetical order; no hierarchy is implied). *Option (Evidence Strength-Grades B, B, C, and B)*
• DMSO, heparin, or lidocaine may be administered intravesically (listed in alphabetical order; no hierarchy is implied). *Option (Evidence strength-grades C, C, and B)*
Third-line treatment
• Cystoscopy under anesthesia with short-duration, low-pressure hydrodistention. *Option (Evidence strength-grade C)*
• If Hunner's lesions are present, the fulguration (with laser or electrocautery) and/or injection of triamcinolone should be performed. *Recommendation (Evidence strength-grade C)*
Fourth-line treatment
• A trial of neurostimulation may be performed. *Option (Evidence strength-grade C)*

(continued)

Table 13.6 (continued)

Fifth-line treatment
• Cyclosporine A. *Option (Evidence strength-grade C)*
• Intradetrusor botulinum toxin A (BTX-A). *Option (Evidence strength-grade C)*
Sixth-line treatment
• Major surgery (e.g., substitution cystoplasty, urinary diversion with or without cystectomy) may be undertaken in carefully selected patients. *Option (Evidence strength-grade C)*
Treatments that should **not** be offered
• Long-term oral antibiotics. *Standard*
• Intravesical instillation of bacillus Calmette–Guerin (BCG). *Standard*
• Intravesical instillation of resiniferatoxin (RTX). *Standard*
• High-pressure, long-duration hydrodistention. *Recommendation*
• Long-term oral glucocorticoids. *Recommendation*

Summarized from Hanno PM, Burks DA, Clemens JQ, et al. AUA guideline for the diagnosis and treatment of interstitial cystitis/bladder pain syndrome. J Urol. Jun 2011;185(6):2162–2170

findings related to chronic inflammation often overlap with other pathophysiology [58, 65]. Though not recommended as a diagnostic test, bladder biopsy has been shown to be somewhat advantageous in determining the severity of the disease when associated with subjective symptoms [66]. The significance of mast cells on biopsy remains controversial [67–69] and research continues in this area.

Bladder biopsy is warranted if a questionable lesion is found or to rule out carcinoma in situ.

AUA Guidelines

In 2011, the American Urological Association (AUA) published the first set of guidelines for BPS. The guidelines, based on empirical data, provide a framework to aid clinicians in recognizing, diagnosing, and treating BPS (Table 13.6) [70].

References

1. Hanno PM. Painful bladder syndrome/interstitial cystitis and related disorders. In: Wein AJ Kavoussi LR, Novick AC, Partin AW, Peters CA, editors. Campell-Walsh urology. 9th ed. Philadelphia: Saunders; 2007. p. 330–70.
2. Butrick CW, Howard FM, Sand PK. Diagnosis and treatment of interstitial cystitis/painful bladder syndrome: a review. J Womens Health (Larchmt). 2010;19(6):1185–93.
3. Bogart LM, Berry SH, Clemens JQ. Symptoms of interstitial cystitis, painful bladder syndrome and similar diseases in women: a systematic review. J Urol. 2007;177(2):450–6.
4. Held PJ, Hanno P, Wein J, et al. Epidemiology of interstitial cysitis. In: Hanno PM, Staskin D, Krane RJ, et al., editors. Interstitial cystitis. New York: Springer; 1990. p. 29–48.
5. Nickel JC, Kaufman DM, Zhang HF, Wan GJ, Sand PK. Time to initiation of pentosan polysulfate sodium treatment after interstitial cystitis diagnosis: effect on symptom improvement. Urology. 2008;71(1):57–61.

6. Forrest JB, Sebastyanski P, O'Brien-Westbrook M. Observations on the clinical factors affecting the outcomes of interstitial cystitis. Chicago: International Pelvic Pain Society (IPPS); 2004.
7. Hanno PM, Landis JR, Matthews-Cook Y, Kusek J, Nyberg Jr L. The diagnosis of interstitial cystitis revisited: lessons learned from the National Institutes of Health Interstitial Cystitis Database study. J Urol. 1999;161(2):553–7.
8. Driscoll A, Teichman JM. How do patients with interstitial cystitis present? J Urol. 2001;166(6):2118–20.
9. Teichman JM, Parsons CL. Contemporary clinical presentation of interstitial cystitis. Urology. 2007;69(4 Suppl):41–7.
10. Ito T, Ueda T, Honma Y, Takei M. Recent trends in patient characteristics and therapeutic choices for interstitial cystitis: analysis of 282 Japanese patients. Int J Urol. 2007;14(12):1068–70.
11. Warren JW, Brown J, Tracy JK, Langenberg P, Wesselmann U, Greenberg P. Evidence-based criteria for pain of interstitial cystitis/painful bladder syndrome in women. Urology. 2008;71(3):444–8.
12. Peters KM, Carrico DJ, Diokno AC. Characterization of a clinical cohort of 87 women with interstitial cystitis/painful bladder syndrome. Urology. 2008;71(4):634–40.
13. Carr LK, Corcos J, Nickel JC, Teichman J. Diagnosis of interstitial cystitis June 2007. Can Urol Assoc J. 2009;3(1):81–6.
14. Nordling J, Anjum FH, Bade JJ, et al. Primary evaluation of patients suspected of having interstitial cystitis (IC). Eur Urol. 2004;45(5):662–9.
15. Mazurick CA, Landis JR. Evaluation of repeat daily voiding measures in the National Interstitial Cystitis Data Base Study. J Urol. 2000;163(4):1208–11.
16. O'Leary MP, Sant GR, Fowler Jr FJ, Whitmore KE, Spolarich-Kroll J. The interstitial cystitis symptom index and problem index. Urology. 1997;49(5A Suppl):58–63.
17. Evans RJ, Sant GR. Current diagnosis of interstitial cystitis: an evolving paradigm. Urology. 2007;69(4 Suppl):64–72.
18. Propert KJ, Mayer RD, Wang Y, et al. Responsiveness of symptom scales for interstitial cystitis. Urology. 2006;67(1):55–9.
19. Lubeck DP, Whitmore K, Sant GR, Alvarez-Horine S, Lai C. Psychometric validation of the O'leary-Sant interstitial cystitis symptom index in a clinical trial of pentosan polysulfate sodium. Urology. 2001;57(6 Suppl 1):62–6.
20. Parsons CL, Dell J, Stanford EJ, et al. Increased prevalence of interstitial cystitis: previously unrecognized urologic and gynecologic cases identified using a new symptom questionnaire and intravesical potassium sensitivity. Urology. 2002;60(4):573–8.
21. Parsons CL, Rosenberg MT, Sassani P, Ebrahimi K, Koziol JA, Zupkas P. Quantifying symptoms in men with interstitial cystitis/prostatitis, and its correlation with potassium-sensitivity testing. BJU Int. 2005;95(1):86–90.
22. Kushner L, Moldwin RM. Efficiency of questionnaires used to screen for interstitial cystitis. J Urol. 2006;176(2):587–92.
23. Bijur PE, Silver W, Gallagher EJ. Reliability of the visual analog scale for measurement of acute pain. Acad Emerg Med. 2001;8(12):1153–7.
24. Gallagher EJ, Bijur PE, Latimer C, Silver W. Reliability and validity of a visual analog scale for acute abdominal pain in the ED. Am J Emerg Med. 2002;20(4):287–90.
25. McCormack HM, Horne DJ, Sheather S. Clinical applications of visual analogue scales: a critical review. Psychol Med. 1988;18(4):1007–19.
26. Todd KH, Funk KG, Funk JP, Bonacci R. Clinical significance of reported changes in pain severity. Ann Emerg Med. 1996;27(4):485–9.
27. Kelly AM. Does the clinically significant difference in visual analog scale pain scores vary with gender, age, or cause of pain? Acad Emerg Med. 1998;5(11):1086–90.
28. Gardella B, Porru D, Ferdeghini F, et al. Insight into urogynecologic features of women with interstitial cystitis/painful bladder syndrome. Eur Urol. 2008;54(5):1145–51.
29. Whitmore K, Siegel JF, Kellogg-Spadt S. Interstitial cystitis/painful bladder syndrome as a cause of sexual pain in women: a diagnosis to consider. J Sex Med. 2007;4(3):720–7.

30. Myers DL, Aguilar VC. Gynecologic manifestations of interstitial cystitis. Clin Obstet Gynecol. 2002;45(1):233–41.
31. Moore K. The developing human: clinically oriented embryology. 4th ed. Philadelphia: Saunders; 1998.
32. Lukban JC, Whitmore KE. Pelvic floor muscle re-education treatment of the overactive bladder and painful bladder syndrome. Clin Obstet Gynecol. 2002;45(1):273–85.
33. Isherwood PJ, Rane A. Comparative assessment of pelvic floor strength using a perineometer and digital examination. BJOG. 2000;107(8):1007–11.
34. Messing EM, Stamey TA. Interstitial cystitis: early diagnosis, pathology, and treatment. Urology. 1978;12(4):381–92.
35. Dodd LG, Tello J. Cytologic examination of urine from patients with interstitial cystitis. Acta Cytol. 1998;42(4):923–7.
36. Gomes CM, Sanchez-Ortiz RF, Harris C, Wein AJ, Rovner ES. Significance of hematuria in patients with interstitial cystitis: review of radiographic and endoscopic findings. Urology. 2001;57(2):262–5.
37. Stanford EJ, Mattox TF, Parsons JK, McMurphy C. Prevalence of benign microscopic hematuria among women with interstitial cystitis: implications for evaluation of genitourinary malignancy. Urology. 2006;67(5):946–9.
38. Rashid HH, Reeder JE, O'Connell MJ, Zhang CO, Messing EM, Keay SK. Interstitial cystitis antiproliferative factor (APF) as a cell-cycle modulator. BMC Urol. 2004;4:3.
39. Keay SK, Zhang CO, Shoenfelt J, et al. Sensitivity and specificity of antiproliferative factor, heparin-binding epidermal growth factor-like growth factor, and epidermal growth factor as urine markers for interstitial cystitis. Urology. 2001;57(6 Suppl 1):9–14.
40. Keay S, Zhang CO, Chai T, et al. Antiproliferative factor, heparin-binding epidermal growth factor-like growth factor, and epidermal growth factor in men with interstitial cystitis versus chronic pelvic pain syndrome. Urology. 2004;63(1):22–6.
41. Bates JM, Raffi HM, Prasadan K, et al. Tamm–Horsfall protein knockout mice are more prone to urinary tract infection: rapid communication. Kidney Int. 2004;65(3):791–7.
42. Parsons CL, Stein P, Zupkas P, et al. Defective Tamm–Horsfall protein in patients with interstitial cystitis. J Urol. 2007;178(6):2665–70.
43. Argade SP, Vanichsarn C, Chenoweth M, Parsons CL. Abnormal glycosylation of Tamm–Horsfall protein in patients with interstitial cystitis. BJU Int. 2009;103(8):1085–9.
44. Parsons CL, Greenberger M, Gabal L, Bidair M, Barme G. The role of urinary potassium in the pathogenesis and diagnosis of interstitial cystitis. J Urol. 1998;159(6):1862–6. discussion 1866-1867.
45. Parsons CL, Zupkas P, Parsons JK. Intravesical potassium sensitivity in patients with interstitial cystitis and urethral syndrome. Urology. 2001;57(3):428–32. discussion 432-423.
46. Liandier F, Gregoire M, Naud A, et al. Profile of interstitial cystitis patients: a review of 189 cases at L'Hotel-Dieu de Quebec. J Urol. 2001;165(Suppl):70.
47. Teichman J. Potassium sensitivity testing in the diagnosis and treatment of interstitial cystitis. Infect Urol. 2003;16:87–94.
48. Forrest JB, Moldwin R. Diagnostic options for early identification and management of interstitial cystitis/painful bladder syndrome. Int J Clin Pract. 2008;62(12):1926–34.
49. Chambers GK, Fenster HN, Cripps S, Jens M, Taylor D. An assessment of the use of intravesical potassium in the diagnosis of interstitial cystitis. J Urol. 1999;162(3 Pt 1):699–701.
50. Moldwin R, Brettschneider N. The use of intravesical anesthetics to aid in the diagnosis of interstitial cystitis. Paper presented at: research insights into interstitial cystitis: a basic and clinical science symposium. October/November, 2003, Alexandria, VA.
51. Parsons CL. Successful downregulation of bladder sensory nerves with combination of heparin and alkalinized lidocaine in patients with interstitial cystitis. Urology. 2005;65(1):45–8.
52. Kirkemo A, Peabody M, Diokno AC, et al. Associations among urodynamic findings and symptoms in women enrolled in the Interstitial Cystitis Data Base (ICDB) Study. Urology. 1997;49(5A Suppl):76–80.

53. Nickel JC. Interstitial cystitis: a chronic pelvic pain syndrome. Med Clin North Am. 2004;88(2):467–81. xii.
54. Sastry DN, Hunter KM, Whitmore KE. Urodynamic testing and interstitial cystitis/painful bladder syndrome. Int Urogynecol J. 2010;21:157–61.
55. Nigro DA, Wein AJ, Foy M, et al. Associations among cystoscopic and urodynamic findings for women enrolled in the Interstitial Cystitis Data Base (ICDB) Study. Urology. 1997;49(5A Suppl):86–92.
56. Kim SH, Kim TB, Kim SW, Oh SJ. Urodynamic findings of the painful bladder syndrome/ interstitial cystitis: a comparison with idiopathic overactive bladder. J Urol. 2009;181(6):2550–4.
57. Wein AJ, Hanno PM, Gillenwater JY. Interstitial cystitis: an introduction to the problem. In: Hanno PM, Staskin DR, Krane RJ, Wein AJ, editors. Interstitial cystitis. London: Springer; 1990. p. 3–15.
58. Denson MA, Griebling TL, Cohen MB, Kreder KJ. Comparison of cystoscopic and histological findings in patients with suspected interstitial cystitis. J Urol. 2000;164(6):1908–11.
59. Waxman JA, Sulak PJ, Kuehl TJ. Cystoscopic findings consistent with interstitial cystitis in normal women undergoing tubal ligation. J Urol. 1998;160(5):1663–7.
60. Erickson DR, Tomaszewski JE, Kunselman AR, et al. Do the National Institute of Diabetes and Digestive and Kidney Diseases cystoscopic criteria associate with other clinical and objective features of interstitial cystitis? J Urol. 2005;173(1):93–7.
61. Braunstein R, Shapiro E, Kaye J, Moldwin R. The role of cystoscopy in the diagnosis of Hunner's ulcer disease. J Urol. 2008;180(4):1383–6.
62. Chai TC. Diagnosis of the painful bladder syndrome: current approaches to diagnosis. Clin Obstet Gynecol. 2002;45(1):250–8.
63. Ottem DP, Teichman JM. What is the value of cystoscopy with hydrodistension for interstitial cystitis? Urology. 2005;66(3):494–9.
64. Aihara K, Hirayama A, Tanaka N, Fujimoto K, Yoshida K, Hirao Y. Hydrodistension under local anesthesia for patients with suspected painful bladder syndrome/interstitial cystitis: safety, diagnostic potential and therapeutic efficacy. Int J Urol. 2009;16(12):947–52.
65. Sant GR. Etiology, pathogenesis, and diagnosis of interstitial cystitis. Rev Urol. 2002;4 Suppl 1:S9–S15.
66. Tomaszewski JE, Landis JR, Russack V, et al. Biopsy features are associated with primary symptoms in interstitial cystitis: results from the interstitial cystitis database study. Urology. 2001;57(6 Suppl 1):67–81.
67. Dundore PA, Schwartz AM, Semerjian H. Mast cell counts are not useful in the diagnosis of nonulcerative interstitial cystitis. J Urol. 1996;155(3):885–7.
68. Teichman JM, Moldwin R. The role of the bladder surface in interstitial cystitis/painful bladder syndrome. Can J Urol. 2007;14(4):3599–607.
69. Larsen MS, Mortensen S, Nordling J, Horn T. Quantifying mast cells in bladder pain syndrome by immunohistochemical analysis. BJU Int. 2008;102(2):204–7. discussion 207.
70. Hanno PM, Burks DA, Clemens JQ, et al. AUA guideline for the diagnosis and treatment of bladder pain syndrome. J Urol. 2011;185(6):2162–70.

Chapter 14
Urine Biomarkers and Bladder Pain Syndrome

Pierre Bouchelouche and Kirsten Bouchelouche

Introduction

Biomarkers are important tools in the diagnostic and therapeutic armamentarium. By definition a biomarker is a biological characteristic that is measured and evaluated objectively as an indicator of normal biological or pathogenic processes (a diagnostic biomarker), or a pharmacological response to therapeutic intervention (a therapeutic biomarker) [1]. Biomarkers may be any patient parameter that can be measured, for example, mRNA expression profiles, proteomic signatures, protein or lipid levels, imaging methods, or electrical signals. The best biomarkers are accurate, relatively noninvasive, and easy-to-perform tests that can be done at the bedside or in the outpatient setting. Biomarkers are useful as a diagnostic tool for identifying those patients with a disease, classifying, or grading the severity of disease in both laboratory and clinical settings. These tests involve a blood or spot urine specimen, can be measured serially, and have a fast turnaround. Most efforts had focused on discovering tissue and urinary biomarkers. Proper biomarker discovery requires detailed knowledge of the disease in question, including the definition, differential diagnosis, disease subsets, and local or systemic responses [2–4]. The lack of universally accepted clinical diagnostic criteria for bladder pain syndrome (BPS) affects all aspects of making progress in understanding this disease. Efforts continue to be made to find objective, specific findings to diagnose BPS. The development of sensitive and specific markers could assist in establishing an etiologic mechanism, generating definitive and reproducible diagnostic criteria, identifying patient subsets, and predicting treatment responses. This chapter focuses on urine biomarkers in BPS.

P. Bouchelouche, M.D. (✉) • K. Bouchelouche, M.D., DMSc.
Smooth Muscle Research Center, Department of Clinical Biochemistry, Koege Hospital,
University of Copenhagen, Copenhagen, Denmark
e-mail: pnb@regionsjaelland.dk

J. Nordling et al. (eds.), *Bladder Pain Syndrome: A Guide for Clinicians*,
DOI 10.1007/978-1-4419-6929-3_14, © Springer Science+Business Media New York 2013

Criteria for Biomarker Selection

Since BPS is a heterogeneous syndrome of pluricausal etiology, it is unlikely that a single biomarker can be identified which will serve to diagnose or exclude the entire spectrum of the disease. Many urine components decrease or increase in some BPS patients and may serve as objective BPS markers. Valid objective markers would be useful for several different purposes [5]:

- To diagnose some of the patients with BPS definitively.
- To identify subsets of patients with different BPS etiologies (high sensitivity and specificity), and to target them for focused research and specific treatments.
- To predict which BPS patients will respond to a specific treatment.
- To provide an objective outcome measurement for BPS treatment trials.

In addition, the biomarker assay needs to be reproducible in many laboratories and ideally the marker should be suitable for use in clinical diagnostic laboratories.

Candidate Biomarkers

The majority of all of the published studies on biomarkers for BPS have been on biomarkers isolated from urine (Table 14.1). Common for all these potential biomarkers for BPS, apart from APF, they have not been well characterized. More importantly the sensitivity/specificity values for BPS have not been studied [6]. Urine diagnostic test would be ideal because it is not invasive and urine is obtained easily. Because no one etiology has been identified as causative in BPS, there have been a myriad of biomarkers (more than two dozen) proposed for its diagnosis. Urine markers usually are biologic molecules found in the bladders of patients with BPS, but not in control subjects or vice versa.

Urine Anti-proliferative Factor and Growth Factors

It has been postulated that factors present in both normal urine and BPS patients' urine are capable of injuring the mucosa and causing increased mucosal permeability. Indirect evidence for a urinary cytotoxin in BPS was first reported by Clemmensen and colleagues in 1988 who demonstrated a toxic or allergic reaction in skin patch tests to a substance present in greater amounts in BPS patients' urine [7]. Parsons and Stein found BPS urine to result in higher cell death of cultured transitional cells than normal urine, suggesting a toxic compound in the urine of some BPS patients [8]. They identified heat-labile, cationic components of low molecular weight that bind to heparin, and that when sepa-

Table 14.1 Selected urinary markers reported in BPS

Urine marker	References
Antiproliferative and growth factors	
Antiproliferative factor (APF)	[10, 15, 16, 19]
Heparin-binding epidermal growth factor-like growth factor (HB-EGF)	[16, 17, 19]
Epidermal growth factor (EGF)	[17, 17, 19]
Insulin-like growth factor (IGF-1)	[17]
Insulin-like growth factor-binding protein (IGFBP-1)	[17]
Nerve growth factor (NGF)	[36, 74–76]
Markers related to urothel/mucus layer	
Glycosaminoglycans	[17, 22–24]
Glycoprotein-51	[20, 21, 25]
MUC-1 glycoprotein	[17]
Hyaluronic acid	[17, 24, 26]
Inflammatory mediators	
Histamine	[31, 37, 38, 51]
Methylhistamine and 1,4-MIAA	[17, 34, 37, 39, 51]
IL-6	[17, 19, 47–49, 51]
IL-8	[17, 19, 49]
IL-1	[17, 50]
IL-2	[49]
Eosinophil cationic protein (ECP)	[45]
Eosinophil protein X (EPX)	[46]
Leukotriene E_4 (LTE_4)	[46]
Substance P	[64, 70]
Major basic protein (MBP)	[33]
PGE_2, PGD_2, $PGF_{2\alpha}$, TNF-α, thromboxane B_2	[33, 47]
Marker of nitric oxide activity	
NO gas	[52–54]
NO synthase	[55–57]
c-GMP	[17, 19, 56]
Others	
Tamm–Horsfall protein	[82–84]
Tryptase	[35]

rated from the bulk of the urinary wastes are cytotoxic to urothelial cells as well as underlying smooth muscle cells [9].

Keay and associates [10] at the University of Maryland reported that urothelial cells of normal controls grow significantly more rapidly in culture than cells from BPS patients [10]. This led to the discovery that the urine of BPS patients specifically contains a factor, antiproliferative factor (APF), that inhibits primary bladder epithelial cell proliferation while simultaneously decreasing the amount of heparin-binding epidermal growth factor-like growth factor (HB-EGF) and increasing levels of epidermal growth factor (EGF) compared with urine from asymptomatic controls and patients with bacterial cystitis. The coexistence of these two processes impedes proper regeneration of damaged areas within the bladder and increases the risk of more injury or insult to occur. Furthermore, APF levels in the urine were found to discriminate between patients with BPS versus those with chronic pelvic pain syndrome or non-bacterial cystitis [11]. The APF appeared to be a low-molecular-weight (<10,000 Da), heat-stable, trypsin-sensitive factor [10]. Later, APF has been purified and proved to be a frizzled eight protein produced by bladder uroepithelial cells of BPS patients [12]. Although some data suggest that the presence of APF may be indicative of BPS, not enough evidence supports the use of APF as a viable definitive diagnostic tool.

Other urine factors that may reflect epithelial abnormalities in the urinary bladder include EGF, HB-EGF, insulin-like growth factor (IGF), and nerve growth factor (NGF). Freeman and colleagues were the first to suggest a physiologic role for HB-EGF in the regulation of urothelial proliferation and regeneration subsequent to mucosal injury [13]. Recent studies have demonstrated that these urine growth factors were significantly different between BPS patients, asymptomatic controls, and patients with acute bacterial cystitis [10, 14, 15]. Furthermore, APF, EGF, and HB-EGF have been shown to be good biomarkers for both ulcerative and nonulcerative BPS [16]. A recent comparative study of 13 different urine markers for BPS performed in a blinded manner in several different laboratories indicated that, of these urine markers, differences in APF activity as well as in levels of HB-EGF and EGF between BPS patients and asymptomatic controls were of greatest significance [17]. However, these same authors have compared these urine markers with bladder biopsy findings [18]. Interestingly, these urine markers (APF, EGF, HB-EGF) did not associate with biopsy findings [18, 19].

APF appeared to be as an ideal candidate for a urine biomarker for symptomatic BPS. However, since its discovery in 1999, findings have not been replicated in other independent laboratories and the assay has to be developed for use in a clinical laboratory before it becomes a standard clinical biomarker. In 2003 Keay et al. wrote that the test for APF activity is currently in the process of undergoing confirmation and possible commercial availability [6]. Unfortunately, these initial promising statements have never been performed.

Urine Glycoconjugates GP51, GAG, MUC-1 Glycoprotein, and Hyaluronic Acid

Markers that may reflect epithelial abnormalities in the urinary bladder include the glycoprotein GP51, Glycosaminoglycans (GAGs), hyaluronic acid, and epitectin. The assumption that a change in urothelial permeability, due to aberrations in bladder surface mucin, can be a pathophysiological factor in patients with BPS led Moskowitz and colleagues to focus on the glycoprotein GP-51, a 51 kDa glycoprotein component of the urothelial mucin lining which is a heterogeneous substance composed of proteoglycans, glycosaminoglycans, and glycoproteins [20]. GP-51 is produced throughout the urinary system. GP-51, a glycoprotein in the urothelium, has been shown to be decreased in bladder biopsies from BPS patients [20]. However, this invasive procedure was not a practical diagnostic tool. Subsequently, these authors examined GP-51 levels in urine specimens from BPS patients and normal controls. Byrne et al. demonstrated significant reduction in urinary excretion of GP51 in BPS patients compared with age-matched normal controls or patients with other urinary tract diseases (including bacterial cystitis, renal calculi, detrusor hyperreflexia, and eosinophilic cystitis [21]). Reduction in GP51 excretion is the strongest evidence so far reported which demonstrates that a specific molecular deficiency in the GAG layer of the bladder exists in BPS. Particularly impressive was how much lower the urinary GP51-to-creatinine ratios were in BPS patients who met the National Institute for Diabetes and Digestive and Kidney Diseases diagnostic criteria than in normal and pathological controls. This finding, if substantiated in larger numbers, particularly because the test can be performed reliably on spot urine, could be valuable in the diagnosis and classification of this syndrome. Additionally, this test may provide a useful marker to monitor therapeutic response and may even serve as a surrogate end point in testing therapies. Finally, if restoration of GP51 excretion to normal is associated with loss of symptoms, this molecule could be the target of genetic, molecular, and intravesical therapeutic strategies. Although, these initial promising studies regarding GP51 specificity for BPS additional studies have not been done on this marker. Thus, considerable additional studies will be required before this measurement becomes clinically useful.

GAG alterations in the urine of patients with BPS have been reported [22, 23]. Hurst et al. originally reported that total GAGs were decreased in BPS urine as compared with healthy subjects [23]. Urinary GAG excretion was found to be elevated significantly in patients with BPS as compared to healthy subjects. In a blinded comparative study, Erickson et al. reported that urine GAG excretion did not differ significantly between these two groups [17]. Another study indicated that the ratio of total to sulfated urine GAGs may be more useful for distinguishing BPS patients from normal controls [24].

In two different reports, BPS urine had significantly decreased MUC-1 glycoprotein (epitectin) [25] or had increased urine hyaluronic acid (HA) [24, 26]. Later studies using different assay methods failed to confirm these previous reports [17]. In conclusion, GAGs or HA may be useful markers in new untreated patients using more reliable assay methods.

Urine Inflammatory Mediators

A number of studies have implicated neuroinflammatory mechanisms, including mast cells and their products with BPS. Mast cells have been considered an important part of the pathogenesis of BPS [27, 28], and their products have been considered potential indicators of the disease first suggested by Simmons in 1950s [29]. The most unusual characteristic in BPS is the activation of bladder mast cells shown by ultrastructural criteria [30] and confirmed by increased urinary levels of mast cell products such as histamine and methylhistamine [31–33], a metabolite of histamine (1,4-MIAA) [34], and the unique mast cell marker tryptase [35, 36] in the urine of patients with BPS. In contrast, the histamine content of either spot or 24-h urine was not different between control and BPS patients [37, 38]. Histamine [38] and methylhistamine [39] were also either elevated or normal in BPS following bladder hydrodistension.

Leukotriene E_4 (LTE_4), the end product of cysteinyl containing leukotrienes, and eosinophil protein X (EPX), eosinophil cationic protein (ECP), and eosinophil peroxidase (EPO) are important mediators of inflammatory diseases. Bladder urothelium and lamina propria of BPS patients contain inflammatory cells including mast cells and eosinophils [40]. The factors responsible for migration and proliferation of these cells in BPS are unknown. Both may be attracted to the bladder wall by means of chemotactic cytokines. Leukotriene D_4, a product of mast cells, has also been shown to attract eosinophils as well [41].

The eosinophil is also a potent inflammatory cell that may release 4 well-characterized cytotoxic proteins, i.e., EPX, ECP, EPO, and major basic protein (MBP) in addition to LTC_4 and platelet-activating factor [42]. Furthermore, eosinophils in the same way as mast cells may release cytokines and IL-8 [43]. Eosinophils and mast cells are the major source of LTE_4 in urine [44]. Increased urinary ECP has been detected in the urine of patients with BPS [45]. BPS patients who have detrusor mastocytosis were shown to have increased urinary LTE_4 and EPX as compared with normal controls [46]. These substances may be useful for assessing the grade of activation of mast cells and eosinophils in patients with BPS and/or for confirming the diagnosis. Additional studies to determine the specificity of these findings for BPS are needed.

Urine Cytokines

Cytokines are small cell-signaling protein molecules that are secreted by numerous cells of the immune system and are a category of signaling molecules used extensively in intercellular communication. Increased urinary levels of cytokines reflect inflammation of the urinary bladder. In urine from BPS patients increased levels of several cytokines have been documented but the results are conflicting [5, 47–49]. Among the cytokines, IL-2, IL-6, and IL-8 were increased in some patients with BPS [17, 47–49] whereas normal levels were found for IL-1, IL-4, IL-10, IL-12, TNF-α, and interferon-γ [17, 49, 50]. Only recently, a combination of IL-6 and methylhistamine has been proposed as a sensitive and specific marker for BPS, with a sensitivity of 70 % and specificity of 72.4 % [51]. Increased urinary excretion of the CXC chemokine IL-8 has been found in some studies but not in others [17, 49]. The strongest association is a positive association between urine IL-8 levels and bladder mast cell count in bladder biopsies from patients with BPS [19].

Urine Markers of Nitric Oxide Activity

A role for nitric oxide (NO) has been suggested in inflammation and host defense. During inflammation NO is produced from the amino acid L-arginine by the enzymatic action of nitric oxide synthase (NOS) which in turn causes an increase in cyclic GMP by activating guanylyl cyclase. In studies where NO levels were measured directly in the urinary bladder increased levels of NO were demonstrated in infectious and noninfectious cystitis [52, 53]. Nitric oxide has also been used to distinguish patients with ulcerative BPS from patients with nonulcerative BPS [54]. Furthermore, long-term oral administration of L-arginine increases nitric oxide-related enzymes and metabolites in the urine of patients with interstitial cystitis, which is associated with a decrease in interstitial cystitis-related symptoms [55]. Urinary levels of NO synthase activity were found to be decreased in BPS patients and increased with urinary tract infections [56]. The increased levels of endogenously formed nitric oxide in patients with BPS correspond to increased inducible NOS mRNA expression and protein levels in these patients [57]. Furthermore, inducible NOS was found to be localized to the urothelium but it was also found in macrophages in the bladder mucosa [57]. Likewise, the urinary levels of cGMP, the end product caused by NO, were decreased in BPS patients [17, 56]. Whether high levels of endogenously formed nitric oxide are a part of the pathogenesis in BPS and whether it has a protective or damaging role remain to be elucidated.

Substance P

Neurogenic inflammation is a process by which sensory nerves may secrete inflammatory mediators, resulting in hyperalgesia and inflammation of BPS and research has demonstrated neurobiological changes in BPS manifested by urothelial dysfunction, sensory nerve-upregulation, mast cell activation, neurogenic inflammation, and spinal cord “wind-up” [58, 59]. Substance P, a short-chain peptide, is a central component of this process [60]. Substance P is an inflammatory mediator that functions as a nociceptive neurotransmitter in the central and peripheral nervous system. When released by peripheral nerves, substance P causes an inflammatory cascade to occur, resulting in such processes as mast cell degranulation and activation of nearby nerve terminals. SP has been implicated in the pathophysiology of pain and has been shown to trigger mast cell secretion [61]. Several studies support this theory, having found increased number of substance P-containing nerves and increased expression of SP receptor-encoding mRNA in bladder biopsies from patients with BPS [61, 62]. The increased number of C-fibers and increased amount of substance P found in IC patients also contribute to the inflammation and pain associated with this condition [61, 63]. In addition, substance P has been found in the urine of women with BPS, with increased concentrations dependent on the severity of pain [64]. Furthermore, urinary SP concentration correlates with urinary frequency and urgency in BPS patients treated with DMSO [65]. However, a recent study revealed no significant increase in substance P in women with BPS when compared to a control group [66], but the control group consisted of women who suffered from symptoms of stress incontinence. Another study found that the number of neurons positive for SP was not significantly different between BPS and controls [67].

Nerve Growth Factor

NGF is a small secreted protein that induces the differentiation and survival of particular target neurons [68]. NGF has also attracted considerable attention as a key player in the link between inflammation and altered pain signaling [68]. NGF is expressed widely in various cells, including urothelial cells, smooth muscle cells, and mast cells, and can activate mast cells to degranulate and proliferate [68]. In patients with BPS increased levels of NGF have been detected in the urine [36, 69–71]. Increased expression of NGF is also present in bladder biopsies from women with BPS [72]. However, also other clinical and experimental reports indicate a direct link between increased levels of NGF in bladder tissue and urine and painful inflammatory conditions in the lower urinary tract, such as bladder outlet obstruction, overactive bladder, BPS, and chronic prostatitis [36, 69–71]. Thus, NGF has been suggested to play a role in urinary bladder dysfunction by mediating inflammation, as well as morphological and functional changes, in sensory and sympathetic neurons innervating the urinary bladder [73].

Future studies are needed to further examine the significance of urinary NGF levels in the pathogenesis of a variety of urologic diseases and whether NGF could be used as a diagnostic or a prognostic marker for specific urologic diseases.

Tamm–Horsfall Protein

Tamm–Horsfall protein (THP) is a high-molecular-weight glycoprotein discovered by Tamm and Horsfall [74]. THP is the most abundant protein in urine of healthy individuals [75]. THP is normally synthesized by thick ascending limb of loop of Henle. THP may accumulate in renal parenchyma, perirenal soft tissue, or bladder with pathologic conditions. THP is deposited in areas of necrosis, inflammation, fibrinous exudates, and ulcer. THP-deficient mice were shown to have difficulty clearing bacteria and may be a host defense factor against bacterial cystitis [76, 77]. Urinary THP protein levels have been investigated in BPS patients and controls [77]. Urinary THP was found to be significantly greater compared with controls [77]. THP is qualitatively different in patients with BPS compared to controls [78]. Abnormal glycosylation of THP in patients with BPS [78] was confirmed by the same research group a couple of years later [79]. Whether THP has a role in the pathophysiology of BPS remains to be elucidated.

Miscellaneous

Other urinary cellular markers of BPS, including tryptase [35, 36], IL-2 inhibitor [80], PGE_2 [33], kallikrein [81], IL-1β [50], IL-2 [49], MBP [33], cortisol [82], autoantibodies [83], and norepinephrine [84], have also been reported although their specificity for BPS is uncertain.

Conclusion and Future Directions in Research

Research is needed. The goal is to develop a simple, noninvasive diagnostic test for BPS. In the future, research on BPS will therefore most likely involve urinary markers which undoubtedly prove to be a valuable tool for determining the diagnosis of BPS in the female population, identifying specific subsets of BPS patients, and differentiating patients with incontinence/overactive bladder syndrome from patients with BPS. Among all the published markers APF appears to be specific to BPS which places APF as the best candidate to date for a biomarker for symptomatic BPS. However, the test has only been evaluated in NIDDK cases and the test requires confirmation in other laboratories around the world. In conclusion, the role of urinary markers remains to be elucidated in large prospective, multi-institutional studies.

References

1. Dimitrakov J. A road map to biomarker discovery and validation in urological chronic pelvic pain syndrome. J Urol. 2008;179:1660–1.
2. Biomarkes Definitions Working Group. Biomarkers and surrogate endpoints: preferred definitions and conceptual framework. Clin Pharmacol Ther. 2001;69:89–95.
3. Hewitt SM, Dear J, Star RA. Discovery of protein biomarkers for renal diseases. J Am Soc Nephrol. 2004;15:1677–89.
4. Holliday EG, Scott RJ, Attia J. Evidence-based medicine in the era of biomarkers: teaching a new dog old tricks? Clin Pharmacol Ther. 2010;88:740–2.
5. Erickson DR. Urine markers of interstitial cystitis. Urology. 2001;57:15–21.
6. Keay S, Takeda M, Tamaki M, Hanno P. Current and future directions in diagnostic markers in interstitial cystitis. Int J Urol. 2003;10(Suppl):S27–30.
7. Clemmensen OJ, Lose G, Holm-Bentzen M, Colstrup H. Skin reactions to urine in patients with interstitial cystitis. Urology. 1988;32:17–20.
8. Parsons CL, Stein P. Role of toxic urine in interstitial cystitis. J Urol. 1990;143:373A.
9. Parsons CL, Bautista SL, Stein PC, Zupkas P. Cyto-injury factors in urine: a possible mechanism for the development of interstitial cystitis. J Urol. 2000;164:1381–4.
10. Keay S, Zhang CO, Trifillis AL, Hise MK, Hebel JR, Jacobs SC, Warren JW. Decreased 3H-thymidine incorporation by human bladder epithelial cells following exposure to urine from interstitial cystitis patients. J Urol. 1996;156:2073–8.

11. Keay S, Zhang CO, Chai T, Warren J, Koch K, Grkovic D, Colville H, Alexander R. Antiproliferative factor, heparin-binding epidermal growth factor-like growth factor, and epidermal growth factor in men with interstitial cystitis versus chronic pelvic pain syndrome. Urology. 2004;63:22–6.
12. Keay SK, Szekely Z, Conrads TP, Veenstra TD, Barchi Jr JJ, Zhang CO, Koch KR, Michejda CJ. An antiproliferative factor from interstitial cystitis patients is a frizzled 8 protein-related sialoglycopeptide. Proc Natl Acad Sci U S A. 2004;101:11803–8.
13. Freeman MR, Yoo JJ, Raab G, Soker S, Adam RM, Schneck FX, Renshaw AA, Klagsbrun M, Atala A. Heparin-binding EGF-like growth factor is an autocrine growth factor for human urothelial cells and is synthesized by epithelial and smooth muscle cells in the human bladder. J Clin Invest. 1997;99:1028–36.
14. Keay S, Zhang CO, Kagen DI, Hise MK, Jacobs SC, Hebel JR, Gordon D, Whitmore K, Bodison S, Warren JW. Concentrations of specific epithelial growth factors in the urine of interstitial cystitis patients and controls. J Urol. 1997;158:1983–8.
15. Keay S, Kleinberg M, Zhang CO, Hise MK, Warren JW. Bladder epithelial cells from patients with interstitial cystitis produce an inhibitor of heparin-binding epidermal growth factor-like growth factor production. J Urol. 2000;164:2112–8.
16. Zhang CO, Li ZL, Kong CZ. APF, HB-EGF, and EGF biomarkers in patients with ulcerative vs. non-ulcerative interstitial cystitis. BMC Urol. 2005;5:7.
17. Erickson DR, Xie SX, Bhavanandan VP, Wheeler MA, Hurst RE, Demers LM, Kushner L, Keay SK. A comparison of multiple urine markers for interstitial cystitis. J Urol. 2002;167:2461–9.
18. Erickson DR, Tomaszewski JE, Kunselman AR, Bentley CM, Peters KM, Rovner ES, Demers LM, Wheeler MA, Keay SK. Do the National Institute of Diabetes and Digestive and Kidney Diseases cystoscopic criteria associate with other clinical and objective features of interstitial cystitis? J Urol. 2005;173:93–7.
19. Erickson DR, Tomaszewski JE, Kunselman AR, Stetter CM, Peters KM, Rovner ES, Demers LM, Wheeler MA, Keay SK. Urine markers do not predict biopsy findings or presence of bladder ulcers in interstitial cystitis/painful bladder syndrome. J Urol. 2008;179:1850–6.
20. Moskowitz MO, Byrne DS, Callahan HJ, Parsons CL, Valderrama E, Moldwin RM. Decreased expression of a glycoprotein component of bladder surface mucin (GP1) in interstitial cystitis. J Urol. 1994;151:343–5.
21. Byrne DS, Sedor JF, Estojak J, Fitzpatrick KJ, Chiura AN, Mulholland SG. The urinary glycoprotein GP51 as a clinical marker for interstitial cystitis. J Urol. 1999;161:1786–90.
22. Akcay T, Konukoglu D. Glycosaminoglycans excretion in interstitial cystitis. Int Urol Nephrol. 1999;31:431–5.
23. Hurst RE, Parsons CL, Roy JB, Young JL. Urinary glycosaminoglycan excretion as a laboratory marker in the diagnosis of interstitial cystitis. J Urol. 1993;149:31–5.
24. Wei DC, Politano VA, Selzer MG, Lokeshwar VB. The association of elevated urinary total to sulfated glycosaminoglycan ratio and high molecular mass hyaluronic acid with interstitial cystitis. J Urol. 2000;163:1577–83.
25. Erickson DR, Mast S, Ordille S, Bhavanandan VP. Urinary epitectin (MUC-1 glycoprotein) in the menstrual cycle and interstitial cystitis. J Urol. 1996;156:938–42.
26. Erickson DR, Sheykhnazari M, Ordille S, Bhavanandan VP. Increased urinary hyaluronic acid and interstitial cystitis. J Urol. 1998;160:1282–4.
27. Sant GR, Kempuraj D, Marchand JE, Theoharides TC. The mast cell in interstitial cystitis: role in pathophysiology and pathogenesis. Urology. 2007;69:34–40.
28. Theoharides TC, Kempuraj D, Sant GR. Mast cell involvement in interstitial cystitis: a review of human and experimental evidence. Urology. 2001;57:47–55.
29. Simmons JL, Bunce PL. On the use of an antihistamine in the treatment of interstitial cystitis. Am Surg. 1958;24:664–7.
30. Theoharides TC, Sant GR, El Mansoury M, Letourneau R, Ucci Jr AA, Meares Jr EM. Activation of bladder mast cells in interstitial cystitis: a light and electron microscopic study. J Urol. 1995;153:629–36.

31. Enerback L, Fall M, Aldenborg F. Histamine and mucosal mast cells in interstitial cystitis. Agents Actions. 1989;27:113–6.
32. Kastrup J, Hald T, Larsen S, Nielsen VG. Histamine content and mast cell count of detrusor muscle in patients with interstitial cystitis and other types of chronic cystitis. Br J Urol. 1983;55:495–500.
33. Lynes WL, Flynn SD, Shortliffe LD, Lemmers M, Zipser R, Roberts LJ, Stamey TA. Mast cell involvement in interstitial cystitis. J Urol. 1987;138:746–52.
34. Holm-Bentzen M, Sondergaard I, Hald T. Urinary excretion of a metabolite of histamine (1,4-methyl-imidazole-acetic-acid) in painful bladder disease. Br J Urol. 1987;59:230–3.
35. Boucher W, El Mansoury M, Pang X, Sant GR, Theoharides TC. Elevated mast cell tryptase in the urine of patients with interstitial cystitis. Br J Urol. 1995;76:94–100.
36. Okragly AJ, Niles AL, Saban R, Schmidt D, Hoffman RL, Warner TF, Moon TD, Uehling DT, Haak-Frendscho M. Elevated tryptase, nerve growth factor, neurotrophin-3 and glial cell line-derived neurotrophic factor levels in the urine of interstitial cystitis and bladder cancer patients. J Urol. 1999;161:438–41.
37. El Mansoury M, Boucher W, Sant GR, Theoharides TC. Increased urine histamine and methylhistamine in interstitial cystitis. J Urol. 1994;152:350–3.
38. Yun SK, Laub DJ, Weese DL, Lad PM, Leach GE, Zimmern PE. Stimulated release of urine histamine in interstitial cystitis. J Urol. 1992;148:1145–8.
39. Erickson DR, Kunselman AR, Bentley CM, Peters KM, Rovner ES, Demers LM, Tomaszewski JE. Is urine methylhistamine a useful marker for interstitial cystitis? J Urol. 2004;172:2256–60.
40. Johansson SL, Fall M. Clinical features and spectrum of light microscopic changes in interstitial cystitis. J Urol. 1990;143:1118–24.
41. Spada CS, Krauss AH, Nieves AL, Woodward DF. Effects of leukotrienes B4 (LTB4) and D4 (LTD4) on motility of isolated normodense human eosinophils and neutrophils. Adv Exp Med Biol. 1997;400B:699–706.
42. Venge P. The human eosinophil in inflammation. Agents Actions. 1990;29:122–6.
43. Desreumaux P, Nutten S, Colombel JF. Activated eosinophils in inflammatory bowel disease: do they matter? Am J Gastroenterol. 1999;94:3396–8.
44. Keppler D, Muller M, Klunemann C, Guhlmann A, Krauss K, Muller J, Berger U, Leier I, Mayatepek E. Transport and in vivo elimination of cysteinyl leukotrienes. Adv Enzyme Regul. 1992;32:107–16.
45. Lose G, Frandsen B, Holm-Bentzen M, Larsen S, Jacobsen F. Urine eosinophil cationic protein in painful bladder disease. Br J Urol. 1987;60:39–42.
46. Bouchelouche K, Kristensen B, Nordling J, Horn T, Bouchelouche P. Increased urinary leukotriene E4 and eosinophil protein X excretion in patients with interstitial cystitis. J Urol. 2001;166:2121–5.
47. Felsen D, Frye S, Trimble LA, Bavendam TG, Parsons CL, Sim Y, Vaughan Jr ED. Inflammatory mediator profile in urine and bladder wash fluid of patients with interstitial cystitis. J Urol. 1994;152:355–61.
48. Lotz M, Villiger P, Hugli T, Koziol J, Zuraw BL. Interleukin-6 and interstitial cystitis. J Urol. 1994;152:869–73.
49. Peters KM, Diokno AC, Steinert BW. Preliminary study on urinary cytokine levels in interstitial cystitis: does intravesical bacille Calmette-Guerin treat interstitial cystitis by altering the immune profile in the bladder? Urology. 1999;54:450–3.
50. Martins SM, Darlin DJ, Lad PM, Zimmern PE. Interleukin-1B: a clinically relevant urinary marker. J Urol. 1994;151:1198–201.
51. Lamale LM, Lutgendorf SK, Zimmerman MB, Kreder KJ. Interleukin-6, histamine, and methylhistamine as diagnostic markers for interstitial cystitis. Urology. 2006;68:702–6.
52. Ehren I, Hosseini A, Lundberg JO, Wiklund NP. Nitric oxide: a useful gas in the detection of lower urinary tract inflammation. J Urol. 1999;162:327–9.

53. Lundberg JO, Ehren I, Jansson O, Adolfsson J, Lundberg JM, Weitzberg E, Alving K, Wiklund NP. Elevated nitric oxide in the urinary bladder in infectious and noninfectious cystitis. Urology. 1996;48:700–2.
54. Logadottir YR, Ehren I, Fall M, Wiklund NP, Peeker R, Hanno PM. Intravesical nitric oxide production discriminates between classic and nonulcer interstitial cystitis. J Urol. 2004;171:1148–50.
55. Wheeler MA, Smith SD, Saito N, Foster Jr HE, Weiss RM. Effect of long-term oral L-arginine on the nitric oxide synthase pathway in the urine from patients with interstitial cystitis. J Urol. 1997;158:2045–50.
56. Smith SD, Wheeler MA, Foster Jr HE, Weiss RM. Urinary nitric oxide synthase activity and cyclic GMP levels are decreased with interstitial cystitis and increased with urinary tract infections. J Urol. 1996;155:1432–5.
57. Koskela LR, Thiel T, Ehren I, De Verdier PJ, Wiklund NP. Localization and expression of inducible nitric oxide synthase in biopsies from patients with interstitial cystitis. J Urol. 2008;180:737–41.
58. Sant GR. Etiology, pathogenesis, and diagnosis of interstitial cystitis. Rev Urol. 2002;4 Suppl 1:S9–S15.
59. Theoharides TC, Pang X, Letourneau R, Sant GR. Interstitial cystitis: a neuroimmunoendocrine disorder. Ann N Y Acad Sci. 1998;840:619–34.
60. Richardson JD, Vasko MR. Cellular mechanisms of neurogenic inflammation. J Pharmacol Exp Ther. 2002;302:839–45.
61. Pang X, Marchand J, Sant GR, Kream RM, Theoharides TC. Increased number of substance P positive nerve fibres in interstitial cystitis. Br J Urol. 1995;75:744–50.
62. Marchand JE, Sant GR, Kream RM. Increased expression of substance P receptor-encoding mRNA in bladder biopsies from patients with interstitial cystitis. Br J Urol. 1998;81:224–8.
63. Burkman RT. Chronic pelvic pain of bladder origin: epidemiology, pathogenesis and quality of life. J Reprod Med. 2004;49:225–9.
64. Chen Y, Varghese R, Lehrer J, Tillem S, Moldwin R, Kusner L. Urinary substance P is elevated in women with interstitial cystitis. J Urol. 1999;161(4):26.
65. Kushner L, Chiu PY, Brettschneider N, Lipstein A, Eisenberg E, Rofeim O, Moldwin R. Urinary substance P concentration correlates with urinary frequency and urgency in interstitial cystitis patients treated with intravesical dimethyl sulfoxide and not intravesical anesthetic cocktail. Urology. 2001;57:129.
66. Campbell DJ, Tenis N, Rosamilia A, Clements JA, Dwyer PL. Urinary levels of substance P and its metabolites are not increased in interstitial cystitis. BJU Int. 2001;87:35–8.
67. Hohenfellner M, Nunes L, Schmidt RA, Lampel A, Thuroff JW, Tanagho EA. Interstitial cystitis: increased sympathetic innervation and related neuropeptide synthesis. J Urol. 1992;147:587–91.
68. Kuo HC, Liu HT, Chancellor MB. Can urinary nerve growth factor be a biomarker for overactive bladder? Rev Urol. 2010;12:e69–77.
69. Jacobs BL, Smaldone MC, Tyagi V, Philips BJ, Jackman SV, Leng WW, Tyagi P. Increased nerve growth factor in neurogenic overactive bladder and interstitial cystitis patients. Can J Urol. 2010;17:4989–94.
70. Liu HT, Tyagi P, Chancellor MB, Kuo HC. Urinary nerve growth factor level is increased in patients with interstitial cystitis/bladder pain syndrome and decreased in responders to treatment. BJU Int. 2009;104:1476–81.
71. Liu HT, Tyagi P, Chancellor MB, Kuo HC. Urinary nerve growth factor but not prostaglandin E2 increases in patients with interstitial cystitis/bladder pain syndrome and detrusor overactivity. BJU Int. 2010;106:1681–5.
72. Lowe EM, Anand P, Terenghi G, Williams-Chestnut RE, Sinicropi DV, Osborne JL. Increased nerve growth factor levels in the urinary bladder of women with idiopathic sensory urgency and interstitial cystitis. Br J Urol. 1997;79:572–7.

73. Schnegelsberg B, Sun TT, Cain G, Bhattacharya A, Nunn PA, Ford AP, Vizzard MA, Cockayne DA. Overexpression of NGF in mouse urothelium leads to neuronal hyperinnervation, pelvic sensitivity, and changes in urinary bladder function. Am J Physiol Regul Integr Comp Physiol. 2010;298:R534–R47.
74. Tamm I, Horsefall Jr FL. A mucoprotein derived from human urine which reacts with influenza, mumps, and Newcastle disease viruses. J Exp Med. 1952;95:71–97.
75. Raffi HS, Bates Jr JM, Laszik Z, Kumar S. Tamm–Horsfall protein acts as a general host-defense factor against bacterial cystitis. Am J Nephrol. 2005;25:570–8.
76. Raffi HS, Bates Jr JM, Laszik Z, Kumar S. Tamm–horsfall protein protects against urinary tract infection by proteus mirabilis. J Urol. 2009;181:2332–8.
77. Bade JJ, Marrink J, Karrenbeld A, van der WL, Mensink HJ. Increased urinary levels of Tamm–Horsfall glycoprotein suggest a systemic etiology of interstitial cystitis. J Urol. 1996;156:943–6.
78. Parsons CL, Stein P, Zupkas P, Chenoweth M, Argade SP, Proctor JG, Datta A, Trotter RN. Defective Tamm–Horsfall protein in patients with interstitial cystitis. J Urol. 2007;178:2665–70.
79. Argade SP, Vanichsarn C, Chenoweth M, Parsons CL. Abnormal glycosylation of Tamm–Horsfall protein in patients with interstitial cystitis. BJU Int. 2009;103:1085–9.
80. Shingleton WB, Fleischmann J. Urinary interleukin-2 inhibitor and the voiding symptoms in women patients with interstitial cystitis. Semin Urol. 1991;9:120–3.
81. Zuraw BL, Sugimoto S, Parsons CL, Hugli T, Lotz M, Koziol J. Activation of urinary kallikrein in patients with interstitial cystitis. J Urol. 1994;152:874–8.
82. Lutgendorf SK, Kreder KJ, Rothrock NE, Hoffman A, Kirschbaum C, Sternberg EM, Zimmerman MB, Ratliff TL. Diurnal cortisol variations and symptoms in patients with interstitial cystitis. J Urol. 2002;167:1338–43.
83. Keay S, Zhang CO, Trifillis AL, Hebel JR, Jacobs SC, Warren JW. Urine autoantibodies in interstitial cystitis. J Urol. 1997;157:1083–7.
84. Stein PC, Torri A, Parsons CL. Elevated urinary norepinephrine in interstitial cystitis. Urology. 1999;53:1140–3.

Chapter 15
Cystoscopy and Hydrodistension in the Diagnosis of Bladder Pain Syndrome

Andrey Zaytsev and Magnus Fall

Introduction

Skene [1] and Hunner [2] are the great pioneers in interstitial cystitis (IC) history. In a disease with disabling bladder symptoms Skene described morphologic changes: destruction of the mucous membrane with extension to the bladder muscle and Hunner peculiar cystoscopic bladder wall changes. For many decades, the understanding of the disease was that of Skene and Hunner. In 1978 Messing and Stamey [3] presented postdistension submucosal petechial bleedings as another cardinal sign, subdividing the disease into an early and a classic (Hunner) form, with possible transition of the first into the other. It was emphasized, though, that the two presentations rather represent separate entities [4]. The two objective endoscopic features were incorporated in the NIDDK criteria together with symptom criteria and a number of exclusions [5], now serving as the established standard for years. Subsequently, the NIDDK criteria were claimed to be too restrictive to be used in clinical practice. When evaluating the National Institutes of Health Interstitial Cystitis Database study, 60% of patients with a clinical diagnosis of IC were found not to fulfil the NIDDK criteria [6]. Obviously at this stage, definitions had changed with less emphasis on objective criteria, and cystoscopy and bladder distension was just an optional measure. Today, not least owing to the activities of the International Society for the Study of Bladder Pain Syndrome (European Society for the Study of

A. Zaytsev, M.D., Ph.D. (✉)
Department of Urology, Moscow State Medical Stomatological University, Vucheticha st., 21, Moscow City Hospital No50, 127206 Moscow, Russian Federation
e-mail: zaitcevandrew@mail.ru

M. Fall, M.D., Ph.D.
Department of Urology, Institute of Clinical Sciences, Sahlgrens Academy at University of Gothenburg, Göteborg, Sweden

J. Nordling et al. (eds.), *Bladder Pain Syndrome: A Guide for Clinicians*, 219
DOI 10.1007/978-1-4419-6929-3_15, © Springer Science+Business Media New York 2013

Interstitial Cystitis, ESSIC), we see a paradigm shift; objective parameters attach greater importance and the value of endoscopy is again upgraded. Herein, we describe techniques and essential findings in the endoscopic diagnosis of bladder pain syndrome (BPS).

Techniques

Local Versus General Anesthesia

To allow an accurate diagnosis, cystoscopy should be performed during anesthesia since sufficient distention is required to visualize lesions characteristic of BPS. Still, cystoscopy using local anesthesia should not be disregarded. Should the communicable patient tolerate several hundred milliliters of fluid in the bladder she probably does not have BPS. Typically, the patient can accept filling with only a very limited volume, irrespective of the true bladder capacity during anesthesia. At the initial office urethrocystoscopy the urethra is examined as to mucosa and caliber. At this stage, palpation allows determination of local tenderness either over the bladder, maybe unilaterally (as may be experienced in unilateral Hunner lesion), or over the urethra, or both. Likewise, graded description of tenderness at examination of the genitalia and the various components of the pelvic floor can be established. Confusable diseases like tumors, stones, inflammations, and metaplasias other than those associated with BPS can be excluded. In the absence of Hunner lesions or scarring, the bladder should have a normal appearance [7, 8]. The presence of submucosal petechial bleedings, the so-called glomerulations, has until now been regarded as one of the endoscopic hallmarks of the disease, present after the bladder has been filled to capacity [3, 9]. Cystoscopy performed under local anesthesia may not reveal the presence or the true extent of glomerulations.

Distension Technique

The use of a rigid cystoscope is preferred to allow rapid rinsing of the bladder, should bleeding occur. General or regional (spinal or epidural) anesthesia is equally useful, the choice depending on the organization of care, ambulatory, or inpatient. Diagnostic hydrodistension is performed using the cystoscopy irrigation fluid. As a standard Cystosol has been suggested, various fluids have varying chemical composition that can influence the result [10]. A superimposed hydrostatic pressure of about 80 cm H_2O above the level of the patient's bladder is applied by increasing the height of the fluid bag, inflow supervised by the use of a dripping chamber [10]. The fluid is allowed to run into the bladder until it stops spontaneously at capacity, as observed when checking the dripping chamber. The intravesical volume is noted when evacuating the bladder. The maximum bladder capacity is often reduced in the classic type of BPS, whereas it is normal or only slightly reduced in the nonulcer variety [11, 12]. The bladder is refilled to approximately 20–50% of capacity and again inspected for lesions and hemorrhages, which will not be conspicuous until the bladder is filled for a second time. The changes typically involve the dome, posterior, and lateral walls of the bladder and spare the trigone.

It is important to note any changes of the bladder mucosa during filling already from the early phase and on. When inflow stops, distension is maintained for approximately 3 min [10]. In the female, especially when regional anesthesia is used, leakage around the cystoscope may occur. To get reproducible results, such leakage is easily prevented by manual compression around the urethra, applying pressure on the anterior vaginal wall on either side of the cystoscope. When there are typical mucosal changes, there is bleeding into the cystoscopy fluid ruining postdistension visibility. By repeated rinsing, clear vision is restored and postdistension changes can be detected. Those findings are the essential ones to note. It should be remembered that the findings are primarily diagnostic and they frequently do not parallel the type or severity of symptoms or the subsequent response to treatment [8, 13, 14].

The bladder should not be "hydrodilated" by syringe-filling or by prolonging filling after the bladder capacity is reached. After the diagnostic examination, i.e., distension followed by rinsing, refilling, and observation, the use of anesthesia further offers the opportunity to carry out a therapeutic distension as well.

Essential Findings

Hunner Lesions

The affirmation of Hunner's lesions is difficult or sometimes even impossible if cystoscopy is performed without hydrodistension. Even with hydrodistension, Hunner's lesions are likely to be reliably detected only by trained urologists; biopsy may be necessary to confirm that it is such a lesion and to exclude carcinoma in situ.

One important misconception caused by its name is that the so-called Hunner's ulcer is a chronic ulcer, while it is rather a distinctive inflammatory lesion with characteristic central fragility, presenting a deep rupture through the mucosa and submucosa when provoked by bladder distension. The word "ulcer" suggests that it can be seen as an ulcer at cystoscopy without hydrodistension which is misleading. Consequently, the name Hunner's ulcer was replaced by Hunner's lesion by the ESSIC [9]. In the ESSIC documents the following definition by M. Fall was accepted: "The Hunner's lesion typically presents as a circumscript, reddened mucosal area with small vessels radiating towards a central scar, with a fibrin deposit or coagulum attached to this area. This site ruptures with increasing bladder distension, with petechial oozing of blood from the lesion and the

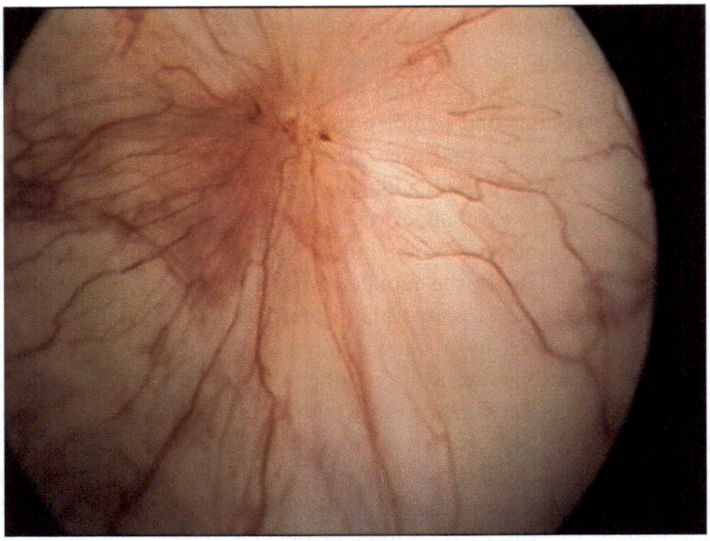

Fig. 15.1 Typical cystoscopic view of Hunner lesion: Circumscript, reddened mucosal area with small vessels radiating towards a central scar

mucosal margins in a waterfall manner. A rather typical edema develops postdistension with varying peripheral extension." (Figs. 15.1, 15.2, and 15.3) [4, 9]. Usually, lesions are multiple but occasionally they may be single. It is not unusual that more lesions are detected at reinspection than seen at the initial phase of distension. The number and location should be noted: lesions on the anterior wall, posterior wall, lateral quadrants, fundus, and trigone in consecutive order. Photographs or video records are recommended but optional. The classic "IC patch" seems to be more prevalent in postmenopausal and in European women [15].

Over the years, controversy has developed as to the actual existence of this kind of lesion. Many urologists maintain that Hunner's lesions are rare, or do not exist, and the fact that they rarely detect them confirms this false impression. The distribution varies from 0 to 50% of cases with BPS in various populations, centers, and series [3, 12]. Detection is a matter of training. Today's urologists are in good company, though already Badenoch speculated that this lesion could be produced by the cystoscope [16], a statement which is not true. Fortunately, the awareness of the indispensability of cystoscopy in BPS/IC diagnostics is increasing [17].

Glomerulations

The most constant endoscopic abnormality following hydrodistension in patients with BPS is punctuate submucosal bleedings or glomerulations (Fig. 15.4)

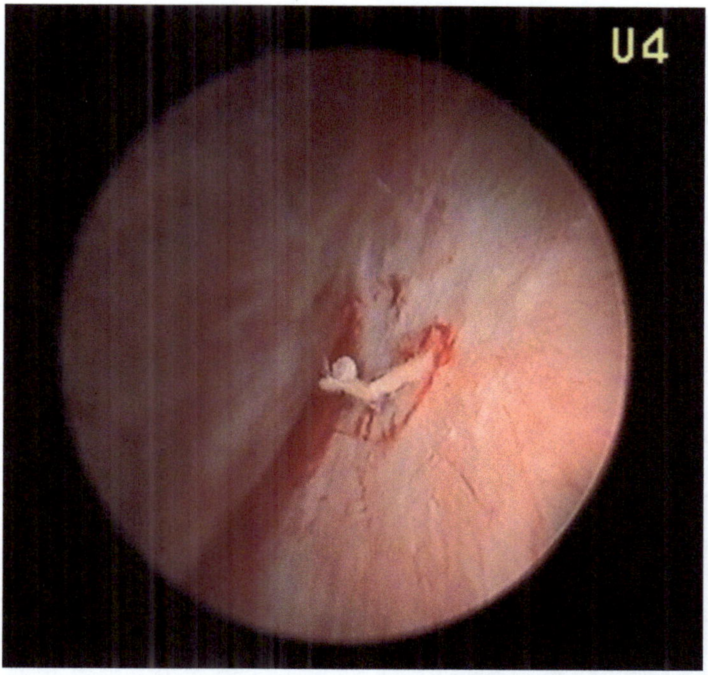

Fig. 15.2 Cystoscopic view of the Hunner lesion with a fibrin deposit attached to this area

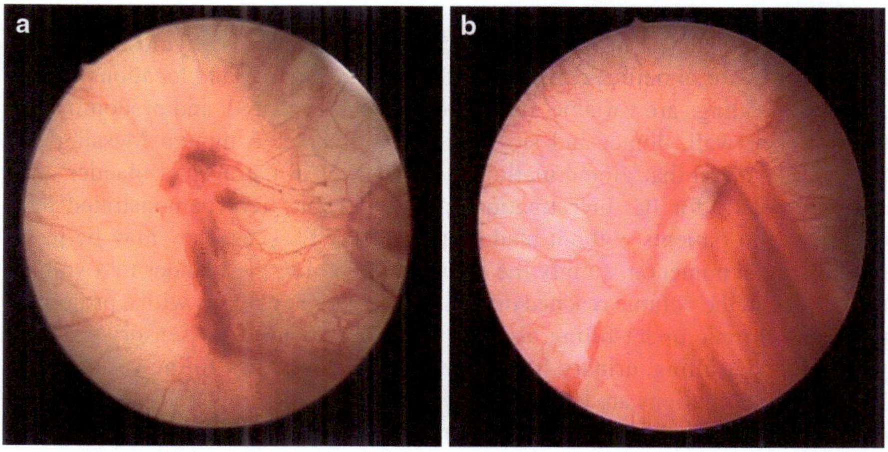

Fig. 15.3 Hunner lesion: (**a**) Petechial oozing of blood from the lesion and (**b**) the mucosal margins in a waterfall-like manner during bladder distension

[3, 9, 10, 18]. Typically, they are present in at least three quadrants of the bladder and not just in the path of the endoscope. The appearance can be a lattice- or checkerboard-type pattern, or they may appear as splotchy areas over a whole

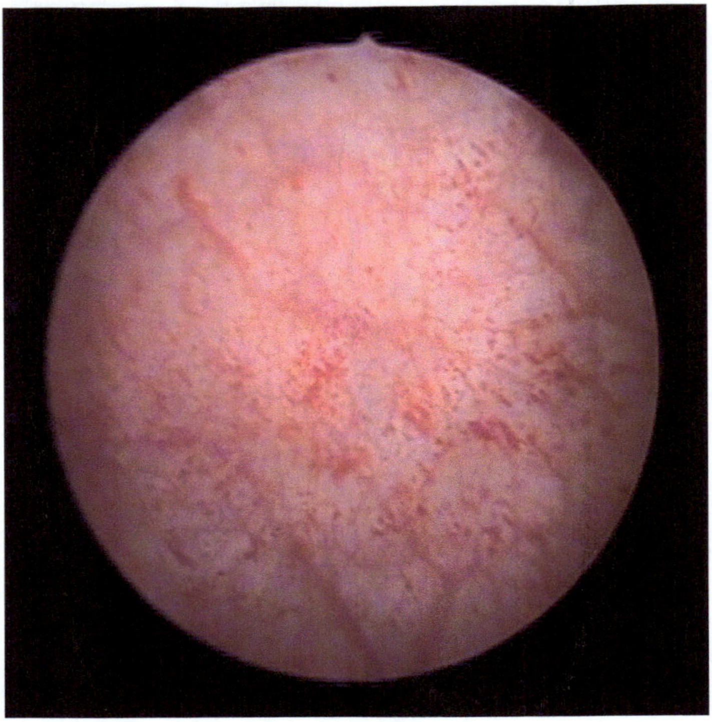

Fig. 15.4 Petechiae in at least two quadrants (grade I according to ESSIC classification)

section of the bladder [3]. More conspicuous changes like ecchymoses or flame hemorrhages are sometimes seen. Even though the quantity and locations of submucosal bleedings are variable, the trigone is usually spared, and predominantly the posterior wall, dome, and side walls are affected. Although Messing and Stamey [3] stated that glomerulations do not occur in the normal bladder, they are not specific for IC. Investigations of a later date have demonstrated their occurrence in patients without bladder pain [19, 20]. Thus, they may be just a secondary phenomenon, simply the result of stretching the bladder to a volume much beyond the volume reached during daily living in patients with a prolonged period of chronic under-filling, as is the case in patients with sensory urgency, pain at bladder filling, urinary frequency, and constantly low filling volumes [4]. In fact, glomerulations are exceptionally found even in completely normal bladders. Furthermore, they have been described in tuberculous cystitis, cyclophosphamide-induced and formalin-induced cystitis, radiation cystitis, distension of the defunctionalized bladder, and carcinoma in situ [13, 21]. Sant also noted them in patients who have received intravesical thiotepa chemotherapy for treatment of recurrent superficial bladder tumors [21]. Despite the doubts as to the specificity of glomerulations, the severity of bleeding might have a positive correlation with BPS symptoms [22].

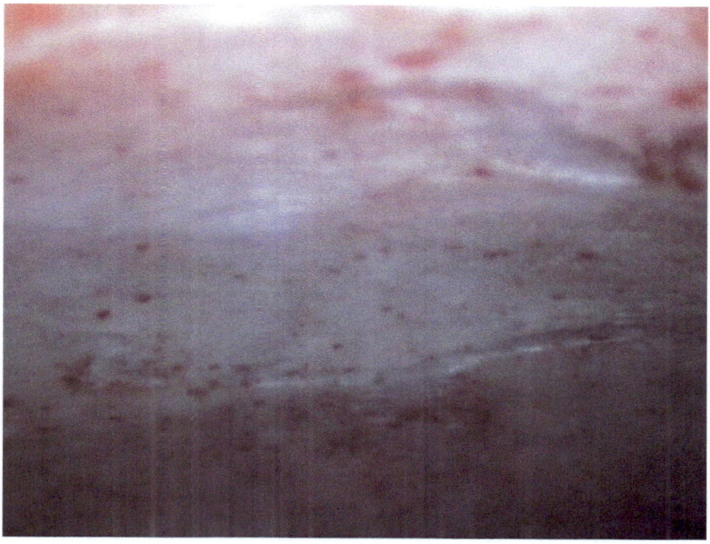

Fig. 15.5 Superficial cracks occurring during bladder distension. From Johansson SL, Fall M. Clinical features and spectrum of light microscopic changes in interstitial cystitis. J Urol, 1990;143(6):1118–24 [23]. Reprinted with permission from Elsevier

Mucosal Splitting and Cracks

Small cracks in the mucosa may appear upon distension but quickly subside, also sometimes observed in normal bladders. In patients with the so-called nonulcer BPS, multiple, superficial, close-set cracks may occur during bladder distention, sometimes in a cobblestone pattern, especially in the bladder dome, resulting in bleeding spots post distension (Fig. 15.5). A more prominent pattern of a similar kind although extending deeper is occasionally seen in patients with the classic Hunner type of disease (Fig. 15.6); these findings represent sign of pathologic mucosal fragility.

Bleeding Provoked by Distension

It is of interest to mark the volume when Hunner lesions start to bleed and when multiple superficial mucosal cracks or glomerulations first appear, subsequently producing bleeding.

Typically, when emptying the bladder after distention, the fluid is clear and then becomes more and more blood-tinged for the last 50–100 cc [13]. Terminal bleeding in the distension fluid is a quite typical sign in BPS/IC.

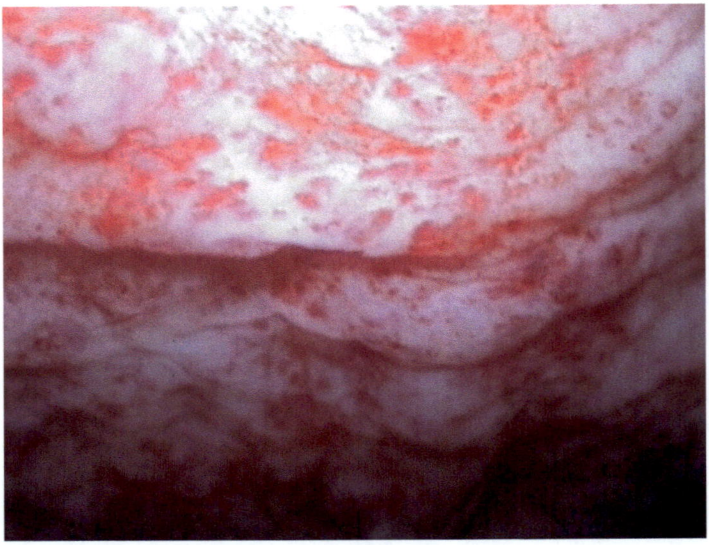

Fig. 15.6 General mucosal edema post distension in nonulcer BPS

Postdistension Edema

A quite characteristic finding at the second filling of the bladder in a patient with the classic Hunner type of lesions is a varying degree of edema extending out in the periphery of the lesion. The reaction is thought to be caused by mast cell degranulation. The edema demarcates the area of more intensive inflammatory involvement of the bladder wall, although microscopically the entire mucosa is to some degree affected [23]. In the nonulcer subtype a general edema of the bladder mucosa is sometimes seen (Fig. 15.7), but just as often there is no edematous reaction, indicating some difference of obscure significance in this category of patients.

Risks of Bladder Distension

Bladder Rupture

The anterior, superior portion of the bladder should be continuously observed for possible rupture during filling. This is a very rare occurrence but should be suspected when the influx of fluid seems too large and the rate of filling shows no sign of decreasing. Only exceptionally, any other measure than catheter drainage for about 3 days would be required. Should bladder distension result in signs of intraperitoneal leakage laparotomy is necessary; however an event at distension is never seen by us.

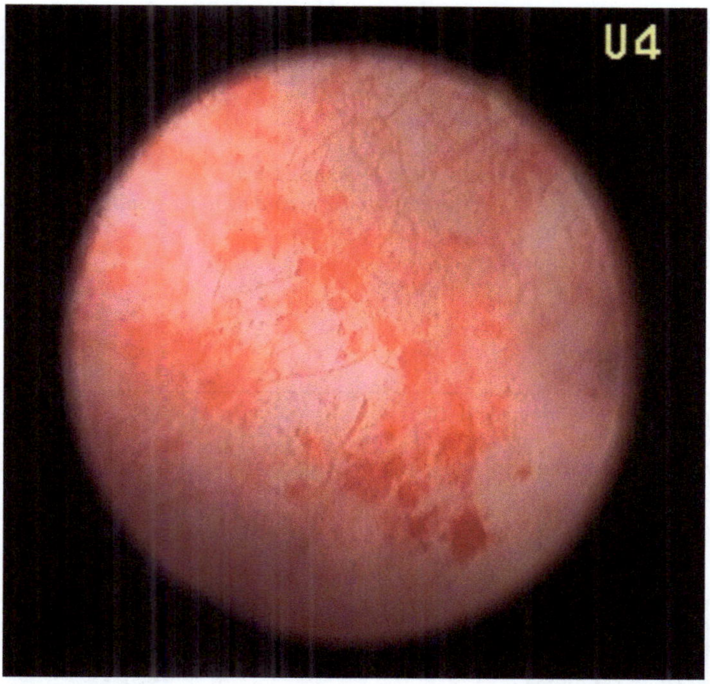

Fig. 15.7 Large submucosal bleeding (ecchymosis) (grade II according to ESSIC classification)

Bladder Necrosis

As example of an as extremely rare as serious complication to bladder distension, bladder necrosis has been mentioned [24], however not within the knowledge of the authors of this chapter.

ESSIC Classification and Cystoscopic Finding

In 2004, the ESSIC published recommendations for the diagnostic workup in patients suspected of having BPS [10]. In addition to history and physical exam, cystoscopy and biopsy have a central role as diagnostic tools in assessing the BPS patient. Standardization of the techniques and description of findings are indispensable to make various studies comparable and translatable [9]. The cystoscopic findings were graded on a scale from I to IV (Table 15.1). A range of mild to severe glomerulations is depicted in Figs. 15.4 and 15.8. As is suggested above it is expected that further work will result in modifications and refinement of categories.

Table 15.1 ESSIC classification of cystoscopic bladder findings following hydrodistention

Grade 0 normal mucosa				
Grade I petechiae in at least two quadrants				
Grade II large submucosal bleeding (ecchymosis)				
Grade III diffuse global mucosal bleeding				
Grade IV mucosal disruption, with or without bleeding/edema				
BPS classification of types of bladder pain syndrome according to the results of cystoscopy with hydrodistension and of biopsies.				
Biopsy/cystoscopy	Not done	[a]	[b]	[c]
Not done	XX	1X	2X	3X
Normal	XA	1A	2A	3A
Inconclusive	XB	1B	2B	3B
Positive	XC	1C	2C	3C

[a]Cystoscopy: Glomerulations grade II–III

[b]With or without glomerulations

[c]Histology showing inflammatory infiltrates, detrusor mastocytosis, granulation tissue, and/or intrafascicular fibrosis

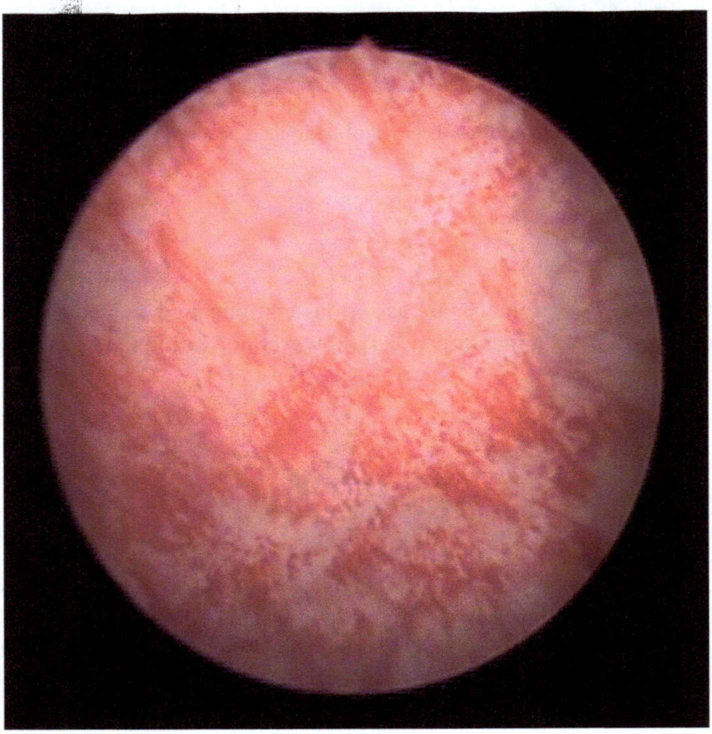

Fig. 15.8 Diffuse global mucosal bleeding (grade III according to ESSIC classification)

References

1. Skene AJC. Diseases of bladder and urethra in women. New York: Wm Wood; 1887. p. 167.
2. Hunner GL. Elusive ulcer of the bladder: further notes on a rare type of bladder ulcer with report of 25 cases. Am J Obstet. 1918;78:374–95.
3. Messing EM, Stamey TA. Interstitial cystitis: early diagnosis, pathology and treatment. Urology. 1978;12:381–92.
4. Fall M, Johansson SL, Aldenborg F. Chronic interstitial cystitis: a heterogeneous syndrome. J Urol. 1987;137:35–8.
5. Gillenwater JY, Wein AJ. Summary of the National Institute of Arthritis, Diabetes, Digestive and Kidney Diseases Workshop on Interstitial Cystitis, National Institutes of Health, Bethesda, Maryland, August 28–29, 1987. J Urol. 1988;140(1):203–6.
6. Hanno P, et al. The diagnosis of interstitial cystitis revisited: lessons learned from the National Institutes of Health Interstitial Cystitis Database study. J Urol. 1999;161:553–7.
7. Oravisto KJ. Epidemiology of interstitial cystitis. Ann Chir Gynaecol Finn. 1975;64:75–7.
8. Wyndaele J, Van Dyck J, Toussaint N. Cystoscopy and bladder biopsies in patients with bladder pain syndrome carried out following ESSIC guidelines. Scand J Urol Nephrol. 2009;25:1–5.
9. van de Merwe J, et al. Diagnostic criteria, classification, and nomenclature for painful bladder syndrome/interstitial cystitis: an ESSIC proposal. Eur Urol. 2008;53:60–7.
10. Nordling J, et al. Primary evaluation of patients suspected of having interstitial cystitis (IC). Eur Urol. 2004;45:662–9.
11. Sant G, Meares EJ. Interstitial cystitis: pathogenesis, diagnosis, and treatment. Infect Urol. 1990;31:24–30.
12. Peeker R, Fall M. Toward a precise definition of interstitial cystitis: further evidence of differences in classic and nonulcer disease. J Urol. 2002;167:2470–2.
13. Messing EM. The diagnosis of interstitial cystitis. Urology. 1987;29(4 Suppl):4–7.
14. Lamale L, et al. Symptoms and cystoscopic findings in patients with untreated interstitial cystitis. Urology. 2006;67:242–5.
15. Herbst RH, Baumrucker GO, German KL. Elusive ulcer (Hunner) of the bladder with an experimental study of the etiology. Am J Surg. 1937;38:152–6.
16. Badenoch AW. Chronic interstitial cystitis. Br J Urol. 1971;43:718–21.
17. Braunstein R, et al. The role of cystoscopy in the diagnosis of Hunner's ulcer disease. J Urol. 2008;180:1383–6.
18. Nigro D, Wein A. Interstitial cystitis: clinical and endoscopic features. In: Sant GR, editor. Interstitial cystitis. Philadelphia: Lippincott-Raven; 1997. p. 137–42.
19. Waxman J, Sulak P, Kuehl T. Cystoscopic findings consistent with interstitial cystitis in normal women undergoing tubal ligation. J Urol. 1998;160:1663–7.
20. Furuya R, et al. Glomerulation observed during transurethral resection of the prostate for patients with lower urinary tract symptoms suggestive of benign prostatic hyperplasia is a common finding but no predictor of clinical outcome. Urology. 2007;70(5):922–6.
21. Sant G. Diagnosis of interstitial cystitis: a clinical, endoscopic and pathologic approach. In: Hanno PM, Staskin DR, Krane RJ, Wein AJ, editors. Interstitial cystitis. London: Springer; 1990. p. 107–14.
22. Messing E, et al. Associations among cystoscopic findings and symptoms and physical examination findings in women enrolled in the Interstitial Cystitis Data Base (ICDB) Study. Urology. 1997;49:81–5.
23. Johansson SL, Fall M. Clinical features and spectrum of light microscopic changes in interstitial cystitis. J Urol. 1990;143(6):1118–24.
24. Zabihi N, Allee T, Maher MG, et al. Bladder necrosis following hydrodistention in patients with interstitial cystitis. J Urol. 2007;177:149–52.

References

Chapter 16
Biopsy Retrieval, Tissue Handling, Morphology, and Histopathological Characteristics

Christina Kåbjörn-Gustafsson and Ralph Peeker

Introduction

The role of histopathology in the diagnosis of BPS is primarily one of excluding other possible diagnoses. Possible confusing and potentially harmful conditions must be ruled out: carcinoma and carcinoma in situ, eosinophilic cystitis, tuberculous cystitis, as well as any other entities with a specific tissue diagnosis, such as enteric metaplasia, cystitis glandularis, squamous cell metaplasia, and nephrogenic metaplasia. Some of these metaplastic conditions have malignant counterparts and in order to rule out such possible malignancies, deep bladder biopsies and sometimes directed immunohistochemical staining may be necessary.

However, biopsy retrieval and histopathological examination may also be of value when it comes to diagnosing BPS. Even though most histopathologic features are not distinctive of BPS in nonulcer disease, certain signs are, for practical clinical purposes, pathognomonic for BPS with Hunner lesion. In recent decades, understanding of the properties of various cell system has developed dramatically and, moreover, the diagnosis with standard staining procedures and light microscopy can now be further refined with immunohistochemistry and even more sophisticated and sensitive amplification techniques such as polymerase chain reaction (PCR) in situ and various blot and array techniques.

C. Kåbjörn-Gustafsson (✉)
Department of Pathology, Sahlgrenska University Hospital,
Gothenburg 413 455, Sweden
e-mail: christina.kabjorn@vgregion.se

R. Peeker
Department of Urology, Sahlgrenska University Hospital,
Bruna Straket 11, Gothenburg 413 45, Sweden
e-mail: ralph.peeker@gu.se

J. Nordling et al. (eds.), *Bladder Pain Syndrome: A Guide for Clinicians*,
DOI 10.1007/978-1-4419-6929-3_16,

Biopsy Retrieval, Fixation, and Staining Procedures

Biopsies may be obtained by transurethral electroresection of large strips of the bladder wall including the detrusor muscle; however cold cup biopsy can also be a feasible option. This is somewhat depending on local tradition but the choice of biopsy retrieval technique can also be governed by which kind of pathology is suspected and what type of pathology the clinician finds important to rule out.

The golden standard of fixating tissue specimens is formaldehyde 4%. Formaldehyde fixation rate is approximately 1 mm per hour; hence small bladder specimens are well fixated by the time they reach the pathology department. In the laboratory the bladder specimen is dehydrated, paraffin or wax embedded, and cut into series of 4 μ(mu)m sections. The specimen is thereafter deparaffinized and stained with hematoxylin/eosin (Htx-Eo) prior to dehydration and mounting with coverslips. Additional stainings are often performed in order to guide the pathologist into a more correct diagnosis. For instance the dye Van Gieson or Sirius may be performed to demonstrate fibrosis. Most antibodies are tested on formaldehyde-fixated tissues and mast cell tryptase may now be visualized using a specific antibody.

Until recently Toluidine blue, a metachromatic dye, was used and may still be used to stain mast cells. The staining procedure with Toluidine blue is, however, somewhat problematic. The method is very dependent on low pH during which circumstances mast cells containing heparin and chondroitin-sulfate are visualized. Chemicals like HCl, citronic acid, and the dye Toluidine blue are unhealthy for the personnel dealing with the dying process. This method has for decades been the routine dye to stain mast cells but it has now been replaced with a mast cell tryptase antibody (Fig. 16.1) because of the mentioned reasons plus the fact that metachromatic staining sometimes may fail to detect mast cells.

Light Microscopic Features

Specimens from patients with BPS type 3C (classic IC) as a rule display striking histologic alterations, from normal mucosa and detrusor musculature (Figs. 16.2 and 16.3) to prominent epithelial denudation (Fig. 16.4) that may be covered by fibrin mixed with inflammatory cells, in particular neutrophils. The inflammatory changes are often wedge shaped and involve the superficial part of the lamina propria, often extending all the way into the lamina muscularis mucosae. Underlying granulation tissue is present in the vast majority of the subjects [1]. These findings tally with those reported already 100 years ago by Hunner, who reported the abundance of granulation tissue formation as well as chronic inflammation involving all coats of the bladder [2].

There is an abnormal microvascularity in the lamina propria which may result in petechial bleeding or glomerulations, and possibly also epithelial denudation as a consequence of ischemia; this in turn may bring about hemorrhage in the entire lamina

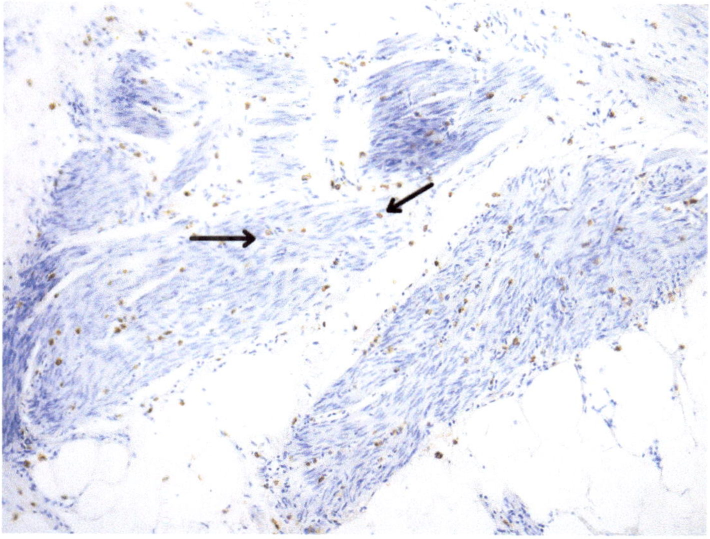

Fig. 16.1 The detrusor muscle. Tryptase in mast cells visualized by immunohistochemistry. Mastocytosis with a high number of mast cells within the muscle bundles (*arrows*), in this case >90 per mm^2

propria. BPS type 3C (classic IC) hence displays marked inflammatory changes in the lamina propria, including the presence of lymphocytes, plasma cells, mast cells, and neutrophils. Eosinophils are generally few. Germinal center formation is frequently seen. In the detrusor muscle fibrosis can frequently be displayed (Fig. 16.5).

The aforementioned light microscopic features differ markedly from what can be seen in BPS type 1 and 2. Lepinard reported that whereas pancystitis affected the three layers of bladder wall, this was not the case in non-Hunner lesion disease [3]. In another report, comprising 64 patients with Hunner lesion and 44 with non-Hunner lesion, Hunner lesion had mucosal epithelial denudation and hemorrhage, granulation tissue, severe inflammatory infiltrates, high mast cell counts, and perineural infiltrates. The non-Hunner lesion group, despite sharing a similar symptomatology and the same chronic course, had an impervious mucosa with a meagre inflammatory response, the main feature being numerous, mucosal ruptures and suburothelial hemorrhages [4]. Frequently biopsies are completely normal in patients with ESSIC type 1 and 2 disease (non Hunner Lesion disease) [5] and, moreover, there has been no report on transition from BPS type 1 or 2 to BPS type 3.

Ultrastructural Studies

Electron microscopy has not been very successful in diagnosing BPS. In an early paper on this topic, Collan et al. stated that there was a considerable similarity of the

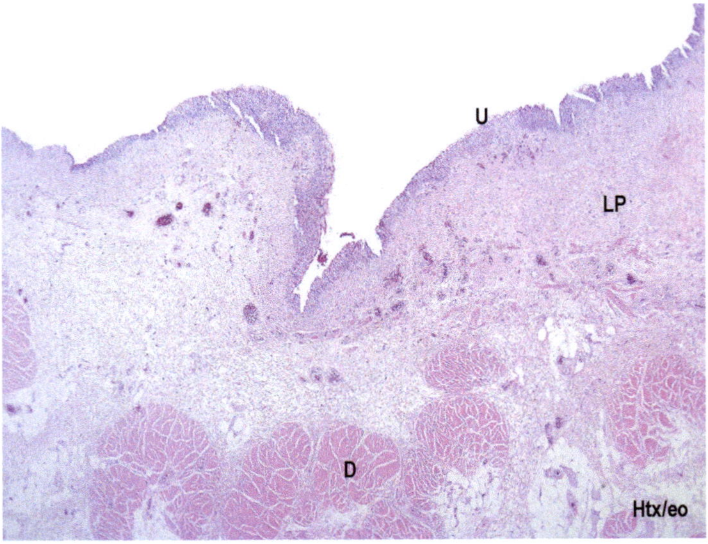

Fig. 16.2 Normal bladder mucosa displaying intact urothelium (U). Beneath the urothelium resides the lamina propria (LP) with, in deeper portions, the detrusor muscle (D)

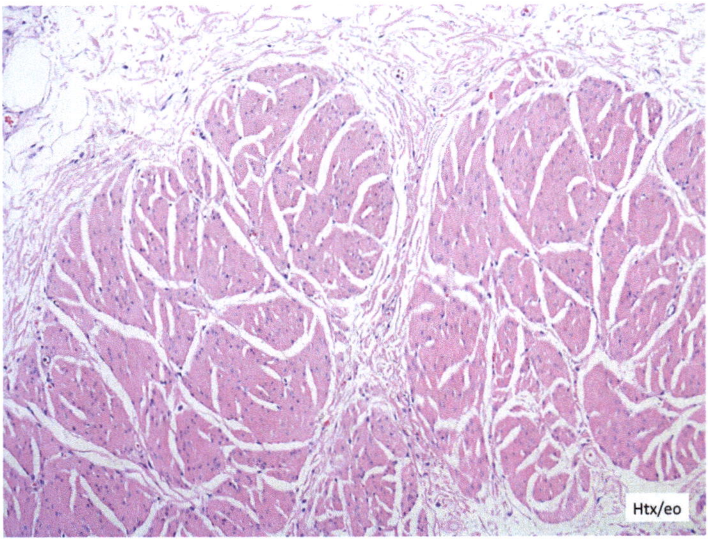

Fig. 16.3 The detrusor muscle. Only loose collagen tissue surrounds the muscle bundles and almost no intrafascicular fibrous tissue is seen

ultrastructure of epithelial cells between controls and BPS patients [6], and some 10 years later Dixon et al. also failed to discover any differences in the morphologic appearances of urothelial cells in patients with BPS as compared to controls [7].

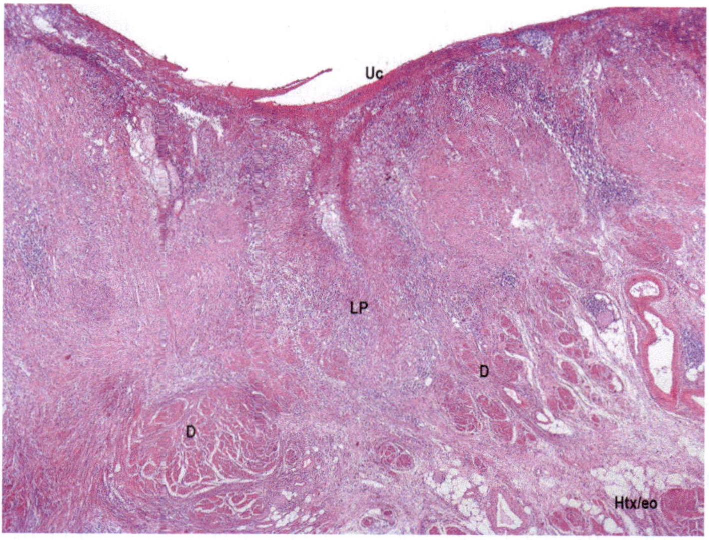

Fig. 16.4 Severe case of bladder pain syndrome. Epithelial denudation with underlying granulation tissue. Heavy inflammatory infiltrate reaching the deeper portions of the lamina propria (LP) and the detrusor muscle compartment (D)

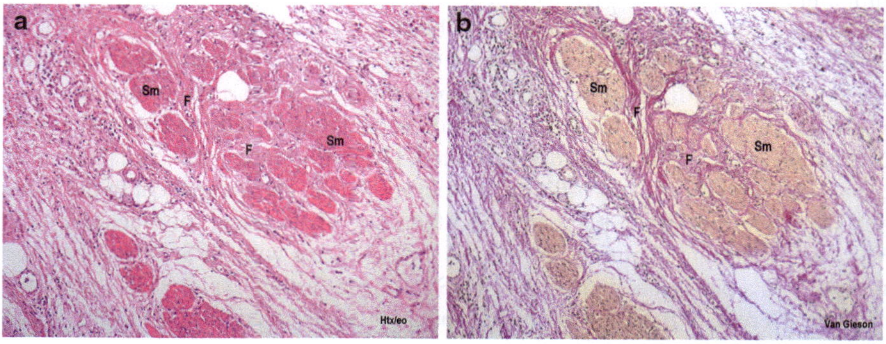

Fig. 16.5 (**a**) Detrusor muscle: Fibrosis (F) within the muscle group separates the smooth muscle bundles (Sm). (**b**) Same case. Van Gieson staining. *Pink* colored collagen (F) separating the smooth muscle bundles (Sm)

Neither could Anderström et al. see any unambiguous ultrastructural surface characteristics for BPS; however, the proportion of cells covered by round, uniform, and pleomorphic microvilli was higher in the BPS patients than in controls [8].

At variance with these reports on lack of diagnostic positive histopathologic signs in BPS type 1 and 2, Elbadawi and Light concluded that ultrastructural changes appear to be sufficiently distinctive to be diagnostic in specimens submitted for pathologic confirmation of BPS type 1 or 2. They performed a detailed ultrastructural study on patients with BPS type 1 or 2 [9]. A distinctive combination of peculiar muscle cell profiles, injury of intrinsic vessels and nerves in muscularis and suburothelium, and discohesive urothelium was observed in lesional and less markedly in nonlesional samples of all specimens. Marked edema of various tissue elements and cells appeared to be a common denominator of many observed changes. Urothelial changes disrupted the true permeability barrier. Neural changes included a combination of degenerative and regenerative features.

Histopathological Detection of Mast Cells in BPS

Accumulated evidence has shown that mast cells circulate as primitive CD117- and CD34-positive lymphocyte-like cells in the blood which upon relevant stimulation migrate into the tissues, where they complete their maturation and acquire phenotypic properties strictly regulated by the local microenvironment [10]. Besides this, there is also a small pool of mitotic mast cells in the tissues [11]. Currently, mast cells are regarded not only as cells involved in allergic tissue reactions but also as multifunctional immunocompetent cells involved in a variety of tissue reactions such as chronic inflammation, examples of which are BPS type 3 and rheumatoid arthritis as well as fibrosis [12]. It has thus been shown that the mast cell, in addition to histamine and heparin, also contains other highly potent inflammatory mediators such as leucotrienes, cytokines, and the angiogenic and fibroblast stimulatory factor, basic fibroblast growth factor (bFGF) [13, 14]. In addition to allergen binding, nerve-derived mediators may also stimulate mast cell secretion. Several lines of evidence support the concept of a neuroimmune connection [15] and morphological association between mast cells and neuropeptide-containing nerves has been demonstrated [16–18]. Since mast cells are also capable to synthesize the pro-fibrotic cytokine TGF-β, and are present in the bladder detrusor, they may play an important role in detrusor fibrogenesis (see Fig. 16.5) resulting in chronicity seen in some patients with BPS. The role of the mast cell as a pathogenetic player in BPS has been further explored in a previous chapter. Herein, we will only briefly address some specific histopathological characteristics.

It was demonstrated, in bladder specimens from patients with BPS type 3, BPS type 1 or 2, and controls, that mast cells were visualized in terms of metachromasia, reflecting glycosaminoglycan content, and immunohistochemically, visualizing tryptase, chymase, and IL-6 as well as the surface markers CD 117 and stem cell factor (SCF) [19]. In this report, BPS type 3 displayed a six to tenfold increase of mast cells in terms of proteinase positivity while BPS type 1 or 2 revealed twice as many mast cells as controls. In contrast to BPS type 1 or 2 and controls, BPS type 3 displayed an abundance of epithelial MC. BPS type 3 also coexpressed SCF and IL-6 in the epithelium.

The proteinase immunostainings yielded higher number of mast cells in BPS mucosal stroma and detrusor musculature as compared to the metachromatic staining mast cells, corroborating what has previously been said about the obvious weakness vin detection ability with metachromatic staining as compared to tryptase immunohistochemistry.

Histopathological Detection of Immunocompetent Cells in BPS

There are numerous reports on autoantibodies in patients with BPS [20–22] and, moreover, some of the common clinical and histopathological characteristics present in BPS patients show certain similarities with other known autoimmune phenomena. This is the background to the theory that BPS may arise from autoimmune disturbances. The role of autoimmunity in BPS is controversial and the disease is not thought to originate from a direct autoimmune attack on the bladder. Rather, some of the autoimmune symptoms and pathologic findings in BPS arise indirectly as a result of tissue destruction and inflammation from other, as yet unknown, causes.

In a study of 47 BPS patients, Mattila et al. found immune deposits in the vessel walls of 33 patients [23] and in a subsequent study, electron microscopy evidence of endothelial injury was found in 14 out of 20 BPS patients [24]. There is, no doubt, an inflammatory response in BPS type 3, of a chronic nature, and this makes it possible that there is a cell-mediated autoimmune response at hand. In a report encompassing 24 BPS type 3 patients, 9 BPS type 1 or 2 patients, and 10 controls [25] it was found that the BPS type 3 patients displayed aggregates of T-cells as well as B-nodules with focal germinal centers. There was a decreased or normal helper/suppressor ratio and suppressor cytotoxic cells were present in the germinal centers. The BPS type 1 or 2 patients, conversely, had only slightly increased number of lymphoid cells, dominated by T-helper cells, the BPS type 1 or 2 group not differing significantly from the controls.

Histopathological Detection of Neurological Alterations in BPS

There has also been emphasis on the neurogenic nature of this BPS. Christmas et al. and Hohenfellner et al. identified nerve fiber sprouting, in particular increase of the sympathetic outflow [26, 27]. Several other authors have also described autonomic nerve changes [26–29] but the findings of patterns are far from uniform.

Tyrosine hydroxylase is the rate-limiting enzyme for all catecholamine synthesis [30]. Scoring the overall presence and density of immunofluorescent nerve fibers by confocal laser scanning microscopy in three different tissue compartments, near epithelial cells, in detrusor muscle tissue, and around vessels, a prominent increase of tyrosine hydroxylase immunoreactivity in bladder tissue in BPS patients was noted, as compared to controls [31]. This can presumably be interpreted as a sign of generally increased sympathetic outflow, which in turn lends further support to the notion of a neurogenic etiology.

References

1. Johansson SL, Ogawa K, Fall M. The pathology of interstitial cystitis. In: Sant GR, editor. Interstitial cystitis. Philadelphia: Lippincott-Raven; 1997. p. 143–52.
2. Hunner GL. Elusive ulcer of the bladder: further notes on a rare type of bladder ulcer with report of 25 cases. Am J Obstet. 1918;78:374–95.
3. Lepinard V, Saint-Andre JP, Rognon LM. Interstitial cystitis. Current aspects. J Urol (Paris). 1984;90(7):455–65.
4. Johansson SL, Fall M. Clinical features and spectrum of light microscopic changes in interstitial cystitis. J Urol. 1990;143(6):1118–24.
5. Johansson SL, Fall M. Pathology of interstitial cystitis. Urol Clin North Am. 1994;21(1):55–62.
6. Collan Y, Alfthan O, Kivilaakso E, Oravisto KJ. Electron microscopic and histological findings on urinary bladder epithelium in interstitial cystitis. Eur Urol. 1976;2(5):242–7.
7. Dixon J, Holm-Bentzen M, Gilpin C. Electrone microscopic investigation of the bladder urothelium and glycocalix in patients with interstitial cystitis. J Urol. 1986;135:621–5.
8. Anderstrom CR, Fall M, Johansson SL. Scanning electron microscopic findings in interstitial cystitis. Br J Urol. 1989;63(3):270–5.
9. Elbadawi A, Light JK. Distinctive ultrastructural pathology of nonulcerative interstitial cystitis. Urol Int. 1996;56:137–62.
10. Galli SJ. New insights into "the riddle of the mast cells": microenvironmental regulation of mast cell development and phenotypic heterogeneity. Lab Invest. 1990;62(1):5–33.
11. Enerbäck L, Rundquist I. DNA distribution of mast cell populations in growing rats. Histochemistry. 1981;71:521–31.
12. Hunt LW, Colby TV, Weiler DA, Sur S, Butterfield JH. Immunofluorescent staining for mast cells in idiopathic pulmonary fibrosis: quantification and evidence for extracellular release of mast cell tryptase [see comments]. Mayo Clin Proc. 1992;67(10):941–8.
13. Qu Z, Liebler JM, Powers MR, Galey T, Ahmadi P, Huang XN, et al. Mast cells are a major source of basic fibroblast growth factor in chronic inflammation and cutaneous hemangioma. Am J Pathol. 1995;147:564–73.
14. Stevens LR, Austen KF. Recent advances in the cellular and molecular biology of mast cells. Immunol Today. 1989;10:381–6.
15. Williams RM, Bienenstock J, Stead RH. Mast cells: the neuroimmune connection. Chem Immunol. 1995;61:208–35.
16. Keith IM, Jin J, Saban R. Nerve-mast cell interaction in normal guinea pig urinary bladder. J Comp Neurol. 1995;363(1):28–36.
17. Naukkarinen A, Harvima IT, Aalto ML, Harvima RJ, Horsmanheimo M. Quantitative analysis of contact sites between mast cells and sensory nerves in cutaneous psoriasis and lichen planus based on a histochemical double staining technique. Arch Dermatol Res. 1991;283(7):433–7.
18. Newson B, Dahlstrom A, Enerback L, Ahlman H. Suggestive evidence for a direct innervation of mucosal mast cells. Neuroscience. 1983;10(2):565–70.
19. Peeker R, Enerbäck L, Fall M, Aldenborg F. Recruitment, distribution and phenotypes of mast cells in interstitial cystitis. J Urol. 2000;163:1009–15.
20. Ochs RL, Stein Jr T, Peebles CL, Gittes RF, Tan EM. Autoantibodies in interstitial cystitis. J Urol. 1994;151(3):587–92.
21. Oravisto KJ. Interstitial cystitis as an autoimmune disease. A review. Eur Urol. 1980;6:10–3.
22. Silk MR. Bladder antibodies in interstitial cystitis. J Urol. 1970;103:307–9.
23. Mattila J, Pitkanen R, Vaalasti T, Seppanen J. Fine-structural evidence for vascular injury in patients with interstitial cystitis. Virchows Arch A Pathol Anat Histopathol. 1983;398(3):347–55.
24. Tan EM. Antinuclear antibodies: diagnostic markers for autoimmune diseases and probes for cell biology. Adv Immunol. 1989;44:93–151.
25. Harrington DS, Fall M, Johansson SL. Interstitial cystitis: bladder mucosa lymphocyte immunophenotyping and peripheral blood flow cytometry analysis. J Urol. 1990;144(4):868–71.

26. Christmas TJ, Rode J, Chapple CR, Milroy EJ, Turner-Warwick RT. Nerve fibre proliferation in interstitial cystitis. Virchows Arch A Pathol Anat Histopathol. 1990;416(5):447–51.
27. Hohenfellner M, Nunes L, Schmidt RA, Lampel A, Thuroff JW, Tanagho EA. Interstitial cystitis: increased sympathetic innervation and related neuropeptide synthesis. J Urol. 1992;147(3):587–91.
28. Palea S, Artibani W, Ostardo E, Trist DG, Pietra C. Evidence for purinergic neurotransmission in human urinary bladder affected by interstitial cystitis. J Urol. 1993;150(6):2007–12.
29. Pang X, Marchand J, Sant GR, Kream RM, Theoharides TC. Increased number of substance P positive nerve fibres in interstitial cystitis. Br J Urol. 1995;75(6):744–50.
30. Goldstein M. Enzymes involved in the catalysis of catecholamine biosynthesis. In: Ubell RN, editor. Methods in neurochemistry. New York: Plenum Press; 1972. p. 317–40.
31. Peeker R, Aldenborg F, Johansson SL, Li J-Y, Dahlström A, Fall M. Increased tyrosine hydroxylase immunoreactivity in bladder tissue from patients with classic and nonulcer interstitial cystitis. J Urol. 2000;163:1112–5.

Chapter 17
Urodynamics in BPS

Paul P. Irwin and Claus Riedl

Introduction

The aim of clinical urodynamics is to reproduce a patient's bladder and micturition symptoms while making precise measurements in order to identify the underlying causes for the symptoms, and to quantify the related pathophysiological processes [1]. The most commonly performed study is the cystometrogram (CMG), in which bladder pressures are recorded during both the filling and voiding phases of micturition.

The role of urodynamic assessment in bladder pain syndrome (BPS) is controversial. Cystometry was once a mandatory investigation as part of the NIDDK diagnostic criteria, but these criteria have since largely been abandoned [2]. The ESSIC diagnostic criteria allow a clinical diagnosis of BPS to be made based on the symptom of pain originating in the bladder associated with at least one other urinary symptom—in the absence of confusable diseases or conditions. On this basis, there is no longer a need to perform CMGs "routinely." Urodynamic studies are only required in order to rule out another pathophysiological process (detrusor overactivity or bladder outlet obstruction) that, if found, might have an implication in a patient's management. Essentially this applies to patients suspected of having BPS but whose symptoms persist despite therapy.

BPS is characterized by increased bladder sensation. However, to date there is no investigation that can quantify bladder sensation. Comparative cystometry, using

P.P. Irwin, M.Ch., F.R.C.S.I(Urol) (✉)
Michael Heal Department of Urology, Mid Cheshire Hospitals NHS Trust, Leighton Hospital, Crewe, Cheshire CW1 4QJ, UK
e-mail: paul.irwin@mcht.nhs.uk

C. Riedl, M.D.
Urology Department, Landesklinikum Thermenregion Baden, Wimmergasse 19, Baden 2500, Austria

J. Nordling et al. (eds.), *Bladder Pain Syndrome: A Guide for Clinicians*, DOI 10.1007/978-1-4419-6929-3_17,

saline and potassium chloride infusions in turn, may have a possible role to play in identifying patients with BPS (or overactive bladder) who may respond to GAG-replacement therapy.

Cystometry

A urodynamic study should only be done in order to answer a specific question. There should be an expectation that an abnormal physiological measurement will correspond with a clinical event—a symptom or a sign. The study should not only aim to reproduce the patient's symptoms, but it should also reproduce his/her physiological bladder volumes—the post-void residual and functional bladder capacity.

The recording of bladder pressures during filling and voiding may be done alone or in conjunction with fluoroscopy and/or electromyography (EMG). It is imperative that the CMG is performed in a standardized and perfect manner. Important points to bear in mind are the following:

1. The patient must complete a frequency–volume record over 2–3 days, recording the times and volumes at each void both day and night. The functional bladder capacity is the maximum voided volume recorded on a frequency–volume diary. The addition of a visual analog scale for pain during a given 24-h period is sometimes helpful in interpreting the diary (Fig. 17.1).
2. The patient is asked to empty the bladder and a dipstick test of a sample is performed, looking for nitrites. If infection is suspected, it should be treated and the CMG deferred until the infection has resolved. The immediate post-void residual is measured by ultrasound. The bladder should not be artificially emptied following this.
3. Once the bladder filling and rectal (or vaginal) pressure lines are inserted and connected to the transducers, the system is balanced to zero by opening the valves to atmospheric air (Fig. 17.2). The transducers' lines are then opened to the bladder and rectal lines before bladder filling begins. Correct placement of the pressure lines should be verified with a cough test at frequent intervals during the filling phase.
4. The bladder should be filled on top of the post-void residual and the filling rate should not exceed 50 ml/min. Throughout filling, the patient is prompted to describe his/her bladder sensation, and specifically to indicate the onset of the pain of which he/she complains.
5. Appropriate prompts, which can be standardized for a given urology department, should be given to the patient throughout filling to indicate "first desire to void" (FDV) and cystometric capacity (C_{max}).
6. The investigator should aim to fill the bladder to at least the functional bladder capacity. If the patient complains of discomfort before functional capacity is reached, it is worth stopping temporarily until the discomfort eases, and then to resume filling. Maximum cystometric capacity (C_{max}) is reached when the patient can no longer tolerate further filling.
7. Pressure monitoring should continue during the voiding phase.

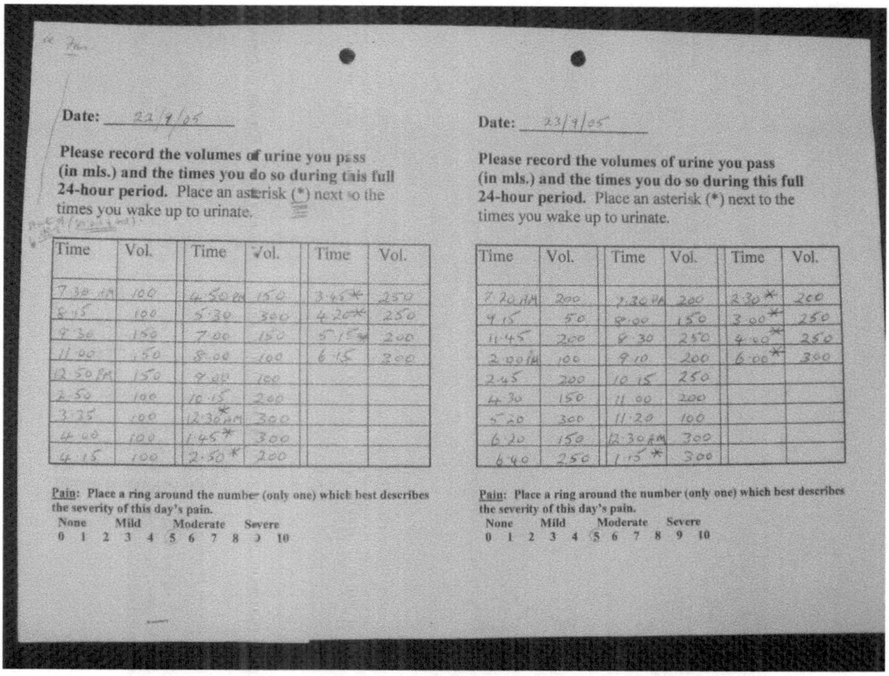

Date: 22/9/05

Please record the volumes of urine you pass (in mls.) and the times you do so during this full 24-hour period. Place an asterisk (*) next to the times you wake up to urinate.

Time	Vol.	Time	Vol.	Time	Vol.
7.30 AM	100	4.50 PM	150	3.45*	250
8.15	100	5.30	300	4.20*	250
9.30	150	7.00	150	5.15*	200
11.00	150	8.00	100	6.15	200
12.50 PM	150	9.00	100		
2.50	100	10.15	200		
3.35	100	12.30 AM*	300		
4.00	100	1.45*	300		
4.15	100	2.50*	200		

Pain: Place a ring around the number (only one) which best describes the severity of this day's pain.
None Mild Moderate Severe
0 1 2 3 4 5 6 7 8 9 10

Date: 23/9/05

Please record the volumes of urine you pass (in mls.) and the times you do so during this full 24-hour period. Place an asterisk (*) next to the times you wake up to urinate.

Time	Vol.	Time	Vol.	Time	Vol.
7.20 AM	200	7.30 PM	200	2.30*	200
9.15	50	8.00	150	3.00*	250
11.45	200	8.30	250	4.00*	250
2.00 PM	100	9.10	200	6.00*	300
2.45	200	10.15	250		
4.30	150	11.00	200		
5.20	300	11.20	100		
6.20	150	12.30 AM	300		
6.40	250	1.15*	300		

Pain: Place a ring around the number (only one) which best describes the severity of this day's pain.
None Mild Moderate Severe
0 1 2 3 4 5 6 7 8 9 10

Fig. 17.1 A typical frequency–volume record of a patient with bladder pain syndrome. The functional bladder capacity is 300 ml

Are Urodynamics Relevant or Useful?

There have been two schools of thought with divergent views on the role of urodynamics in BPS. Those who favor using cystometry in the diagnostic pathway believe that it is essential in ruling out two important "confusable conditions"—detrusor overactivity and bladder outlet obstruction—as a prerequisite to making a diagnosis of BPS [3, 4]. This group believes that abnormal urodynamic findings are relevant and that treating them may alleviate the symptoms of which the patient complains. Indeed, it was a requirement of the NIDDK criteria that the CMG should demonstrate (1) no evidence of detrusor overactivity, (2) sensory urgency (FDV at less than 150 ml), (3) a C_{max} less than 400 ml, and (4) low bladder compliance. These are largely what one would expect in a condition characterized by pain and marked sensory urgency and so rigidly defined by the NIDDK. However, they are not the foundation on which the diagnosis of BPS is made. It must be remembered that urodynamic findings, with the exception of bladder outlet obstruction, are simply that—*findings*. They are not diagnoses in themselves. With the new ESSIC diagnostic criteria, BPS is a clinical diagnosis and it should not matter what the urodynamic study reveals—unless it is going to influence a patient's management. This is the philosophy of the second school of thought with respect to urodynamics. ESSIC believes that urodynamics do have a role in the

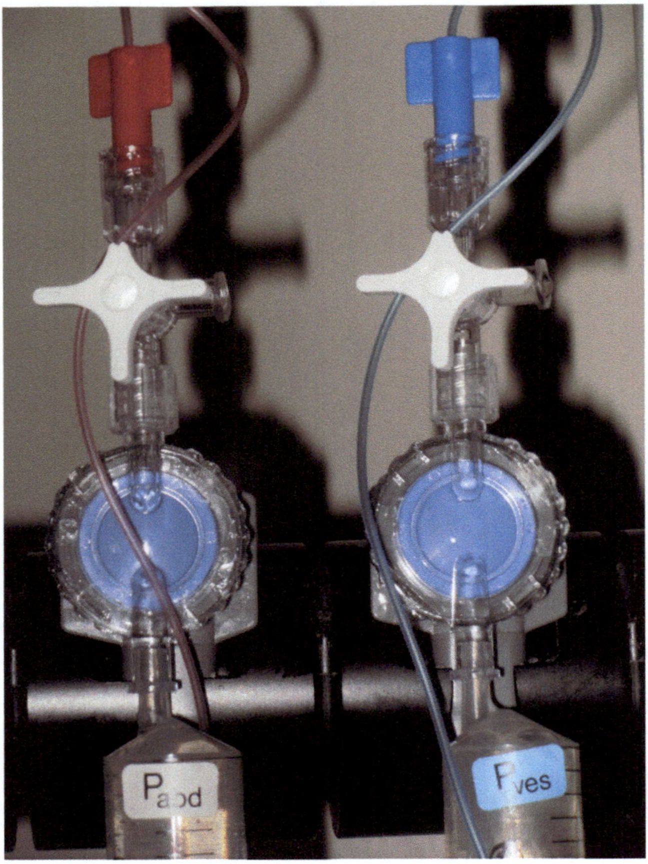

Fig. 17.2 The rectal and vesical pressure transducers are balanced to zero by opening them to atmospheric pressure before starting the CMG

diagnostic pathway, but only for selected patients whose symptoms persist despite a reasonable trial of standard therapy. Between 14 and 30% of "BPS patients" are found to have detrusor overactivity [5]. If this is found, it may certainly be worth treating them with antimuscarinic agents. It could equally be argued that all BPS patients should be started on antimuscarinic agents ab initio.

There is one group of patients who deserve special consideration for urodynamic investigation—men. It is this group who are highly likely to have "confusable conditions" that may masquerade as bladder pain. In a study in which patients with a working diagnosis of BPS were systematically reinvestigated, four out of five male patients had symptoms and uroflowmetric evidence of bladder outlet obstruction. Three of these had bladder outlet obstruction confirmed on urodynamics and all three obtained complete symptomatic relief with alpha-adrenergic blockade [6].

Because BPS is such a rare condition in men, one should have a low threshold for performing cystometry.

Comparative Urodynamics

Comparative urodynamics involves performing consecutive CMGs using normal saline followed by 0.2–0.3 M potassium chloride. The use of potassium as a filling solution is not only more physiological (as urine is potassium-rich)—but it is also a means of performing a potassium sensitivity test (PST) under controlled conditions. The PST was devised by Parsons to help in the diagnosis of BPS. It is based on the hypothesis that, because of increased urothelial permeability in BPS, potassium ions cross through the urothelium and depolarize sensory nerve endings, reproducing the pain of which the BPS patient complains [7, 8]. However, the diagnostic accuracy of the KCl test has received conflicting reports [9–12].

Comparative cystometry using normal saline followed by 0.2 M KCl has shown that the potassium infusion lowers the C_{max} obtained by saline by approximately 30% in over 90% of patients with a diagnosis of BPS [13]. The comparative decrease in C_{max} in a control group of non-BPS patients was only 8.6%. The authors recommended using a 30% decrease in C_{max} with KCl compared to saline as an "indicative" for a disorder at the urine–tissue barrier that is typically found in BPS. These findings were reproduced by other authors [14]. However, a randomized blinded study using 0.3 M KCl versus saline in which BPS patients were compared to those with proven detrusor overactivity showed that KCl produces an even greater reduction in C_{max} in DO [15, 16]. While this might suggest that the two conditions (BPS and DO) may share a similar pathogenesis, it does not support the notion that comparative cystometry can be used to diagnose either IC (as it was previously defined) or BPS (as we now know it).

The logical next step for comparative cystometry was to see if it could be used to predict which patients might respond best to GAG replacement therapy. In a pilot study of 48 BPS patients, who underwent comparative cystometry and subsequently received intravesical hyaluronic acid treatment, all patients obtained symptomatic relief. However, the improvements appeared to be more significant in those who had a reduction in C_{max} of more than 30% with KCl compared to saline [17]. A subsequent study by Daha et al. found that BPS patients who responded to GAG replacement therapy with complete symptomatic remission showed a normalization of the modified potassium test, while potassium sensitivity remained unchanged in the group of nonresponders. This suggests that whatever the nature of the disorder at the urine–tissue barrier is, it may be detected with potassium testing and cured with GAG substitution therapy [18].

It is important to understand that neither the original 0.4 M PST nor the modified 0.2 M (comparative cystometry) test can be used to diagnose BPS: this is still a clinical diagnosis. However it may be useful in predicting which patients have a higher probability of responding to GAG replacement therapy.

References

1. Schafer W, Abrams P, Liao L, Mattiasson A, Pesce F, Spangberg A, Sterling AM, Zinner NR, van Kerrebroeck P. Good urodynamic practices: uroflowmetry, filling cystometry, and pressure-flow studies. Neurourol Urodyn. 2002;21(3):261–74.
2. Gillenwater J, Wein AJ. Summary of the National Institute of Arthritis and Kidney Diseases workshop on Interstitial Cystitis, National Institute of Health, Bethesda, Maryland, 28–29, 1987. J Urol. 1988;140:203–6.
3. Irwin PP. Interstitial cystitis: a time for revision of name and diagnostic criteria in the new millennium? BJU Int. 2002;89:794.
4. Blaivas JG. Urodynamics for the evaluation of painful bladder syndrome/interstitial cystitis. J Urol. 2010;184(1):16–7.
5. Payne C. Urodynamics for the evaluation of painful bladder syndrome/interstitial cystitis. J Urol. 2010;184(1):15–6.
6. Irwin P, Samsudin A. Reinvestigation of patients with a diagnosis of interstitial cystitis: common things are sometimes common. J Urol. 2005;174(6):584–7.
7. Parsons CL, Greenberger M, Gabal L, Bidair M, Barme G. The role of urinary potassium in the pathogenesis and diagnosis of interstitial cystitis. J Urol. 1998;159(6):1862–67.
8. Parsons CL. Diagnosing chronic pelvic pain of bladder origin. J Reprod Med. 2004;49(3):235–42.
9. Chambers GK, Fenster HN, Cripps S, Jens M, Taylor D. An assessment of the use of intravesical potassium in the diagnosis of interstitial cystitis. J Urol. 1999;162(3Pt1):699–701.
10. Teichman JM, Nielsen-Omeis BJ. Potassium leak test predicts outcome in interstitial cystitis. J Urol. 1999;161(6):1791–4.
11. Gregoire M, Liandier F, Naud A, Lacombe L, Fradet Y. Does the potassium stimulation test predict cystometric, cystoscopic outcome in interstitial cystitis? J Urol. 2002;168(2):556–7.
12. Irwin PP, Takei M, Sugino Y. Summary of the urodynamics workshops on IC, Kyoto, Japan. Int J Urol. 2003;10:S19–23.
13. Daha LK, Riedl CR, Hohlbrugger G, Knoll M, Engelhardt PF, Pfluger H. Comparative assessment of maximal bladder capacity, 0.9% NaCl versus 0.2 M KCl, for the diagnosis of interstitial cystitis: a prospective controlled study. J Urol. 2003;170:807–9.
14. da Silveira AB, Riccetto CLZ, Natalin RA, Herrmann V, Dambros M, Palma P. Pilot study on the comparative assessment of maximum bladder capacity for the diagnosis of Interstitial Cystitis: NaCl 0.9% versus 0.2 M KCl. UroToday Int J. 2009;2(4).
15. Philip J, Willmott S, Irwin P. Interstitial cystitis versus detrusor overactivity: a comparative, randomized controlled study of cystometry using saline and 0.3 m potassium chloride. J Urol. 2006;175(2):566–71.
16. Irwin PP, Samsudin A, Philip J. Comparative assessment of maximal bladder capacity, 0.9% NaCl versus 0.2% KCl, for the diagnosis of interstitial cystitis: a prospective controlled study (letter). J Urol. 2003;171(4):1635.
17. Daha LK, Riedl CR, Lazar D, Hohlbrugger G, Pflüger H. Do cystometric findings predict the results of intravesical hyaluronic acid in women with interstitial cystitis? Eur Urol. 2005;47(3):393–7.
18. Daha LK, Riedl CR, Lazar D, Simak R, Pfluger H. Effect of intravesical glycosaminoglycan substitution therapy on bladder pain syndrome/interstitial cystitis, bladder capacity and potassium sensitivity. Scand J Urol Nephrol. 2008;42(4):369–72.

Part IV
Therapy

Chapter 18
Complementary and Alternative Medical Treatments of Bladder Pain Syndrome

Z. Chad Baxter, Helen R. Levey, Jennifer Yonaitis Fariello, and Robert M. Moldwin

Introduction

Bladder pain syndrome (BPS) patients often present with symptoms for which physically invasive therapies have been ineffective [1]. Patients with refractory symptoms may, however, still respond to complementary and alternative medical treatments (CAM).

CAM therapies center upon patient education and encompass a wide variety of methods to address concomitant physical and emotional distress. The goal is to empower patients, augment traditional medical therapy, and ultimately improve quality of life (QOL). CAM therapies are frequently used to complement traditional therapies and provide additional treatment options for patients with refractory BPS. CAM includes behavioral therapy such as bladder retraining, dietary changes, relaxation techniques, acupuncture, yoga, and cognitive-behavioral therapy (CBT). Many of these therapies have been reported to reduce pain and improve QOL in patients with

Z.C. Baxter, M.D.
Urology, Center for Pelvic Health and Reconstructive Surgery, Smith Institute for Urology, North Shore—LIJ School of Medicine, New Hyde Park, NY, USA
e-mail: zbaxter@nshs.edu

H.R. Levey, D.O., M.P.H.
The Arthur Smith Institute for Urology, North Shore—Long Island Jewish Health System, New Hyde Park, NY, USA

J.Y. Fariello, M.S.N., C.R.N.P. (✉)
Urology Division, Department of Obstetrics and Gynecology, FPMRS, The Pelvic and Sexual Health Institute, Drexel University College of Medicine,
207 N. Broad Street, 4th Floor, Philadelphia, PA 19107, USA
e-mail: jfariello@gmail.com

R.M. Moldwin, M.D.
Urology Division, North Shore-Long Island Jewish Health System, The Arthur Smith Institute for Urology, New Hyde Park, NY, USA

Urology Department, The Hofstra University School of Medicine, New Hyde Park, NY, USA

J. Nordling et al. (eds.), *Bladder Pain Syndrome: A Guide for Clinicians*,
DOI 10.1007/978-1-4419-6929-3_18, © Springer Science+Business Media New York 2013

other pain-mediated, chronic conditions such as rheumatoid arthritis, fibromyalgia, back pain, dyspareunia, and vulvodynia [2–5]. Just as they have on patients suffering from other chronic pain syndromes, CAM therapies may have a significant positive clinical impact on BPS patients. This chapter reviews some of the techniques and rationales of the CAM interventions that have been used for the BPS patient.

Bladder Retraining

Voiding commonly lessens the pain and urinary urgency associated with IC/BPS. This, in turn, perpetuates urinary frequency with frequent, low-volume voids, often less than 120 mL [6]. Eventually, a pattern of frequent voiding occurs that may be difficult to reverse, even after successful pain management. Additionally, patients with long-standing BPS or those with Hunner's ulcer disease may have an associated decrease in bladder capacity and compliance. Bladder retraining (BT) is a behavioral therapy intended to treat frequent urination by increasing the time between voiding intervals. Delayed voiding thereby increases bladder capacity and decreases discomfort. BT is most effective when the pain associated with bladder filling has been significantly reduced or controlled through adjuvant treatment [7].

The most common form of bladder retraining described is timed urination. The patient is instructed to void at timed intervals, usually before the urge to urinate. This protocol has been found to be efficacious in patients with overactive bladder (OAB) or stress urinary incontinence (SUI); however the technique has limitations in patients with BPS. For these patients, a more simplistic approach is to routinely defer voiding by a specified period of time, usually 5–30 min. Progressive increases of 15–30 min in the voiding interval every 3–4 weeks resulted in a 50% decrease in frequency, nocturia, and urgency in 71% of BPS patients [8] according to Chaiken et al. who evaluated 42 women with refractory symptoms of BPS for a minimum of 2 years. The women reported symptoms of urgency and frequency of urination at least once every 2 h while awake and persistent pelvic pain and discomfort. They were instructed to keep a voiding diary, control fluid intake, and practice timed voiding and pelvic floor muscle training techniques. After 3 months of treatment the voiding interval increased in all patients by an average of 93 min ($p<0.001$) and 98% of patients experienced a decrease in the number of voids per day by a mean of 9 ($p<0.01$). In addition, 50% of patients reported that their symptoms were markedly improved using a global assessment scale and 71% showed a significant increase in functional bladder capacity on their voiding diaries [9].

Behavioral therapy is a time-consuming process that requires consistent effort by the patient. The process is complicated by patient skepticism about the treatment leading to noncompliance and dissatisfaction. Formal written instructions explaining the program, regular follow-up visits, patient monitoring, and encouragement can aid in patient adherence to behavioral therapy. Success depends on patients seeing their progress over time and accepting the chronic nature of their condition and the treatment.

Behavioral Therapy and Patient Empowerment

Chronic illnesses, particularly those with associated pain, may have a profound effect upon QOL. Feelings of hopelessness and helplessness often result; and their impact can be as distressful to the patients as the illness itself [10]. Catastrophizing is a maladaptive coping behavior characterized by excessive focus and rumination, and is a significant predictor of pain severity and diminished QOL in patients with chronic pelvic pain [11–15]. A recent case-controlled survey demonstrated a correlation between stress, anxiety, depression, and catastrophizing to BPS-specific symptoms and a decreased QOL [16]. Treatments such as supportive psychotherapy and directed psychopharmaceutical agents may assist patients to mentally and emotionally adjust to their condition [17]. The therapeutic goal is for patients to develop a sense of empowerment over their illness. Self-efficacy, the belief that one can achieve success in a situation, is affected by the patient's mental health, cognitive thinking patterns, coping mechanisms, and availability or degree of surrounding support. A strong sense of self-efficacy improves coping skills, empowers the patient, and may lead to better QOL [18]. Conversely, as patients' sense of self-efficacy and control diminishes, they feel more helpless and isolated. Thus, the impact of social support on the patient cannot be overemphasized. Social support theory has demonstrated that patients with stronger social ties have positive health behavior outcomes [19].

An important resource for information and support is the Interstitial Cystitis Association (ICA), http://www.ichelp.org/, which was founded in 1984 [20]. This not-for-profit organization provides advocacy, research funding, and education to patients and clinicians. Additionally, the ICA reviews and recommends numerous Web sites, online databases, telephone hotlines, educational videos, health magazines, journal articles, and support groups that can assist patients in making educated health decisions [20]. Not only does the ICA provide the location and contact information for support groups across the country and around the world, but it also links to several forms of online support. Patients can find help through Facebook, Twitter, chat rooms, or blogs, significantly increasing the accessibility of support.

Beyond supportive psychotherapy, patient empowerment may be achieved by many of the techniques discussed in this chapter. Additionally, the use of other self-applied techniques such as physical therapy, dietary changes, patient-initiated treatment of occasional urinary tract infections, and self-intravesical instillations can foster a sense of mastery over the medical condition.

Cognitive Behavioral Therapy/Psychotherapy

CBT includes a broad category of different treatment regimes consisting of a cognitive (thought) component and an interventional behavior component. CBT is designed to help patients develop better coping strategies, alter their chronic pain beliefs, decrease their catastrophic thinking, and, ultimately, to empower them

[21, 22]. Patients are taught to recognize an irrational or catastrophizing thought and then learn to replace it with a rational thought. This is combined with an accompanying behavior to help alleviate pain or the targeted distressing symptom. CBT is most successful when the patient is meeting with a therapist and practicing thought recognition and replacement and helpful interventional behaviors regularly.

Although it is more difficult to research the efficacy of CBT because it is not as standardized as other treatments, numerous studies have shown that CBT increases perceived control in patients with chronic pain by reducing pain, helplessness, disability, and psychological distress [23–26]. Sinclair et al. enrolled 90 women with rheumatoid arthritis into an interventional CBT program designed to teach pain coping therapies. Significant improvements were observed in self-efficacy, pain coping behaviors, fatigue, and overall psychological well-being after engaging in CBT [27]. A large review by Eccleston et al. examined 52 randomized controlled trials (RCTs) that implemented CBT or other behavioral therapies for the management of chronic pain. It was concluded that, overall, CBT has positive effects on pain, distress, disability, and mood with changes that lasted up to 6 months following the intervention [28].

Sex therapy has been hypothesized as another possible treatment for symptoms of BPS. A review of the literature, however, demonstrated that well-controlled studies examining the relationship of sex therapy and BPS are lacking. Research did show that the techniques used in sex therapy, including CBT, correlated positively with decreased chronic prostatitis/chronic pelvic pain syndrome (CP/CPPS) symptoms and other sexual pain disorders [22].

Nickel et al. developed a CBT program for men with CP/CPPS based on the theory that individuals may learn to respond to either stressful or positive situations similarly based on past experiences [29]. The design of the CBT program developed for CP/CPPS helps patients assess the relationship between their distress due to symptoms, the thoughts that occur when they are distressed, and the emotions and behavioral responses associated with these thoughts. This CBT program is the first comprehensive attempt to target specific evidence-supported biopsychosocial variables (i.e., catastrophizing, mood, social interaction, maladaptive rest as a pain coping strategy) for symptom and QOL improvement in CP/CPPS. Currently, there is a pilot study under way which evaluates how this CBT program may improve QOL as the primary outcome and any decrease in disability and perception of pain severity as secondary outcomes [29].

The link between BPS, pain, and sexual dysfunction has significant implications for clinicians who play a crucial role in initiating and implementing treatments. Psychological approaches to pain management have been shown to decrease pain intensity and improve coping in patients with chronic pain conditions and, in the case of vulvodynia, reduce catastrophizing and improve sexual functioning in women [30, 31]. Prior to 2000, only two published studies investigated the effectiveness of combination sex therapy and CBT [32]. Since then, overall results of subsequent studies have shown that CBT leads to significant improvements in pain and psychosexual functioning, even when delivered in a research context with a short-term treatment duration and group format [3, 33, 34]. CBT, delivered in actual clinical practice, tailored to the patient's needs, and targeting specific biopsychosocial variables, may help break the pain response cycle and maintain improvement of symptoms [32].

Acupuncture

Acupuncture is an alternative treatment thought to achieve beneficial results through neuromodulation. Acupuncture stimulates increased production of endorphins and is thought to diminish pain by stimulating α-delta fibers while inhibiting unmyelinated sensory C-fibers [35, 36]. A pilot study of 12 men with refractory CP/CPPS who received a minimum of twice-weekly acupuncture for 6 weeks showed that 92% of patients had a greater than 50% reduction in their NIH-Chronic Prostatitis Symptom Index (NIH-CPSI) total score (28.2–8.5), and 83% of patients had more than 75% subjective global improvement. The response rate was unchanged during 33 weeks of follow-up [37].

The NIH funded the first randomized study of acupuncture versus sham acupuncture for CP/CPPS. Ninety patients were divided between two groups and received treatment for 30 min twice weekly for 10 weeks, with an additional 24-week follow-up. Using NIH-CPSI as the validated symptom tool, acupuncture was found to be twice as effective as sham acupuncture, a greater number of acupuncture patients had a complete resolution of symptoms, and those in the acupuncture cohort had better long-term response rates at 20 weeks after treatment compared to the sham acupuncture group [36].

Most recently, Lee et al. evaluated the effects of acupuncture, exercise, and advice on the NIH-CPSI scores of men with CP/CPPS. The men were divided into three cohorts ($n=13$). The first group received treatment advice and exercise; the second received treatment advice, exercise, and sham acupuncture; and the third, treatment advice, exercise, and acupuncture. Results showed that the NIH-CPSI scores of men who received acupuncture reported a significant decrease in pain compared to the men who received sham or no acupuncture. However, there was no reported change in urinary symptoms or QOL from pretreatment to posttreatment scores [38].

A systematic review and meta-analysis evaluating the analgesic effect of acupuncture in three-armed, randomized clinical trials comparing acupuncture with no acupuncture and with placebo acupuncture concluded that while a small analgesic effect was found with acupuncture, it could not be clearly distinguished from bias [35]. Other studies have shown that penetration of a needle through the skin, whether at an acupuncture point or not, does in fact have physiological effects [35].

Guided Imagery

Guided Imagery (GI) uses words to direct one's thoughts or focus to imagined visual, auditory, tactile, or even olfactory sensation in order to elicit the physiological effects of relaxation [39]. Several theories attempt to describe the physiologic and psychological effects seen with guided imagery. The Gate Control Theory suggests that only one impulse can travel up the spinal cord to the brain at a time. If that pathway is occupied by the thought produced from GI, the pain sensation impulses are unable to be carried to the brain, thereby reducing pain sensation [39]. An alternative theory postulates that endorphins are released in response to GI by activating the parasympathetic nervous system, thus lowering blood pressure and decreasing pulse and respiratory rates while increasing the pain threshold [39]. Regardless of the mechanism, GI has been documented to reduce pain in many conditions such as cancer, chronic low-back pain, and postoperative pain [40–42]. In one study, 30 women with IC were randomized into two groups: one group listened to a 25-min GI compact disc (CD) specifically designed for BPS patients, twice a day for 8 weeks, and the other group was instructed to rest during that same time interval. At the end of the study, over 45% of the treatment group noted subjective moderate or marked improvements on the global response assessment. Mean pain scores showed significant improvement pre- and post-treatment (from 5.50 to 2.57, $p=0.039$), and episodes of urgency decreased significantly as reported via a voiding diary (from 16 to 12, $p=0.02$) [39]. Furthermore, the treatment group showed significant reductions in BPS symptoms, as defined by responses on the Interstitial Cystitis Symptom Index and Problem Index (IC-SIPI) questionnaire (problem index from 11.13 to 9.45, $p=0.006$, and symptom index from 13.4 to 11.6, $p=0.004$). Comparatively, the nontreatment group remained essentially the same with no change in pain levels pre- to post-treatment (from 4.9 to 4.4, $p=0.187$), episodes of urgency (from 9.8 to 9, $p=0.684$), or their change in their IC-SIPI scores (problem index 11.6–9.85, symptom index 12.26–10.71) [39]. While larger RCTs need to be conducted, GI has shown to be a promising option to reduce stress and pain in otherwise refractory chronic pain conditions.

Hatha Yoga

Hatha Yoga has been promoted for centuries to reduce stress and is potentially useful in the BPS population. Hatha Yoga uses body positions and deep-breathing techniques to provide beneficial results in patients afflicted with numerous chronic disorders. Through the incorporation of over 200 individual exercises, all with various patient-specific modifications, it is universally adaptable to fit almost any patient's medical condition [43]. Pelvic floor hypertonicity is a comorbid condition seen in as many as 85–87% of BPS patients [44] that can be targeted for treatment through Hatha Yoga. Pelvic floor hypertonicity can be improved by specific positions, termed "asanas," which promote relaxation of the levator ani and the superficial layer of the urethral and anal sphincters. Rotation or dysfunction in the spine, pelvic floor, bony pelvis, or sacroiliac joint can create additional musculoskeletal compromise and aggravate chronic urological conditions such as BPS, prostatitis, chronic orchitis, vulvodynia, and chronic epididymitis. Yoga programs have been designed to treat those structural dysfunctions in the pelvis and improve chronic urological conditions [43]. Hatha Yoga is not an alternative to traditional treatments such as medical and physical therapy and caution should be used before beginning any exercise or yoga program. However, the regular practice of yoga has been shown to increase endorphin release, improve muscle strength, aerobic capacity, and pain control and decrease stress and fatigue. There have also been reports of improved psychological and emotional well-being [43, 45–47].

Diaphragmatic Breathing

Diaphragmatic breathing, used alone or with yoga, can considerably reduce stress and anxiety. In times of stress, we subconsciously tend to inhale and hold our breath. The most significant and therapeutic advantage of diaphragmatic breathing is in the exhalation, which lasts twice as long as the inhalation. The exhalation notifies the body that it can relax and resume essential body functions by ameliorating the "fight or flight" state [48, 49].

Diaphragmatic breathing is deep, abdominal breathing, rather than shallow breathing from the chest. The patient is taught to take slow, deep inhalations allowing for sequentially deeper relaxation with each breath. Diaphragmatic breathing is often used for treatment of hypoventilation, anxiety, or stuttering disorders [49]. In a small study by Mendelowitz et al. 19 patients with BPS and pelvic floor dysfunction were given therapy consisting of sitz baths, 2 mg of diazepam (three times a day), and relaxation therapy which included diaphragmatic breathing and progressive relaxation techniques. After 3 months of therapy, patients reported a significant reduction in pain and urgency scores as demonstrated on visual analog scales [50].

Paradoxical Relaxation

The primary support for the pelvic organs comes from the levator ani muscles which are often hypertonic, thus producing pain and urinary symptoms in patients with BPS and CP/CPPS [44, 51]. Certain types of chronic pelvic pain may reflect a self-perpetuating state of tension in the pelvic floor. Cycles of tension, anxiety, stress, or pain induced pelvic floor muscle hypertonicity, tension, spasms, and myofascial trigger points that are sensitive to palpation [44, 52, 53]. This is more commonly known as pelvic floor dysfunction and is prevalent in men and women with BPS.

Paradoxical relaxation (PR) is a technique in which manual therapy is used to teach the pelvic floor muscles to contract and relax, thereby decreasing the resting tone of the muscles and breaking the cycle of pain and spasm [51]. Anderson et al. treated 138 men with refractory CP/CPPS for 1 month using PR and myofascial trigger point release therapy (MFRT). 72% of patients reported "moderate" or "marked improvement" based on global response assessments, with over 50% of patients having a 25% or greater reduction in pain and urinary symptom scores as scored by the pelvic pain symptom survey (PPSS). In patients with a 50% or greater improvement level, median pain and urinary symptom scores decreased by 69% and 80%, respectively [53]. When used repetitively and with proper technique, the practice of PR reduces hypertonicity of the pelvic floor muscles and provides significant relief to patients with BPS and comorbid pelvic floor dysfunction.

Conclusion

Complementary and alternative therapies have demonstrable benefits for patients suffering from chronic pain syndromes and may likely be effective, adjunctive therapies appropriate for many patients suffering from BPS. CAM therapies are a broad and diverse group of treatments that may be individualized to each patient. Further research is needed to determine if and which CAM therapy is suitable for a given patient, but there is mounting evidence that alternative treatment modalities may be beneficial to many patients both today and in the future.

References

1. Ottem DP, Carr LK, Perks AE, Lee P, Teichman JM. Interstitial cystitis and female sexual dysfunction. Urology. 2007;69(4):608–10.
2. van Tulder MW, Ostelo R, Vlaeyen JW, Linton SJ, Morley SJ, Assendelft WJ. Behavioral treatment for chronic low back pain: a systematic review within the framework of the Cochrane Back Review Group. Spine (Phila Pa 1976). 2000;25(20):2688–99.
3. Bergeron S, Binik YM, Khalife S, et al. A randomized comparison of group cognitive–behavioral therapy, surface electromyographic biofeedback, and vestibulectomy in the treatment of dyspareunia resulting from vulvar vestibulitis. Pain. 2001;91(3):297–306.
4. Breton A, Miller CM, Fisher K. Enhancing the sexual function of women living with chronic pain: a cognitive-behavioural treatment group. Pain Res Manag. 2008;13(3):219–24.
5. McCracken LM, MacKichan F, Eccleston C. Contextual cognitive-behavioral therapy for severely disabled chronic pain sufferers: effectiveness and clinically significant change. Eur J Pain. 2007;11(3):314–22.
6. Butrick CW, Howard FM, Sand PK. Diagnosis and treatment of interstitial cystitis/painful bladder syndrome: a review. J Womens Health (Larchmt). 2010;19(6):1185–93.
7. Whitmore KE. Complementary and alternative therapies as treatment approaches for interstitial cystitis. Rev Urol. 2002;4 Suppl 1:S28–35.
8. Parsons CL, Koprowski PF. Interstitial cystitis: successful management by increasing urinary voiding intervals. Urology. 1991;37(3):207–12.
9. Chaiken DC, Blaivas JG, Blaivas ST. Behavioral therapy for the treatment of refractory interstitial cystitis. J Urol. 1993;149(6):1445–8.
10. McNaughton Collins M, Pontari MA, O'Leary MP. Quality of life is impaired in men with chronic prostatitis: the Chronic Prostatitis Collaborative Research Network. J Gen Intern Med. 2001;16(10):656–62.
11. Sullivan MJ, Thorn B, Haythornthwaite JA, et al. Theoretical perspectives on the relation between catastrophizing and pain. Clin J Pain. 2001;17(1):52–64.

12. Tripp DA, Nickel JC, Wang Y, et al. Catastrophizing and pain-contingent rest predict patient adjustment in men with chronic prostatitis/chronic pelvic pain syndrome. J Pain. 2006;7(10):697–708.
13. Nickel JC, Tripp DA, Chuai S, et al. Psychosocial variables affect the quality of life of men diagnosed with chronic prostatitis/chronic pelvic pain syndrome. BJU Int. 2008;101(1):59–64.
14. Nickel JC, Tripp DA, Pontari M, et al. Psychosocial phenotyping in women with interstitial cystitis/painful bladder syndrome: a case control study. J Urol. 2010;183(1):167–72.
15. Rothrock NE, Lutgendorf SK, Kreder KJ. Coping strategies in patients with interstitial cystitis: relationships with quality of life and depression. J Urol. 2003;169(1):233–6.
16. Nickel JC, Tripp DA, Pontari M, et al. Interstitial cystitis/painful bladder syndrome and associated medical conditions with an emphasis on irritable bowel syndrome, fibromyalgia and chronic fatigue syndrome. J Urol. 2010;184(4):1358–63.
17. Rapkin AJ, Kames LD. The pain management approach to chronic pelvic pain. J Reprod Med. 1987;32(5):323–7.
18. Groysman V. Vulvodynia: new concepts and review of the literature. Dermatol Clin. 2010;28(4):681–96.
19. Hupcey JE. Clarifying the social support theory-research linkage. J Adv Nurs. 1998;27(6):1231–41.
20. Association IC. October 7, 2010; http://www.ichelp.org/Page.aspx id=329. Accessed 6 Nov 2010.
21. Jensen MP. Psychosocial approaches to pain management: an organizational framework. Pain. 2010;152:717–25.
22. Wehbe SA, Fariello JY, Whitmore K. Minimally invasive therapies for chronic pelvic pain syndrome. Curr Urol Rep. 2010;11(4):276–85.
23. McCracken LM, Turk DC. Behavioral and cognitive-behavioral treatment for chronic pain: outcome, predictors of outcome, and treatment process. Spine (Phila Pa 1976). 2002;27(22):2564–73.
24. Lopez-Martinez AE, Esteve-Zarazaga R, Ramirez-Maestre C. Perceived social support and coping responses are independent variables explaining pain adjustment among chronic pain patients. J Pain. 2008;9(4):373–9.
25. Sinclair VG, Wallston KA. Predictors of improvement in a cognitive-behavioral intervention for women with rheumatoid arthritis. Ann Behav Med. 2001;23(4):291–7.
26. Evers AW, Kraaimaat FW, van Riel PL, de Jong AJ. Tailored cognitive-behavioral therapy in early rheumatoid arthritis for patients at risk: a randomized controlled trial. Pain. 2002;100(1–2):141–53.
27. Sinclair VG. Predictors of pain catastrophizing in women with rheumatoid arthritis. Arch Psychiatr Nurs. 2001;15(6):279–88.
28. Eccleston C, Palermo TM, Williams AC, Lewandowski A, Morley S. Psychological therapies for the management of chronic and recurrent pain in children and adolescents. Cochrane Database Syst Rev. 2009;(2):CD003968.
29. Nickel JC, Mullins C, Tripp DA. Development of an evidence-based cognitive behavioral treatment program for men with chronic prostatitis/chronic pelvic pain syndrome. World J Urol. 2008;26(2):167–72.
30. Morley S, Eccleston C, Williams A. Systematic review and meta-analysis of randomized controlled trials of cognitive behaviour therapy and behaviour therapy for chronic pain in adults, excluding headache. Pain. 1999;80(1–2):1–13.
31. Landry T, Bergeron S, Dupuis MJ, Desrochers G. The treatment of provoked vestibulodynia: a critical review. Clin J Pain. 2008;24(2):155–71.
32. Bergeron S, Landry T, Leclerc B. Cognitive-behavioral, physical therapy and alternative treatments for dyspareunia. In: Goldstein AT, Pukall C, Goldstein I, editors. Female sexual pain disorders. 1st ed. Hoboken: Wiley-Blackwell; 2008.
33. Bergeron S, Khalife S, Glazer HI, Binik YM. Surgical and behavioral treatments for vestibulodynia: two-and-one-half year follow-up and predictors of outcome. Obstet Gynecol. 2008;111(1):159–66.

34. ter Kuile MM, Weijenborg PT. A cognitive-behavioral group program for women with vulvar vestibulitis syndrome (VVS): factors associated with treatment success. J Sex Marital Ther. 2006;32(3):199–213.
35. Madsen MV, Gotzsche PC, Hrobjartsson A. Acupuncture treatment for pain: systematic review of randomised clinical trials with acupuncture, placebo acupuncture, and no acupuncture groups. BMJ. 2009;338:a3115.
36. Lee SW, Liong ML, Yuen KH, et al. Acupuncture versus sham acupuncture for chronic prostatitis/chronic pelvic pain. Am J Med. 2008;121(1):79.e71–7.
37. Chen R, Nickel JC. Acupuncture ameliorates symptoms in men with chronic prostatitis/chronic pelvic pain syndrome. Urology. 2003;61(6):1156–9. discussion 1159.
38. Lee SH, Lee BC. Electroacupuncture relieves pain in men with chronic prostatitis/chronic pelvic pain syndrome: three-arm randomized trial. Urology. 2009;73(5):1036–41.
39. Carrico DJ, Peters KM, Diokno AC. Guided imagery for women with interstitial cystitis: results of a prospective, randomized controlled pilot study. J Altern Complement Med. 2008;14(1):53–60.
40. Syrjala KL, Donaldson GW, Davis MW, Kippes ME, Carr JE. Relaxation and imagery and cognitive-behavioral training reduce pain during cancer treatment: a controlled clinical trial. Pain. 1995;63(2):189–98.
41. Turner JA, Jensen MP. Efficacy of cognitive therapy for chronic low back pain. Pain. 1993;52(2):169–77.
42. Manyande A, Berg S, Gettins D, et al. Preoperative rehearsal of active coping imagery influences subjective and hormonal responses to abdominal surgery. Psychosom Med. 1995;57(2):177–82.
43. Ripoll E, Mahowald D. Hatha Yoga therapy management of urologic disorders. World J Urol. 2002;20(5):306–9.
44. Peters KM, Carrico DJ, Kalinowski SE, Ibrahim IA, Diokno AC. Prevalence of pelvic floor dysfunction in patients with interstitial cystitis. Urology. 2007;70(1):16–8.
45. Ulger O, Yagli NV. Effects of yoga on balance and gait properties in women with musculoskeletal problems: a pilot study. Complement Ther Clin Pract. 2011;17(1):13–5.
46. Bower JE, Garet D, Sternlieb B. Yoga for persistent fatigue in breast cancer survivors: results of a pilot study. Evid Based Complement Alternat Med. 2011;2011:623168.
47. Wren AA, Wright MA, Carson JW, Keefe FJ. Yoga for persistent pain: new findings and directions for an ancient practice. Pain. 2011;152:477–80.
48. Cohen L, Parker PA, Vence L, et al. Presurgical stress management improves postoperative immune function in men with prostate cancer undergoing radical prostatectomy. Psychosom Med. 2011;73:218–25.
49. Jefferson LL. Exploring effects of therapeutic massage and patient teaching in the practice of diaphragmatic breathing on blood pressure, stress, and anxiety in hypertensive African-American women: an intervention study. J Natl Black Nurses Assoc. 2010;21(1):17–24.
50. Mendelowitz F, Moldwin R. Complementary therapies in the management of interstitial cystitis. In: Sant G, editor. Interstitial cystitis. Philadelphia: Lippincott-Raven; 1997. p. 235–9.
51. Srinivasan AK, Kaye JD, Moldwin R. Myofascial dysfunction associated with chronic pelvic floor pain: management strategies. Curr Pain Headache Rep. 2007;11(5):359–64.
52. Anderson RU, Sawyer T, Wise D, Morey A, Nathanson BH. Painful myofascial trigger points and pain sites in men with chronic prostatitis/chronic pelvic pain syndrome. J Urol. 2009;182(6):2753–8.
53. Anderson RU, Wise D, Sawyer T, Chan C. Integration of myofascial trigger point release and paradoxical relaxation training treatment of chronic pelvic pain in men. J Urol. 2005;174(1):155–60.

Chapter 19
Diet and Its Role in Bladder Pain Syndrome and Comorbid Conditions

Justin I. Friedlander, Barbara Shorter, and Robert M. Moldwin

Abbreviations

BPS	Bladder pain syndrome
CFS	Chronic fatigue syndrome
FMS	Fibromyalgia syndrome
GAG	Glycosaminoglycan
IBS	Irritable bowel syndrome
IC	Interstitial cystitis
ICA	Interstitial Cystitis Association
OSPI	O'Leary–Sant pain index
PUF	Pain urgency, frequency scale

J.I. Friedlander (✉)
The Arthur Smith Institute for Urology, North Shore-Long Island Jewish Health System, 450 Lakeville Rd, Suite M-41, New Hyde Park, NY 11042, USA
e-mail: jfriedland@nshs.edu

B. Shorter
Didactic Program in Dietetics, Department of Nutrition, Long Island University, Brookville, NY, USA

R.M. Moldwin
Urology Division, The Arthur Smith Institute for Urology, North Shore-Long Island Jewish Health System, New Hyde Park, NY, USA

Urology Department, The Hofstra University School of Medicine, New Hyde Park, NY, USA

J. Nordling et al. (eds.), *Bladder Pain Syndrome: A Guide for Clinicians*, DOI 10.1007/978-1-4419-6929-3_19, © Springer Science+Business Media New York 2013

Introduction

While the pathophysiology of Bladder Pain Syndrome (BPS) remains uncertain, many theories exist linking dietary intake and symptoms, including alterations in urothelial barrier protection, organ-cross talk, neural upregulation, neurogenic inflammation, and others. Most of the studies performed to assess the role of diet on BPS have been anecdotal reports and questionnaire-based studies, but what they do suggest is that there is a high prevalence of food and beverage sensitivity in this patient population. Unfortunately, therapy for this condition is frequently suboptimal due to often-encountered comorbid medical disorders such as irritable bowel syndrome, migraine headaches, vulvodynia, and fibromyalgia [1–4]. This poses a particular challenge for clinicians wishing to make dietary recommendations for patients. The remainder of this chapter discusses links between diet and bladder pain, as well as dietary considerations among BPS and its comorbid conditions.

The Link Between Diet and BPS-Related Pain

The exact pathogenic mechanism of BPS remains to be established; however promising hypotheses do exist to explain how diet may alter associated symptoms. One commonly held theory is that a dysregulated or disrupted bladder urothelial barrier is responsible. Studies suggest that epithelial dysfunction can lead to the migration of urinary solutes across the urothelium with subsequent provocation of BPS symptoms [5]. Barrier disruption is believed to be due to abnormal protein expression, specifically with alterations of the glycosaminoglycan (GAG) layer [6]; dysregulation of other proteoglycans, cell adhesion, and tight junction proteins; and bacterial defense molecules [7]. Taken together, an altered urothelial barrier would allow normally innocuous substances, perhaps dietary metabolites, the opportunity to become noxious stimuli. Another mechanism that might contribute to urologic symptom production is organ "cross talk." Animal studies have demonstrated that colonic irritation and cross-afferent pelvic stimulation can lead to bladder cross-sensitization via integrated sensory pathways [8]. Hence, diet's influence on the bowel may modulate the pelvic pain seen in BPS [9]. Neural upregulation, either centrally or peripherally, is thought to amplify the effect of diet upon symptoms produced by other pathological mechanisms [10]. Neural upregulation may occur via neurogenic inflammation, by which mediators are directly released from sensory nerves resulting in various inflammatory changes [11].

BPS patients often report altered symptoms with certain foods, beverages, and dietary supplements; however, this association is not seen in all patients. Additionally, sensitivity to individual comestibles may vary between patients [12]. Historically, one of the early tenets of dietary modification with BPS was dietary restriction. Some of the evidence for this intervention was based on the observation that alcohol and foods high in acid and arylalkylamines increased discomfort in some individuals [13].

Another early study demonstrated that BPS-related pain was increased in more than half of the study population by acidic and spicy foods, alcoholic or carbonated beverages, and coffee and tea [14]. The following sections discuss these findings.

The Effect of Acid Foods

Recent studies suggest that acidic foods exacerbate bladder pain [15–17], and ingestion of alkalinizing agents such as sodium bicarbonate or agents that neutralize acid in food such as calcium glycerophosphate [18, 19] may provide symptomatic relief. Outside of cranberries, other acidic foods do not necessarily produce a change in urine pH or a corresponding change in the physiologic state of the bladder [20]. However, with reference to the possibility that alterations in urinary pH lead to alteration of symptoms, one prospective, randomized, double-blind study was performed [15]. The study involved 26 women with BPS, and consisted of crossover intravesical instillations of urine at a physiological pH (5.0) and neutral buffered pH (7.5). No statistically significant difference in pain scores was noted in patients with BPS upon instillation of urine at physiological pH or sodium-buffered saline; and no significant change from baseline scores was seen after instillation in either group. Although the study did suggest that urine pH has little direct sensory effect on the bladder surface, it does not preclude other mechanisms by which acidic foods may affect bladder symptoms. Dietary lists for BPS patients suggest acidic comestibles such as grapefruit and oranges as triggers for bladder inflammation and should be used with caution [21].

The Effect of High-Potassium Foods

Dietary information for BPS patients includes limiting high-potassium foods to avoid increasing bladder symptoms. Potassium levels in the urine are typically high with a range from 24 to 133 mEq/L [22]. Many studies have demonstrated the phenomenon of epithelial leak with increased urinary potassium absorption and exacerbation of bladder pain; however, the studies were small, underpowered investigations with a limited number of subjects [22–24]. In addition, these studies used intravesical "KCl challenges" and did not quantify or record food-related potassium intake. The recommendation of limiting dietary potassium is further complicated by the fact that surveys of foods that worsen bladder symptoms indicate that BPS patients do not typically experience food sensitivities when consuming certain high-potassium foods including white or sweet potatoes and milk [12]. What is missing is a better understanding of how changes in dietary potassium lead to changes in urinary levels of potassium, and if the changes in dietary intake are significant enough to cause symptoms as demonstrated with potassium sensitivity testing. Clearly there is no consensus regarding dietary potassium intake, and additional work is needed before any conclusions should be drawn.

The Effect of Caffeine

Surveys on food sensitivities indicate that when patients report that they are food sensitive, some of the most problematic comestibles are coffee, tea, and chocolate [12–14, 25]. Although the ingredient responsible for triggering flares has not been established, a common denominator for these products is caffeine. A study of caffeine ingestion in healthy volunteers demonstrated that caffeine caused an initial increase in voiding frequency [26]. Ultimately, the volunteers appeared to develop a tolerance to the caffeine, resulting in no overall difference in voiding frequency over the course of the study.

The Effect of Alcohol

Alcohol use as a possible trigger for BPS symptoms was investigated by a survey conducted by the IC Network. They found that 94% of 535 patients responding reported that their bladder symptoms increased when drinking various alcoholic beverages [27]. While only 5% of patients reported flares lasting longer than 1 week, 75% of patients stated that they had an increase in pain after drinking alcohol. Responses varied widely, but results suggested that alcoholic beverage tolerance from worst to best included wines (white wines provoking fewer reactions than red wines); mixed drinks; beers (with lighter beers being easier to tolerate); and "hard liquor" alcohol (scotch and brandy being better tolerated than tequila and vodka). In guiding decision-making, the study advocated patient avoidance of all alcohols when symptoms are active, and if alcohol is to be consumed, that it be followed by water to dilute the effect of alcohol in the urine.

New Directions Regarding Comestibles

More rigorous studies have only recently been undertaken to better assess diet's role in BPS. In a study by Shorter et al., a validated questionnaire was used to determine the incidence of women who feel that foods, beverages, and dietary supplements have an effect on bladder symptoms, as well as to determine which foods and beverages exacerbate or ameliorate the symptoms of BPS [12]. Results of this survey indicated that of 104 respondents who met the National Institute for Diabetes and Digestive Kidney Diseases criteria for BPS 90% felt that edibles did affect bladder symptoms. Furthermore, out of 175 individual items listed, 35 comestibles were found to be the chief offenders including caffeinated, carbonated, and alcoholic beverages, certain fruits and fruit juices, artificial sweeteners, and spicy foods. Patients who reported that specific foods worsened symptoms tended to have higher O'Leary–Sant Pain Index (OSPI) and Pain, Urgency, Frequency (PUF) scale scores.

A study recently published out of the University of South Florida surveyed members of the Interstitial Cystitis Association (ICA) with a Web-based questionnaire [28]. The goal was to better define what truly exacerbates or improves BPS symptoms, using a symptom-based Likert scale to assess the effect of 344 consumable items on urinary frequency, urgency, and/or pelvic pain symptoms. Of the 598 completed surveys, 95.8% of respondents noted that certain foods/beverages affected symptoms. Most items were found to have no effect on symptoms, but the biggest offenders were similar to those previously reported: citrus fruits, tomatoes, vitamin C, artificial sweeteners, coffee, tea, carbonated and alcoholic beverages, and spicy foods [12]. Again as found in other studies, both calcium glycerophosphate and sodium bicarbonate appeared to lead to improvement or symptomatic relief. Studies such as these are inherently subject to selection bias, but do help focus further investigative efforts given that the findings are not so disparate from what have been demonstrated by others.

Based upon these observations, many clinicians caring for patients with BPS advocate an elimination diet [21]. This diet entails the avoidance of potentially noxious foods/beverages for 2 weeks; these items are then reintroduced one at a time to determine whether or not a specific item provokes an exacerbation of symptoms. This intervention is often successful at alleviating symptoms. Care should be taken to avoid an overly restrictive diet as this can have a negative impact on overall health. Table 19.1 shows current dietary recommendations for patients with BPS.

Co-morbidities of Bladder Pain Syndrome and Diet

The management of BPS is made all the more difficult when clinicians must take into consideration co-morbidities often associated with this syndrome. Many of these conditions pose as additional pain generators. Furthermore, the symptoms of many of these comorbid conditions may be altered by diet. In one case–control study, some conditions commonly found to exist along with chronic pelvic pain included irritable bowel syndrome (IBS)/gastrointestinal symptoms, vulvar/vaginal pain, fibromyalgia, and headache [29]. Taken a step further, one study identified 25 publications with significant data linking urological conditions such as BPS and non-urological unexplained clinical conditions, some of which are mentioned above [30]. When trying to reconcile all of these conditions, it is clear that dietary advice must take into account comorbid conditions.

Irritable Bowel Syndrome

IBS is the second most common comorbid disease found in BPS patients. It is characterized by chronic symptoms that may include abdominal discomfort, altered intestinal motility, abdominal pain and distension, feelings of incomplete evacua-

Table 19.1 BPS dietary recommendations [12]

Foods identified as most bothersome to BPS patients	Foods identified as least bothersome to BPS patients
Coffee (caffeinated)	Water
Coffee (decaffeinated)	Milk, low-fat
Tea (caffeinated)	Milk, whole
Cola soda	Bananas
Noncola soda	Blueberries
Diet soda	Honeydew melon
Caffeine free soda	Pears
Beer	Raisins
Red wine	Watermelon
White wine	Broccoli
Champagne	Brussels sprouts
Grapefruit	Cabbage
Lemons	Carrots
Oranges	Cauliflower
Pineapple	Celery
Cranberry juice	Cucumber
Grapefruit juice	Mushrooms
Orange juice	Peas
Pineapple juice	Radishes
Tomato	Squash
Tomato products	Zucchini
Hot peppers	White potatoes
Spicy foods	Sweet potatoes/yams
Chili	Chicken
Horseradish	Eggs
Vinegar	Turkey
MSG	Beef
Nutrasweet	Pork
Sweet and Low	Lamb
Equal	Shrimp
Saccharin	Tuna fish
Mexican food	Salmon
Thai food	Oat
Indian food	Rice
	Pretzels
	Popcorn

tion, mucous in the stool, straining or urgency, and associated psychosocial distress [31]. As with BPS, the cause of IBS is unknown, yet these patients share many epidemiological, clinical, and pathophysiological findings [32].

Diet therapy must be tailored to address the specific gastrointestinal symptoms experienced. Modifications of nutritional intake that have been successful in IBS include such limitations as dietary fats to no more than 50 g/day, caffeine, sugars (particularly fructose in all forms), lactose, sugar alcohols, alcohol, wheat, citrus, corn, and gas-forming foods such as legumes and certain vegetables [33]. Although many physicians recommend bran in the management of constipation, this therapy has been found to worsen symptoms in patients with IBS. Soluble verses insoluble fibers (bulk forming laxatives such as psyllium fiber) with adequate liquids are recommended, as well as small versus large meals [34]. Similar to BPS patients, IBS patients often feel anxious about food and consume unnecessarily restrictive diets, resulting in poor nutrition status, increased anxiety, and worsened symptoms [35, 36].

Fibromyalgia Syndrome

Fibromyalgia syndrome is defined by the American College of Rheumatology as a history of widespread pain persisting for greater than 3 months in 11 of 18 well-defined tender point sites found on digital palpation [37]. An estimated 19% of patients with BPS also have FMS, with a large overlap in symptoms even if patients do not share both diagnoses [38]. Unfortunately despite high prevalence among BPS patients, the dietary information for FMS is rather generic.

A review of studies determining the effect of dietary modifications on patients with rheumatic conditions including FMS indicated that 40% of the participants felt that dietary modifications, without listing specific items, had an influence on mitigation of their symptoms [39]. A separate review on diet and FMS drew the conclusion that patients express a desire to maintain dietary interventions in their quest for pain relief [40]. This study was focused on a vegetarian diet but was not well constructed. A recent review article on diet and FMS suggested that the benefit of a vegetarian-based diet may be due to increased antioxidant intake, and weight control was an effective tool at controlling symptoms [41].

Chronic Fatigue Syndrome

Chronic Fatigue Syndrome is associated with BPS in roughly 9% of BPS patients [42]. It is defined as a persistent or relapsing fatigue of at least a 6-month duration that is not alleviated by rest and that causes substantial reduction in activities. The fatigue cannot be explained by medical or psychiatric conditions and must be accompanied by four of the eight case-defining symptoms (unusual post-exertional fatigue, impaired memory or concentration, un-refreshing sleep, headaches, muscle pain, joint pain, sore throat, and tender cervical nodes) [43].

The etiology of CFS has not been determined; however, an impaired immune system has been implicated, or possibly abnormal or insufficient response to oxidative stress [44]. Various treatments such as consuming a balanced diet, limiting caffeine intake, and drinking adequate fluids, along with medications, are sometimes effective. There exists no consensus for the use of dietary supplementation with vitamins and minerals as a treatment for CFS [45]; however, D-ribose, a form of sugar, seems promising in decreasing pain associated with CFS [46]. An example of the dietary management dilemma is seen with BPS patients who avoid food groups such as fruits, and end up lacking in powerful antioxidants including beta-carotene and Vitamin C, important for a properly functioning immune system and potentially beneficial for CFS.

Vulvodynia

Vulvodynia, a condition of chronic vulvar pain with no apparent etiology, is frequently found in the BPS population [47–50]. The first report of diet's influence upon vulvodynia centered upon the use of calcium citrate for a patient with high levels of urinary oxalate. The result was the cessation of her bladder pain symptoms [51], and a possible new intervention for these patients. Baggish et al. took a closer look, comparing urinary oxalate excretion in patients with vulvodynia versus that of controls and evaluated the role of dietary intervention in vulvodynia patients [52]. They found no difference in the 24-h excretion of oxalate between the two groups. Fifty-nine of the patients with vulvodynia and elevated oxalate concentrations were treated with a low-oxalate diet and calcium citrate supplementation. Only 14/49 (24%) had erythema or pain but there was no placebo group for comparison; hence no substantial conclusions regarding dietary intervention can be drawn. Another group examined the link between dietary oxalates and the development of vulvodynia [53]. This was a population-based, case–control study of women with and without vulvodynia. They found no increased risk of developing vulvodynia with increased oxalate intake. Taken together, it appears that the link between vulvodynia and dietary oxalate is at best anecdotal.

Depression

Depression is frequently identified in the BPS population [54]. While it is well documented that antidepressant medications are often helpful in the management of depression, promising evidence indicates that essential fatty acids, specifically omega 3-fatty acids, found in cold water fish, play an essential role in brain structure and function and that inadequate amounts of these essential fatty acids may be implicated in depression [55]. Specifically, work is ongoing to better understand the association between depression and a pro-inflammatory cytokine profile that can be seen in patients with a higher omega-6 fatty acid-to-omega-3 fatty acid ratio [56]. Whether there is a role for dietary intervention remains to be determined.

Neuropathic Pain

Neuropathic pain is defined as pain arising from a lesion or disease affecting the somatosensory system [57]. Patients with BPS often have coexisting neuropathic pain that is difficult to treat [29]. A recent case series examined five patients, all with different neuropathic pain conditions (cervical radiculopathy, thoracic outlet syndrome, fibromyalgia, carpal tunnel syndrome, burn injury), treated with high oral doses of omega-3 fish oil [58]. Outcome measures were measured pre- and post-treatment with various validated surveys. These patients had clinically significant pain reduction and improved function, such as grip strength, based on both subjective and objective measures up to as many as 19 months post treatment. A randomized control trial would be beneficial to investigate this further. Neuropathic pain also frequently coexists with depression. Perhaps the treatment of one disorder may be beneficial for the other as there may be a shared neurogenic pathophysiology [59]. As stated previously, work is needed to understand the role of omega-3 fatty acids in depression.

Headache

Many BPS patients present with a review of systems significant for headache [2]. Historically, foods such as cheese, alcohol, chocolate, and citrus fruits were thought to be triggers for migraines; yet this theory has not been borne out by the literature [60]. Two beneficial supplements in the battle against headache appear to be riboflavin and coenzyme Q10, both proving efficacious in reducing the frequency and duration of headache days, particularly for migraine headache [61]. Another study, recently published by the International Headache Society, showed that dietary restriction based on IgG antibodies might be an effective strategy to reduce the frequency of migraine headache attacks [62].

Conclusion

The prevalence of sensitivities to varied comestibles appears to be high amongst BPS patients. Sensitivities to foods and beverages may be derived from varied pathologic mechanisms. Based upon mainly anecdotal findings and survey studies, certain food types affect symptoms of BPS and comorbid conditions more than others, suggesting that a controlled method to determine dietary sensitivities, such as the elimination diet, may play an important first-line role in the management of the BPS patient. Consideration of the effect of diet on comorbid conditions may also need to be taken into account when counseling patients.

References

1. Buffington CA. Comorbidity of interstitial cystitis with other unexplained clinical conditions. J Urol. 2004;172:1242.
2. Erickson DR, Morgan KC, Ordille S, et al. Nonbladder related symptoms in patients with interstitial cystitis. J Urol. 2001;166:557.
3. Jones CA, Nyberg L. Epidemiology of interstitial cystitis. Urology. 1997;49:2.

4. Rodríguez MB, Afari N, Buchwald DS. Evidence for overlap between urological and nonurological unexplained clinical conditions. J Urol. 2009;182:2123.
5. Parsons CL. The role of the urinary epithelium in the pathogenesis of interstitial cystitis/prostatitis/urethritis. Urology. 2007;69:9.
6. Hauser PJ, Dozmorov MG, Bane BL, et al. Abnormal expression of differentiation related proteins in the urothelium of patients with interstitial cystitis. J Urol. 2008;179:764.
7. Hurst RE, Moldwin RM, Mulholland SG. Bladder defense molecules, urothelial differentiation, urinary biomarkers, and interstitial cystitis. Urology. 2007;69:17.
8. Ustinova EE, Fraser MO, Pezzone MA. Cross-talk and sensitization of bladder afferent nerves. Neurourol Urodyn. 2010;29:77.
9. Rudick CN, Chen MC, Monglu AK, et al. Organ cross talk modulates pelvic pain. Am J Physiol Regul Integr Comp Physiol. 2007;293:R1191.
10. Nazif O, Teichman JM, Gebhart GF. Neural upregulation in interstitial cystitis. Urology. 2007;69:24.
11. Wesselmann U. Neurogenic inflammation and chronic pelvic pain. World J Urol. 2001;3:180.
12. Shorter B, Lesser M, Moldwin R, et al. Effect of comestibles on symptoms of interstitial cystitis. J Urol. 2007;178:145.
13. Gillespie L. You don't have to live with cystitis! New York: Rawson Associates; 1996.
14. Koziol JA, Clark DC, Gittes RF, et al. The natural history of interstitial cystitis: a survey of 374 patients. J Urol. 1993;149:465.
15. Nguan C, Franciosi LG, Butterfield N, et al. A prospective, double-blind, randomized crossover study evaluating changes in urinary pH for relieving the symptoms of interstitial cystitis. BJU Int. 2005;95:91.
16. Clemens JQ, Brown SO, Kosloff L, et al. Predictors of symptoms severity in patients with chronic prostatitis and interstitial cystitis. J Urol. 2006;175:963.
17. Yamada T. Significance of complications of allergic diseases in young patients with interstitial cystitis. Int J Urol. 2003;10:S56.
18. Bologna RA, Gomelsky A, Lukban JC, Whitmore KE, et al. The efficacy of calcium glycerophosphate in the prevention of food-related flares in interstitial cystitis. Urology. 2001;57(6):119.
19. Theoharides TC, Sant GR. A pilot open label study of cystoprotek in interstitial cystitis. Int J Immunopathol Pharmacol. 2005;18:183.
20. Gettman MT, Ogan K, Brinkley LJ, et al. Effect of cranberry juice consumption on urinary stone risk factors. J Urol. 2005;174:590.
21. Marinkovic SP, Moldwin R, Gillen LM, et al. The management of interstitial cystitis or painful bladder syndrome in women. BMJ. 2009;339:337.
22. Parsons CL, Greene RA, Chung M, et al. Abnormal urinary potassium metabolism in patients with interstitial cystitis. J Urol. 2005;173:1182.
23. Parsons CL, Greenberger M, Gabal L, et al. The role of urinary potassium in the pathogenesis and diagnosis of interstitial cystitis. J Urol. 1998;159:1862.
24. Parsons CL, Zupkas P, Parsons JK. Intravesical potassium sensitivity in patients with interstitial cystitis and urethral syndrome. Urology. 2001;57:428.
25. Gillespie L. Metabolic appraisal of the effects of dietary modifications on hypersensitive bladder symptoms. Br J Urol. 1992;72:293.
26. Bird ET, Parker BD, Kim HS, et al. Caffeine ingestion and lower urinary tract symptoms in healthy volunteers. Neurourol Urodyn. 2005;24:611.
27. Osborne J. Wine, beer & spirits – do they trigger IC flares? A patient survey reveals surprising results. IC Optimist. 2010;7:15.
28. Bassaly R, Downes K, Hart S. Dietary consumption triggers in interstitial cystitis/bladder pain syndrome patients. Female Pelvic Med Reconstr Surg. 2011;17:36.
29. Clemens JQ, Meenan RT, O'KeeffeRosetti MC, et al. Case–control study of medical comorbidities in women with interstitial cystitis. J Urol. 2008;179(6):2222.

30. Rodríguez MA, Afari N, Buchwald DS, National Institute of Diabetes and Digestive and Kidney Diseases Working Group on Urological Chronic Pelvic Pain. Evidence for overlap between urological and nonurological unexplained clinical conditions. J Urol. 2009;182:2123.
31. Mahan L, Escott-Stump S. Krause's food and nutrition therapy. St. Louis: Saunders; 2008.
32. Theoharides TC, Cochrane DE. Critical role of mast cells in inflammatory diseases and the effect of acute stress. J Neuroimmunol. 2004;146:1.
33. Heizer WD, Southern S, McGovern S. The role of diet in symptoms of irritable bowel syndrome in adults: a narrative review. J Am Diet Assoc. 2009;109:1204.
34. Bijkerk CJ, de Wit NJ, Muris JW, et al. Soluble or insoluble fibre in irritable bowel syndrome in primary care? Randomised placebo controlled trial. BMJ. 2009;339:b3154.
35. Warren JW, Howard FM, Cross RK, et al. Antecedent nonbladder syndromes in case–control study of interstitial cystitis/painful bladder syndrome. Urology. 2009;73:52.
36. Heitkemper M, Jarrett M. Overlapping conditions in women with irritable bowel syndrome. Urol Nurs. 2005;25:25.
37. Wolfe F, Smythe HA, Yunus MB, et al. The American College of Rheumatology 1990 criteria for the classification of fibromyalgia: report of the Multicenter Criteria Committee. Arthritis Rheum. 1990;33:160.
38. Nimnuan C, Rabe-Hesketh S, Wessely S, et al. How many functional somatic syndromes? J Psychosom Res. 2001;51:549.
39. Haugen M, Kjeldsen-Kragh J, Nordvåg BY, et al. Diet and disease symptoms in rheumatic diseases–results of a questionnaire based survey. Clin Rheumatol. 1991;10:401.
40. Holton KF, Kindler LL, Jones KD. Potential dietary links to central sensitization in fibromyalgia: past reports and future directions. Rheum Dis Clin North Am. 2009;35:409.
41. Arranz LI, Canela MA, Rafecas M. Fibromyalgia and nutrition, what do we know? Rheumatol Int. 2010;30:1417.
42. Nickel JC, Tripp DA, Pontari M, et al. Interstitial cystitis/painful bladder syndrome and associated medical conditions with an emphasis on irritable bowel syndrome, fibromyalgia and chronic fatigue syndrome. J Urol. 2010;184:1358.
43. Fukuda K, Straus SE, Hickle I, et al. The chronic fatigue syndrome; a comprehensive approach to its definition and study. Ann Intern Med. 1994;121:953.
44. Logan AC, Wong C. Chronic fatigue syndrome: oxidative stress and dietary modifications. Altern Med Rev. 2001;6:450.
45. Brouwers FM, Van Der Wef S, Bleijenberg G, et al. The effect of a polynutrient supplement on fatigue and physical activity of patients with chronic fatigue syndrome: a double-blind randomized controlled trial. Q J Med. 2002;95:677.
46. Teitelbaum JE, Johnson C, St Cyr J. The use of d-ribose in chronic fatigue syndrome and fibromyalgia: a pilot study. J Altern Complement Med. 2006;12:857.
47. Moldwin R. The interstitial cystitis survival guide. Oakland: New Harbinger; 2000.
48. Dell JR, Mokrzycki ML, Jayne CJ. Differentiating interstitial cystitis from similar conditions commonly seen in gynecologic practice. Eur J Obstet Gynecol Reprod Biol. 2009;144:105.
49. Carrico DJ, Sherer KL, Peters KM. The relationship of interstitial cystitis/painful bladder syndrome to vulvodynia. Urol Nurs. 2009;29:233.
50. Moyal-Barracco M, Lynch PJ. 2003 ISSVD terminology and classification of vulvodynia; a historical perspective. J Reprod Med. 2004;49:772.
51. Solomons CC, Melmed MH, Heitler SM. Calcium citrate for vulvar vestibulitis. A case report. J Reprod Med. 1991;36:379.
52. Baggish MS, Sze EH, Johnson R. Urinary oxalate excretion and its role in vulvar pain syndrome. Am J Obstet Gynecol. 1997;177:509.
53. Harlow BL, Abenhaim HA, Vitonis AF, et al. Influence of dietary oxalates on the risk of adult-onset vulvodynia. J Reprod Med. 2008;53:171.
54. Novi JM, Jeronis S, Srinivas S, et al. Risk of irritable bowel syndrome and depression in women with interstitial cystitis: a case–control study. J Urol. 2005;174:937.

55. Stahl LA, Begg DP, Weisinger RE, et al. The role of omega-3 fatty acids in mood disorders. Curr Opin Investig Drugs. 2008;9:57.
56. Dinan T, Siggins L, Scully P, et al. Investigating the inflammatory phenotype of major depression: focus on cytokines and polyunsaturated fatty acids. J Psychiatr Res. 2009;43:471.
57. Treede RD, Jensen TS, Campbell JN, et al. Redefinition of neuropathic pain and a grading system for clinical use; consensus statement on clnical and research diagnostic criteria. Neurology. 2008;70:1630.
58. Ko GD, Nowacki NB, Arseneau L, et al. Omega-3 fatty acids for neuropathic pain: case series. Clin J Pain. 2010;26:168.
59. Gormsen L, Rosenberg R, Bach FW, et al. Depression, anxiety, health-related quality of life and pain in patients with chronic fibromyalgia and neuropathic pain. Eur J Pain. 2010;14:127.
60. Jansen SC, van Dusseldorp M, Botterna KC, et al. Intolerance to dietary biogenic amines: a review. Ann Allergy Asthma Immunol. 2003;91:233.
61. Schiapparelli P, Allais G, Castagnoli Gabellari I, et al. Non-pharmacological approach to migraine prophylaxs: part II. Neurol Sci. 2010;31:S137.
62. Alpay K, Ertas M, Orhan EK, et al. Diet restriction in migraine, based on IgG against foods: a clinical double-blind, randomised, cross-over trial. Cephalalgia. 2010;30:829.

Chapter 20
Physiotherapy

Amy Rejba Hoffmann, Hina M. Sheth, and Kristene E. Whitmore

Introduction

Traditionally in urology, the term pelvic floor dysfunction has referred to low-tone or laxity. The majority of research has focused on proper diagnosis and treatment of lax pelvic floor muscles (PFM) and resultant disorders such as pelvic organ prolapse and incontinence. Physiotherapist-based treatment has been demonstrated to be effective for urinary incontinence via pelvic floor strengthening [1, 2] and physiotherapy is a mainstay of the treatment of urinary stress incontinence [3].

More recently, clinicians have recognized the hypertonic pelvic floor and its relationship to bladder pain syndrome (BPS). As with low-tone pelvic floor dysfunction, clinicians rely on collaboration with physiotherapists to treat high-tone dysfunction and other musculoskeletal abnormalities that accompany BPS. The Bladder Pain Syndrome International Consultation on Incontinence recommends referring BPS patients to a physiotherapist as a first-line therapy [4].

In 2005, the International Continence Society developed the term overactive pelvic floor muscles (OPFM). This is defined as: "a situation in which the pelvic floor muscles do not relax or may even contract when relaxation is functionally needed, for example during micturition or defecation. This condition is based on symptoms such as voiding problems, obstructed defecation, or dyspareunia and on signs like the absence of voluntary pelvic floor muscle relaxation" [5]. A variety of terms have

A.R. Hoffmann, M.S.N. (✉)
The Pelvic and Sexual Health Institute, 207 No Broad St., 4th Floor, Philadelphia, PA, 19107, USA
e-mail: amyrejba@yahoo.com

H.M. Sheth, M.S., P.T., O.C.S., M.T.C.
Rebalance Physical Therapy, Philadelphia, PA, USA

K.E. Whitmore, M.D.
Urology, Obstetrics/Gynecology and Female Pelvic Medicine and Reconstructive Surgery, Drexel University
College of Medicine, Philadelphia, PA, USA

J. Nordling et al. (eds.), *Bladder Pain Syndrome: A Guide for Clinicians*, 271
DOI 10.1007/978-1-4419-6929-3_20, © Springer Science+Business Media New York 2013

been used for this condition in the last 30 years. More recently, OPFM has been described as high-tone pelvic floor dysfunction [6], short pelvic floor [7], and pelvic floor hypertonic disorder [8].

There has also been a developing body of literature focusing on treatment of the pelvic floor of male patients with chronic prostatitis/chronic pelvic pain syndrome (CP/CPPS). Both BPS and CP/CPPS are conditions with similar patient symptoms and proposed similar pathophysiology. Due to the lack of differentiating criteria, BPS and CP/CPPS recently have been combined and described as urologic chronic pelvic pain syndromes (UCPPS) in recent literature and research. Therefore, UCPPS may be used in this chapter when referring to both conditions.

Prevalence

There is extensive descriptive literature regarding the abnormalities detected in the PFM and the pelvic girdle of the BPS patient but there is limited research on their prevalence. Lack of common terminology across disciplines and lack of validated diagnostic measures of the pelvic floor present barriers to determining the prevalence of OPFM. Though generally accepted that tenderness and hypertonus on palpation as well as the inability to properly relax the pelvic floor are diagnostic, there are no accepted diagnostic values for OPFM on manometry, EMG, or imaging.

One study found the prevalence of OPFM in BPS patients to be 50–87% [9]. Another study examining voiding symptoms of BPS patients found that 76% have voiding dysfunction and elevated urethral closure pressures suggestive of OPFM [10]. A recent study of 231 BPS patients demonstrated that 48% of women with BPS met the criteria for bladder outlet obstruction. Further urologic testing performed on these patients allowed the authors to conclude that this is due to voiding dysfunction, also suggestive of OPFM [11]. Hetrick et al. compared 62 men with CPPS to 89 healthy controls and found significant difference in pelvic floor findings [12]. Increased muscle tone was found in 57% compared to 12% in the control group, and the incidence of pain with PFM palpation was 73% in the CPPS group compared to 15% in the control patients.

Sacro-iliac (SI) joint dysfunction, myofascial trigger points, and myofascial pain syndromes of the external musculature have been observed in the CPP patients [12–15], but there is limited data on these findings specifically in the BPS patient.

Etiology

The complex pathophysiology of the development of OPFM in relationship to BPS is detailed in the Pelvic Floor chapter of this book. The excessive visceral afferents that are activated in the BPS patient can lead to hypertonus of the PFM via viscerosomatic neuropathic reflexes [16]. However, this explanation of PFD development as a physiologic reaction to BPS does not take into account that hypertonus might develop concurrently with UCPPS or even precede UCPPS in some cases. Therefore, this chapter focuses on the development of OPFM in the context of the rest of the musculoskeletal system.

Abnormal voiding behaviors, psychological distress, and direct neuromuscular injury to the pelvic floor have all been cited as causative for OPFM [16]. Though OPFM may develop secondary to a visceral pain disorder or multiple visceral pain disorders, it may also develop secondary to another adjacent myofascial pain syndrome. A myofascial pain syndrome is a myalgic condition characterized by local and referred pain that originates in a myofascial trigger point (MTrP). A myofascial trigger point is defined as a hyperirritable spot, usually within a taut band of skeletal muscle or the muscle fascia that is painful on compression and causes characteristic referred pain, local tenderness, autonomic phenomena, and proprioceptive disturbances [17]. The PFM can have MTrPs; therefore in some cases overactive pelvic floor is a myofascial pain syndrome. The development of an MTrP, as described comprehensively by Gerwin, can be caused by acute overuse, direct trauma, persistent muscular trauma, prolonged immobility, systemic biochemical imbalance, associated trigger points in adjacent tissue, afferent input from joints, afferent input from internal organs, or stress [18].

The pelvic floor is vulnerable to dysfunction as it coordinates with muscles of the back, abdomen, buttocks, and thighs to maintain skeletal position as well as those of the upper pelvis, vagina, and rectum to provide local support to the pelvic organs. Several authors have associated poor posture with pelvic floor hypertonus, including Baker's description of "typical pelvic pain posture," which involves thoracic kyphosis and excessive lumbar lordosis [19]. Thiele proposed that excessive flexion of the coccyx in sitting posture results in OPFM [20]. The presence of SI joint dysfunction, even without prolonged poor posture, may serve as an impetus for the development of the OPFM. Voluntary behaviors may worsen hypertonus. This is seen in the patient that actively contracts the PFM in order to suppress urge or mistakenly performs PFM-strengthening exercises as a proposed panacea for bladder symptoms.

Physiotherapy for UCPPS

Few studies have been completed examining the effects of manual therapy techniques upon patients with UCCPS symptoms. Weiss reported on the use of manual therapy of the pelvic floor in 10 patients with BPS and 42 patients with frequency/urgency [21]. Seven of the ten BPS patients reported moderate to marked improvement in symptoms. Oyama et al. treated 21 patients with BPS and OPFM biweekly with transvaginal Thiele massage [22]. Though the sample size was small there was statistically significant improvement in BPS symptoms and a decrease in pelvic floor hypertonus.

Fitzgerald et al. have completed and published the only prospective study of manual therapy of the pelvic floor [23]. It was a feasibility trial comparing myofascial physical therapy to global therapeutic massage in 23 men and 24 women. Patients randomized to the myofascial physical therapy arm reported a global assessment response rate of 57%, which was significantly higher than the rate of improvement reported by the global therapeutic massage treatment group (21%).

Evaluation of the Patient

Though the limited prevalence data indicates that many BPS patients have pelvic floor dysfunction, not all BPS patients have PFD or require a referral to a physiotherapist. A focused patient history and physical exam can help the clinician identify an appropriate patient for physiotherapy.

History

A musculoskeletal history is necessary for all BPS patients. It is important to assess events that have happened throughout the course of the lifetime not just the immediate past. Conditions including medical procedures and child/adulthood sports injuries should be addressed. A detailed orthopedic and trauma history is important, as many events could be predisposing factors that the patient may not consider relevant. Many musculoskeletal injuries, in particular lower-limb or gait abnormalities, are important. Details of daily exercise routines (new sport or attempting to lose weight), common postural strains (excessive driving, carrying a child), and occupational detail (prolonged sitting, limited bathroom access) should be ascertained.

Confirmation of events associated with acute symptom exacerbation including urinary tract infections, yeast infections, kidney stones, or ruptured ovarian cysts can be difficult to obtain. It is important to determine what steps were taken to medically confirm such events. Some of these diagnoses are treated without sufficient evidence via phone or without proper follow-up. Some musculoskeletal and myofascial abnormalities can trigger similar symptoms, confusing patients about the origin of their pain. It is also possible that these are real events and can aggravate musculoskeletal symptoms through viscero-somatic reflexes or viscero-cutaneous reflexes.

A patient's history will often reveal a series of precipitating events leading up to their pain syndrome. It is important to relay this to patients, as they often struggle to make sense of their insidious onset of pain.

Symptoms

The pelvic floor can affect multiple organ systems; therefore it is important to interview the patient about bowel, bladder, and vaginal function and sexual and pain symptoms [5]. PFM can affect the lower urinary tract causing symptoms of urgency and frequency. However slow/intermittent stream or straining to void is a hallmark symptom of OPFM. It is important to note that incontinence and prolapse can occur in the patient with hypertonus, as an overactive pelvic floor is dysfunctional and often weak.

The clinician should inquire about the patient's experience of pain over a 24-h period from awakening to bedtime, as some musculoskeletal complaints will abate with rest or worsen as the day progresses. Determine if the pain awakens the patient from sleep; this may help differentiate pain of a visceral origin versus one that is musculoskeletal. Triggering events such as bowel movements, micturition, and intercourse should be also evaluated.

Physical Exam

The purpose of this musculoskeletal-focused exam is to determine the extent of external sources of pain and dysfunction in the BPS patient, establish a diagnosis of OPFM, and discern the need for a physical therapy referral. A more detailed musculoskeletal exam, as performed by a physiotherapist, is covered in the next section of this chapter.

The exam should focus on the external pelvis if a patient presents with a history of specific lumbosacral pain or orthopedic surgery. A rudimentary examination of bony landmarks of the pelvis to check for misalignment and palpation of pelvic girdle musculature for tenderness is often all that is needed to screen a patient for physiotherapy referral. In detail, the exam includes standing and/or sitting examination of the height of the iliac crest, posterior superior iliac spine (PSIS), and anterior superior iliac spine (ASIS), palpation of the SI joint for tenderness, and palpation of the coccyx for position and tenderness. In the supine position the clinician can examine the ASIS for height and symmetry, the pubic symphysis for symmetry and tenderness, and the iliopsoas and rectus abdominus for tenderness and trigger points (TrPs). In side-lying position the Gluteus maximus, Gluteus medius, Gluteus minimus, piriformis, obturator, and greater trochanter can be examined for tenderness or TrPs.

Exam of the PFM should focus on tone, tenderness, and identification of TrPs. Male patients can be evaluated during digital rectal exam; however the female patient is commonly more comfortably assessed transvaginally. The pubococcygeus, iliococcygeus, and obturator internus should be assessed bilaterally. In some patients, the coccygeus can be palpable. In our practice we use the modified oxford hypertonus scale, assigning a 0–4 score for each muscle.

The Physiotherapist's Perspective

The remainder of this chapter details the evaluation and treatment of the BPS patient from the physiotherapist's perspective. It is imperative for a clinician to understand the treatment techniques available in order to critically evaluate the ability of a physiotherapist when referring a BPS patient. Physiotherapists have a wide range of training and expertise in techniques. Therefore when establishing a referral relationship it is important to ascertain the skill level of the physiotherapist. It is also important for the clinician to be familiar with treatments in order to provide expectations to the patient and allay anxiety the patient may have about painful treatments or internal therapy.

Detailed Physiotherapy Evaluation

A physiotherapy evaluation consists of assessment of patient history, orthopedic/biomechanics, connective tissue, internal PFM, and lastly a biofeedback exam. Examination of all these components may not be appropriate on the patient's first visit and may extend out to several visits.

Orthopedic/Biomechanical Examination

The components of a basic external musculoskeletal exam are (a) postural and structural screening noting head and neck position, spinal curvatures (i.e., scoliosis, excessive lordosis, or kyphosis), pelvic, hip positions, and any leg length discrepancies; (b) range of motion and muscle length assessment of the trunk and lower extremities; (c) muscle strength and motor control specifically for Assessing lumbo-pelvic-hip complex; and (d) gait analysis and functional movement tests [24].

Specific tests and measures may be necessary to further assess impairments found during the basic musculoskeletal exam. Particular attention should be given to sacral torsions, ilial rotations, pubic symphysis asymmetries, and coccyx deviations, as these landmarks serve as attachment sites for the PFM. In patients with a history of low back or sacroiliac joint pain, performing provocation tests may be necessary [25], motor control of the spinal and pelvic stabilizers includes testing transverse abdominus, multifudi, and gluteals.

Common orthopedic and biomechanical dysfunctions in chronic pelvic pain patients include thoracic and lumbar spine positional faults especially at the junctional zone of T12 and L1, presence of a diastasis recti, paradoxical breathing pattern, hip internal rotation restrictions, sacroiliac joint torsion, rotations and instabilities, and weakness of the trunk and hip stabilizers [14, 19].

The presence of a diastasis recti (separation of the rectus abdominus) must also be assessed as many abdominal trigger points arise due to anterior wall instability. The clinician measures between the rectus abdominus muscle above and below the umbilicus with the patient at rest and in a flexed position. Anything greater than approximately two finger widths is considered significant [7].

Another common finding in this patient population is a paradoxical breathing pattern which has been highly correlated to the high-tone pelvic floor [13]. Normally on inhalation the abdomen should expand and the chest should remain still; however the opposite is typically seen in this patient population.

Connective Tissue Assessment

Connective tissue encompasses a broad variety of structures from the dermis of the skin down to the osseous structures. For purposes of this assessment, three general areas of connective tissue are commonly assessed: the subcutaneous tissue, muscles, and the visceral fascia.

The subcutaneous tissue of the abdominal wall, lower back, buttocks, thighs, and perineum are assessed by a method called skin or pinch rolling. Attention is focused in this region because research has demonstrated that vasoconstriction in these areas is associated with uterine and bladder inflammation [26]. The tissue between the skin and the muscle is rolled between the examining fingers to assess for mobility and any areas of restrictions, also known as subcutaneous panniculosis. In areas of severely restricted tissue it is common for patients to report intense sharp pain even with minimal pressure. Specifically, abdominal surgical scars tend to coincide with cutaneous reflex zones of the bladder and pelvic organs [7].

The muscles are examined for the presence of MTrPs via manual palpation. Once a TrP is located, patients may report exquisite localized tenderness and even pain referral into the areas of their subjective complaints. Muscles containing the TrP can present with weakness, loss of motor function, and inability to adequately lengthen. Patients with BPS commonly present with TrPs in the abdominal muscles, iliopsoas, adductors, quadratus lumborum, obturator internus, piriformis, and gluteals as well as within the PFM [27].

The visceral fascia is assessed using specific manual forces known as "listening," to examine mobility and motion of the connective tissue surrounding the viscera. It is believed that all organs have a normal physiologic motion. Restrictions, fixations, or adhesions can impair the mobility of an organ, therefore compromising optimal function of that organ and surrounding structures. BPS patients often have visceral fascial restrictions surrounding the bladder, urethra, kidney, and intestines [28].

Internal Pelvic Floor Exam (Transvaginal/Transrectal)

Similar to the pelvic floor screening performed by the clinician, the physiotherapist inserts one lubricated finger into the vagina or rectum to assess for strength, tone, and tenderness of the pelvic floor. However, more specificity is used to identify TrPs in each individual layer of the pelvic floor. In addition, the physical therapist will examine urethral, bladder, and coccygeal mobility.

Accuracy in locating the individual muscles is best performed via bony landmark palpation and contraction of each individual muscle. The most superficial layer is palpated by inserting the examining finger up to the first distal interphalangeal joint to assess the superficial transverse perineum, bulbospongiosus, and ischiocavernosus muscles via the pubic rami. The middle layer is assessed by inserting the finger up to the proximal interphalangeal joint to examine the sphincter urethra and deep transverse perineal muscles. The transverse abdominus and this pelvic floor layer form a continuous connection. The patient is asked to exhale as if blowing out a flame. A tension should develop under the therapist's finger for confirmation. The third layer is assessed by fully inserting the finger up to the metacarpal joint to assess the levator ani, coccygeus, and obturator internus muscles. The obturator internus muscle is easily palpated by asking the patient to resist external rotation of the hip during examination.

The urethra, bladder, and coccyx can be restricted in BPS patients [28]. Mobility of the urethra is assessed by inserting two fingers along each side of the urethra and guided into various planes to determine the direction of restriction. Bladder mobility is assessed by directing two fingers to distract the trigone while the external hand distracts the bladder superiorly. Note any tension or restrictions to this area of the bladder. The coccyx serves as an important attachment site for many of the PFM. Any excessive or limited mobility can impact pelvic floor function. There are several methods to assess coccygeal mobility. Typically the therapist grasps the coccyx internally with the index finger and externally with the thumb, and motion is assessed in all three planes [28].

Determining motor control of the pelvic floor is essential. The BPS patient will present with difficulty in lengthening the pelvic floor. The patient is asked to "drop" the pelvic floor by mimicking initiating urination. In a healthy pelvic floor, the clinician should feel an excursion or bulge of the muscles. Instead, these patients demonstrate little to no movement or even a contraction of the pelvic floor.

Biofeedback Testing

Biofeedback testing has been traditionally used to assess strength and motor control of the PFM. A pressure probe measures internal pressure at rest, and during contractions. Typically, patients with BPS will present with an elevated tone at rest, gradual loss of peak contractions with subsequent quick contractions, and an inability to maintain pelvic floor endurance during their 10-s contractions [24]. Biofeedback testing has limitations in that it cannot make bilateral comparisons of strength and tone. Biofeedback should not be used as a stand-alone exam to determine pelvic floor function, but should be used to further confirm the findings found manually.

Treatment

This section concentrates on connective tissue and internal pelvic floor treatment of the BPS patient. Orthopedic techniques will not be addressed as basic physiotherapy

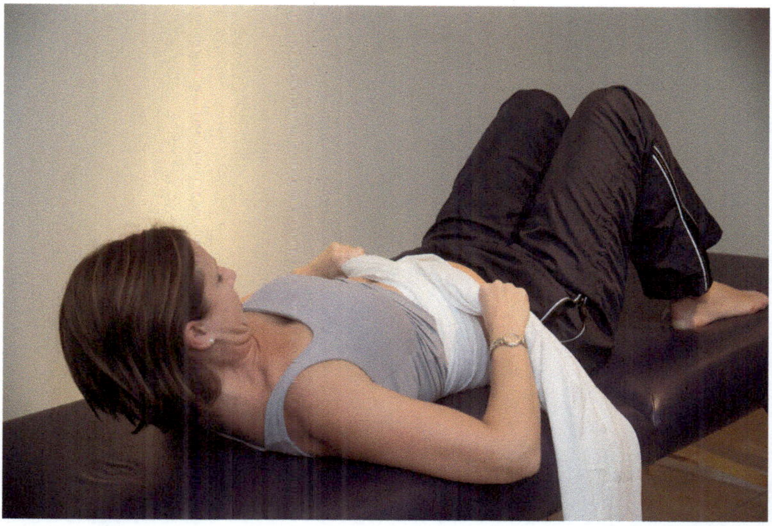

Fig. 20.1 Diastasis recti is a common biomechanical dysfunction that contributes to pelvic instability and dysfunction. This photo demonstrates a self-correction exercise for diastasis recti

texts specifically address orthopedic corrections in detail. Application of a particular technique can have a profound effect and may eliminate the need to use others. Ultimately it will be at the physiotherapist's discretion as to which therapeutic regimen is appropriate. The following sequence is only intended as a general guideline to treatment and does not indicate the scope of practice of the treating physiotherapist.

Orthopedic and Biomechanical Treatment

Orthopedic and biomechanical problems should be addressed in conjunction with connective tissue and internal pelvic floor treatment. Failure to address any of these impairments could prolong or hinder improvement in other areas. Early intervention includes correction of a diastasis recti and normalizing a paradoxical breathing pattern.

Diastasis correction is performed with the patient in a hook-lying position with a towel wrapped tightly around the mid-section of the rectus abdominus. The patient is asked to perform a series of head and chin lifts twice daily until adequate closure is achieved (Fig. 20.1) [24].

Proper diaphragmatic breathing is established by having the patient place one hand on the chest and one hand on the abdomen. The patient is asked to breathe in while keeping the chest quiet but allowing the belly to expand. On exhalation the belly should passively fall. The patient should perform this breathing several times a day, especially when the urge is present.

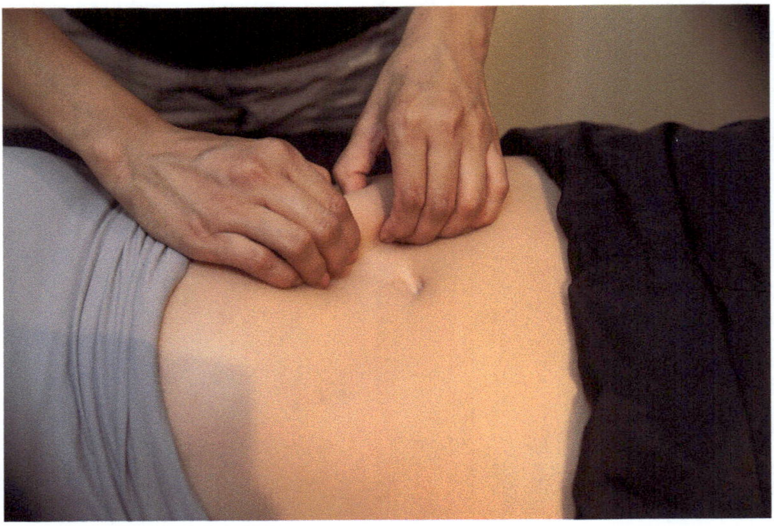

Fig. 20.2 Skin rolling can be used as both evaluation and treatment of connective tissue restriction. The photo demonstrates the skin rolling technique on the abdomen

Connective Tissue Treatment

The subcutaneous tissue is addressed using the same technique used during evaluation. Using minimal lubrication, skin rolling and/or dragging is applied to the restricted tissue, from all angles, until mobility is felt to improve (Fig. 20.2). Initially the patient may report severe discomfort during and after treatment, especially in areas of restrictions. Treatment will become less painful and the clinician will be able to work deeper as tissue fluidity improves. Skin rolling improves circulation, lessens tissue hypersensitivity, and decreases reflexive effects on the surrounding muscles, nerves, and viscera [29].

Muscular trigger points, found during evaluation, can be treated with several techniques. Commonly they include ischemic compression, strumming and strain–counterstrain. Ischemic compression involves applying graduated pressure directly on the trigger point for 30–90 s. Strumming or fractioning involves stroking across the fibers of the TrP 6–12 times or until release is appreciated. Strain–counterstrain is a technique in which the involved muscle is guided into a shortened position and held for 30–90 s in order to promote relaxation (Fig. 20.3).

The visceral fascia is addressed by using a technique called visceral manipulation. Specific directed pressures are used to engage the fascia around the visceral organs. Externally, this technique is useful for addressing restrictions around the obturator membrane, urachus, and pubovesical ligaments to improve bladder mobility and filling [28].

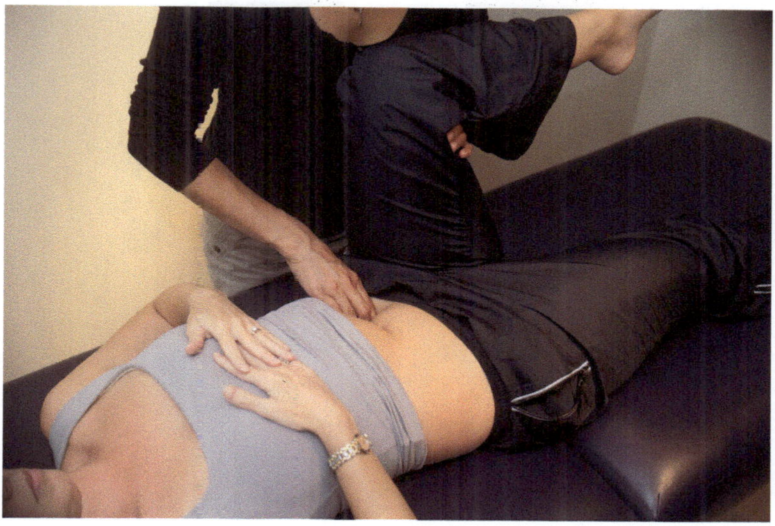

Fig. 20.3 Myofascial trigger points in the Psoas contribute to chronic pelvic pain. Strain–counterstrain technique, illustrated in the photo, may be used as a correction to release the Psoas

Internal Pelvic Floor Treatment

The ultimate goal of internal pelvic floor treatment is to reduce tone, eliminate TrPs, normalize urethral, bladder, and coccygeal mobility, and improve motor control of the pelvic floor. The internal pelvic floor is treated transvaginally or transrectally. Tone and TrPs are addressed with the same techniques used to treat external TrPs as described above. The urethra, bladder, and coccyx can be treated with specific visceral and joint manipulation techniques aimed at restoring normal mobility and motility. The structures are guided into their restrictive zones, similar to the evaluation, and followed until release is noted. In cases of coccygeal instability, taping and strengthening of the gluteal muscles may be appropriate.

Motor control techniques can be initiated once some reduction in tone and symptoms is achieved. Proprioceptive neuromuscular re-education techniques should be considered to facilitate lengthening of the PFM. The patient is asked to resist hip flexion, abduction, and internal rotation for 5 s and this is repeated up to five times. This induces relaxation of the pelvic floor and is a useful exercise for patients to perform as a home exercise program (Fig. 20.4). As the patient gains proprioceptive awareness, pelvic drops can be initiated throughout the day, in various positions, to help maintain tone established in the clinic. Biofeedback, with emphasis on relaxation, may assist in development of this skill [24].

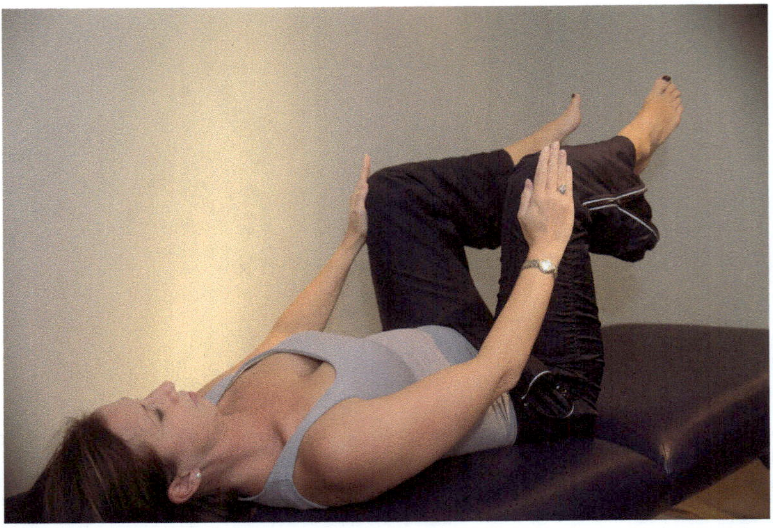

Fig. 20.4 This photo illustrates home exercise to facilitate lengthening of the PFM. The patient is asked to resist hip flexion, abduction, and internal rotation for 5s

Frequency of Treatment

Typical treatment sessions are 30–60 min with the patient being seen 1–2 times per week. Duration is highly variable from 12 weeks up to 1 year or more depending on severity of symptoms, patient tolerance, response to treatment, and compliance.

References

1. Bo K, Talseth T, Holme I. Single blind, randomized controlled trial of pelvic floor excercises, electrical stimulation, vaginal cones, and no treatment in the management of genuine stress incontinence in women. BMJ. 1999;318:487–93.
2. Burns PA, Pranikoff K, Nochaski T, et al. Treatement of stress urinary incontinence with pelvic floor exercises and biofeedback. J Am Geriatr Soc. 1990;38:341–4.
3. Abrams P, Anderson KE, Birder L, et al. Fourth International Consulation on Incontinence recommendations of the International Scientific Committee: evaluation and treatment of urinary incontinence, pelvic organ prolapse, and fecal incontinence. Neurourol Urodyn. 2010;29:213–40.
4. Hanno P, Lin A, Nordling J, et al. Bladder pain syndome International Consulation on Incontinence. Neurourol Urodyn. 2010;29:191–8.
5. Messelink B, Benson T, Berghmans B, et al. Standardization of the terminology of the pelvic floor muscle function and dysfunction: report form the pelvic floor clinical assessment group of the International Continence Society. Neurourol Urodyn. 2005;24:374–80.
6. Whitmore K, Kellogg-Spadt S, Fletcher E. Comprehensive assessment of pelvic floor dysfunction. Issues in Incont. 1998;Fall: 1–2, 10.
7. Fitzgerald MP, Kotarinos R, Fitzgerald MP, Kotarinos R. Rehabilitation of the short pelvic floor. I: background and patient evaluation. Int Urogynecol J. 2003;14:261–8.

8. Butrick CW. Pelvic floor hypetonic disorders: identification and management. Obstet Gynecol Clin North Am. 2009;36:707–22.
9. Peters KM, Carrico DJ, Kalinowski SE, et al. Prevalence of pelvic floor dysfunction in patients with interstitial cystitis. Urology. 2007;70:16–8.
10. Butrick CW, Sanford D, Hou Q, et al. Chronic pelvic pain syndromes: clinical urodynamic and urothelial observations. Int Urogynecol J Pelvic Floor Dysfucnt. 2009;20:1047–53.
11. Cameron A, Gajewski J. Bladder outlet obstruction in painful bladder syndrome/interstitial cystitis. Neurourol Urodyn. 2009;28:944–8.
12. Hetrick DC, Ciol MA, Rothman I, et al. Musculoskeletal dysfunction in men with chronic pelvic pain syndrome type III: a case–control study. J Urol. 2003;170:828–31.
13. Chaitow, Leon ND. Chronic pelvic pain: pelvic floor problems, sacroiliac dysfunction and the trigger point connection. 6th Interdisciplinary World Congress on Low Back and Pelvic Pain Barcelona November 2007; 42–52.
14. Tu FF, Hold J, Gonzales J, Fitzgerald CM. Physical Therapy evaluation of patients with chronic pelvic pain: a controlled study. Am J Obstet Gynecol. 2008;198:272e1–7.
15. Anderson RU, Sawyer T, Wise D, et al. Painful Myofascial trigger points and pain sites in men with chronic prostatis/chronic pelvic pain syndrome. J Urol. 2009;182:2753–8.
16. Butrick CW. Pathophysiology of the pelvic floor hypertonic disorders. Obstet Gynecol Clin North Am. 2009;36:699–705.
17. Simons DG, Travell JG, Simons LS. Myofascial pain and dysfunction: the trigger point manual, vol. 1. Baltimore: Lippincot Williams and Wilkins; 1999.
18. Gerwin RD. Classification, epidemiology, and natural history of myofascial pain syndrome. Curr Pain Headache Rep. 2001;5:412–20.
19. Baker PK. Musculoskeletal origins of chronic pelvic pain. Obstet Gynecol Clin North Am. 1993;20:719–41.
20. Thiele GH. Coccygodynia: cause and treatment. Dis Colon Rectum. 1963;6:422–36.
21. Weiss J. Pelvic floor myofascial trigger points: manual therapy for interstitial cystitis and the urgency-frequency syndrome. J Urol. 2001;166:2226–31.
22. Oyama IA, Rejba A, Lukban JC, et al. Modified thiele massage as therapeutic intervention for female patients with interstitial cystitic and high-tone pelvic floor dysfunction. Urology. 2004;64:862–5.
23. Fitzgerald MP, Anderson RU, Potts J, et al. Randomized multicenter feasibility trial of myofascial physical therapy for the treatment of urologic chronic pelvic pain syndromes. J Urol. 2009;182:570–80.
24. Fitzgerald MP, Kotarinos R. Rehabilitation of the short pelvic floor. II: treatment of the patient with the short pelvic floor. Int Urogynecol J Pelvic Floor Dysfunct. 2003;14:269.
25. Laslett M. Evidenced-based diagnosis and treatment of the painful sacroiliac joint. J Man Manip Ther. 2008;16:142–52.
26. Wesselmann U, Lai J. Mechanisms of referral visceral pain: uterine inflammation in the adult virgin rat results in plasma extravasation in the skin. Pain. 1997;73:309–17.
27. Prendergast SA, Weiss JM. Screening for musculoskeletal causes of pelvic pain. Clin Obstet Gynecol. 2003;46:4.
28. Barral J-P. Urogenital manipulation. Seattle: Eastland Press; 2003.
29. Prendergast, S, Kotarinos, R. Treating vulodynia with manual physical therapy. National Vulvodynia Association News. 2008;Fall:2–6.

Chapter 21
Oral Therapy for Bladder Pain Syndrome Directed at the Bladder

Philip M. Hanno

Few of the oral therapies commonly used for the treatment of BPS have unequivocal evidence of efficacy in large, multicenter, randomized controlled clinical trials. There is little evidence that any change the natural history of the disease, though many seem to be effective in relieving symptoms in individual patients. Tachyphylaxis may be a problem.

Sodium Pentosan Polysulfate

Parson's suggestion that a defect in the epithelial permeability barrier, the glycosaminoglycan (GAG) layer, contributes to the pathogenesis of BPS has led to an attempt to correct such a defect with the synthetic sulfated polysaccharide sodium pentosan polysulfate (PPS), a heparin analogue available in an oral formulation, 3–6% of which is excreted into the urine [1]. It is sold under the trade name *Elmiron*™. It is the only oral medication approved by the Food and Drug Administration for the pain associated with interstitial cystitis. Studies have been contradictory.

Fritjofsson treated 87 patients in an open multicenter trial in Sweden and Finland [2]. Bladder volume with and without anesthesia was unchanged. Relief of pain was complete in 35% and partial in 23% of patients. Daytime frequency decreased from 16.5 to 13 and nocturia decreased from 4.5 to 3.5. Mean voided volumes increased by less than a tablespoon in the nonulcer group.

Holm-Bentzen studied 115 patients in a double-blind, placebo-controlled trial [3]. Symptoms, urodynamic parameters, cystoscopic appearance, and mast cell counts were unchanged after 4 months. Bladder capacity under anesthesia increased significantly in the group with mastocytosis, but this had no bearing on symptoms or awake capacity.

P.M. Hanno, M.D., M.P.H. (✉)
Division of Surgery, Department of Urology, Hospital of the University of Pennsylvania, Philadelphia, PA, USA
e-mail: hannop@uphs.upenn.edu

J. Nordling et al. (eds.), *Bladder Pain Syndrome: A Guide for Clinicians*, 285
DOI 10.1007/978-1-4419-6929-3_21, © Springer Science+Business Media New York 2013

Parsons had a more encouraging initial experience [4], and subsequently the results of two pivotal placebo-controlled multicenter trials in the United States were published [5, 6]. In the initial study, overall improvement of greater than 25% was reported by 28% of the PPS-treated group versus 13% in the placebo group. In the latter study the respective figures were 32% on drug versus 16% on placebo. Average voided volume on PPS increased by 20 cc. No other objective improvements were documented.

A Finnish study comparing PPS to cyclosporine A over a 6-month period showed a global response assessment rate to PPS of 16% in 26 women and 6 men meeting NIDDK research criteria [7].

An underpowered National Institutes of Health 2×2 factorial study to evaluate PPS and hydroxyzine looked at each drug used alone and in combination and compared results to a placebo group [8]. Patients were treated for 6 months. No statistically significant response to either medication was documented. No significant trend was seen in the PPS treatment groups (34%) compared to non-PPS groups (18%). Of the 29 patients on PPS alone, 28% had global response (the primary endpoint) of moderately or markedly improved versus 13% on placebo, a number remarkably similar to the results in the 3-month pivotal trials, although not reaching statistical significance in the 6-month study. A subsequent industry-sponsored trial showed no dose-related efficacy response in the range of 300–900 mg daily; however adverse events *were* dose related [9].

Long-term experience with PPS is consistent with efficacy in a subset of patients that may drop below 30% of those initially treated [10]. Tachyphylaxis seems to be uncommon in responders. Adverse events with PPS occurred in less than 4% of patients at the dose of 100 mg three times daily [11] and include reversible alopecia, diarrhea, nausea, and rash. Rare bleeding problems have been reported [12]. The drug promotes cellular proliferation in vitro in the MCF-7 breast cancer cell line, and caution has been suggested in prescribing it in groups at high risk for breast cancer and premenopausal females [13]. A 3–6-month treatment trial is generally required to see symptom improvement. In a small trial, PPS has shown efficacy when administered intravesically [14]. It may be of value in the management of radiation cystitis [15, 16] and cyclophosphamide cystitis [17], but its value in the treatment of BPS seems marginal.

Amitriptyline

Amitriptyline, a tricyclic antidepressant, has become a staple of oral treatment for BPS. The tricyclics possess varying degrees of at least three major pharmacologic actions: (1) they have central and peripheral anticholinergic actions at some but not all sites; (2) they block the active transport system in the presynaptic nerve ending that is responsible for the reuptake of the released amine neurotransmitters serotonin and noradrenaline; and (3) they are sedatives, an action that occurs presumably on a central basis but perhaps is related to their antihistaminic properties.

Amitriptyline, in fact, is one of the most potent tricyclic antidepressants in terms of blocking H1-histaminergic receptors [18]. There is also evidence that it desensitizes alpha2 receptors on central noradrenergic neurons. Paradoxically, it also has been shown to block alpha-adrenergic receptors and serotonin receptors. Theoretically, tricyclic agents have actions that might tend to stimulate predominantly beta-adrenergic receptors in bladder body smooth musculature, an action that would further facilitate urine storage by decreasing the excitability of smooth muscle in that area [19].

Hanno and Wein first reported a therapeutic response in interstitial cystitis after noting a "serendipitous" response to amitriptyline in one of their patients concurrently being treated for depression [20]. The following year a similar report appeared relating a response to desipramine hydrochloride [21]. Reasoning that a drug used successfully at relatively low dosages for many types of chronic pain syndromes, which would also have anticholinergic properties, beta-adrenergic bladder effects, sedative characteristics, and strong H1 antihistaminic activity, would seem to be ideal for interstitial cystitis, the first clinical trial was carried out with promising results [22]. A subsequent follow-up study [23] reported that 28 of 43 patients could tolerate therapy for at least a 3-week trial at a dosage of 25 mg before bed gradually increasing to 75 mg nightly over 2 weeks, 18 had total remission of symptoms with a mean follow-up of 14.4 months, 5 dropped out because of side effects, and 5 derived no clinical benefit. Benefits were apparent within 4 weeks. All patients had failed hydrodistention and intravesical dimethyl sulfoxide therapy. Sedation was the main side effect. Kirkemo and colleagues treated 30 patients and had a 90% subjective improvement rate at 8 weeks [24]. Both studies noted that patients with bladder capacities over 450–600 cc under anesthesia seemed to have the best results. Another uncontrolled study of 11 patients with urinary frequency and pelvic pain [25] related success in 9 of the patients, with 5 reporting complete resolution of symptoms and four significant relief. Two patients could not tolerate the medication. In a 4-month intent to treat placebo-controlled double-blind trial of 50 patients, 63% on amitriptyline at doses of 25–75 mg (dose as tolerated) before bed reported good or excellent satisfaction versus 4% on placebo [26]. At 19-month follow-up there was little tachyphylaxis and good response rates were observed in the entire spectrum of BPS/IC symptoms [27, 28].

The large, double-blind, randomized controlled trial by the National Institute of Diabetes and Digestive and Kidney Diseases comparing education and behavioral modification with and without oral amitriptyline showed a 55% response to the arm that included both medication and conservative therapy compared to a 45% response to education and behavioral therapy alone [29]. The difference was not statistically significant. However, if only patients who could tolerate 25 mg or more of medication or placebo are included, the success compared to conservative therapy alone was 73% compared to 53% at 12 weeks. Frequency, O'Leary–Sant symptom and problem scores also showed significant improvement. Thus, on an intent-to-treat basis, there was no significant benefit from amitriptyline, but in the 62% of patients who could tolerate the relatively low doses of drug, the benefits appear substantial. Patients should be cautioned about fatigue, constipation, dry mouth, increased appetite, and dizziness. Slowly titrating the dose on a weekly basis, beginning at 10 mg before bed and increasing by 10 mg weekly to a maximum tolerated dose of 50–75 mg before bed, seems to minimize side effects.

Amitriptyline has proven analgesic efficacy with a median preferred dose of 50 mg in a range of 25–150 mg daily. This range is lower than traditional doses for depression of 150–300 mg. The speed of the onset of effect is much faster (1–7 weeks) than reported in depression, and the analgesic effect is distinct from any effect on mood [30]. Tricyclic antidepressants are contraindicated in patients with long QT syndrome or significant conduction system disease (bifascicular or trifascicular block) after recent myocardial infarction (within 6 months), unstable angina, congestive heart failure, frequent premature ventricular contractions, or a history of sustained ventricular arrhythmias. They should be used with caution in patients with orthostatic hypotension [31]. Doses greater than 100 mg are associated with increased relative risk of sudden cardiac death [32].

Other Antidepressants

Other tricyclic antidepressants have been used for bladder pain syndrome. One trial employed the combination of doxepin and piroxicam, a cox-2 inhibitor. Twenty-six of 32 patients (81%) experienced remission of symptoms [33]. Another study reported satisfactory outcome with desipramine [21]. The safety and efficacy of duloxetine, a serotonin and norepinephrine reuptake inhibitor, for BPS were assessed in an observational study with 48 women [34]. Patients were prospectively treated for 2 months following an uptitration protocol to the target dose of 40 mg duloxetine twice daily. Five patients were identified as responders and 17 patients dropped out due to side effects including nausea in all 17 patients. No severe adverse events were reported. In the five responders, the 40 mg twice-daily dose was required to see efficacy. Overall, duloxetine did not result in clinically meaningful improvement of symptoms.

Antihistamines

The use of antihistamines goes back to the late 1950s and stems from work by Simmons who postulated that the local release of histamine may be responsible for, or may accompany the development of, interstitial cystitis [35]. He reported on six patients treated with pyribenzamine. The results were far from dramatic, with only half of the patients showing some response. The therapy is notable for this disease in that it was very logically conceived. It has been Theoharides who has spearheaded mast cell research in this field and been a major modern proponent of antihistamine therapy [36]. He has used the unique piperazine H1-receptor antagonist hydroxyzine, a first-generation antihistamine [37], which can block neuronal activation of mast cells [38]. In 40 patients treated with 25 mg before bed increasing over

2 weeks (if sedation was not a problem) to 50 mg at night and 25 mg in the morning, virtually every symptom evaluated improved by 30%. Only three patients had absolutely no response. As with many IC drug reports, these responses were evaluated subjectively and without being blinded or placebo controlled. A subsequent study suggested improved efficacy in patients with documented allergies and/or evidence of bladder mast cell activation [39, 40]. No significant response to hydroxyzine was found in an NIDDK placebo-controlled trial [8].

Why an H2-antagonist would be effective is unclear, but uncontrolled studies show improvement of symptoms in two-thirds of patients taking cimetidine in divided doses totaling 600 mg [41, 42]. It proved effective in a double-blind, placebo-controlled trial [43], but histologic studies show the bladder mucosa to be unchanged before and after treatment, and the mechanism of any efficacy remains unexplained [44]. All told, only 40 patients comprise all clinical published efficacy database on this over-the-counter medication when used for BPS/IC. Cimetidine is a common treatment in the United Kingdom where over a third of patients reported having used it [45]. Long-term follow-up data is lacking.

Immunosuppressant Drugs

Cyclosporine

Cyclosporine, a widely used immunosuppressive drug in organ transplantation, was the subject of a novel bladder pain syndrome trial [46]. Eleven patients received cyclosporine for 3–6 months at an initial dose of 2.5–5 mg/kg daily and a maintenance dose of 1.5–3 mg/kg daily. Micturition frequency decreased, and mean and maximum voided volumes increased significantly. Bladder pain decreased or disappeared in ten patients. After cessation of treatment, symptoms recurred in the majority of patients.

In a longer term follow-up study, 20 of 23 refractory IC patients on cyclosporine therapy followed for a mean of 60.8 months became free of bladder pain. Bladder capacity more than doubled. Eleven patients subsequently stopped therapy, and in 9, symptoms recurred within months, but responded to reinitiating cyclosporine [47]. Sairanen et al. further found that cyclosporine A was far superior to sodium PPS in all clinical outcome parameters measured at 6 months [48]. Global response assessment showed a 75% response to the immune modulator. Patients who responded to cyclosporine A had a significant reduction of urinary levels of epidermal growth factor (EGF) [7].

Suplatast Tosilate

Suplatast Tosilate (IPD-1151T) is an immunoregulator that selectively suppresses IgE production and eosinophilia via suppression of helper T cells that produce IL-4 and -5.

It is used in Japan to treat allergic disorders including asthma, atopic dermatitis, and rhinitis. Ueda et al. reported a small study in 14 women with interstitial cystitis [49]. Treatment for 1 year resulted in a significantly increased bladder capacity and decreased urinary urgency, frequency, and lower abdominal pain in ten women. Concomitant changes occurred in blood and urine markers suggesting an immune system response. Larger, multicenter, randomized controlled trials (unpublished) in the United States and Japan by Taiho Pharmaceuticals and Astellas Pharmaceuticals have not led to the governmental approval of the BPS indication, and the medication has yet to be approved for use in the United States.

Azathioprine and Chloroquine Derivatives

In a single report in 1976, Oravisto et al. used azathioprine or chloroquine derivatives for BPS patients not responding to other treatments [50]. About 50% patients responded.

Mycophenolate Mofetil

In an aborted multicenter randomized placebo-controlled NIDDK trial, Mycophenolate Mofetil (Cellcept™) 1–2 g daily in divided doses failed to show efficacy in the treatment of symptoms of refractory BPS/IC, http://www.clinicaltrial.gov/ct2/show/NCT00451867. The trial, which included 59 patients randomized 2:1 to the active arm, was halted when the FDA issued a new black box warning for the drug (*miscarriage and congenital malformations have been associated with its use*), and an interim analysis showed no benefit.

Miscellaneous Agents

L-Arginine

Foster and Weiss were the original proponents of L-arginine in the therapy of interstitial cystitis [51]. Eight patients with IC were given 500 mg of L-arginine three times daily. After 1 month, urinary nitric oxide synthase activity increased eightfold and seven of the eight patients noticed improvement in symptoms. An open-label study of 11 patients showed improvement in all 10 of the patients who remained on L-arginine for 6 months [52].

An open-label study of nine women in Sweden failed to find any change in symptom scores or in nitric oxide production in the bladder [53]. A placebo-controlled randomized trial of 53 BPS patients could find no difference on an intention to treat analysis between drug- and placebo-treated patients [54]. A smaller randomized placebo-controlled crossover trial of 16 BPS patients found no clinically significant improvement with L-arginine and concluded that it could not be recommended for IC(BPS) treatment [55].

The body of evidence does not support the use of L-arginine for the relief of symptoms of Bladder Pain Syndrome.

Quercetin

Quercetin, a bioflavonoid available in many over-the-counter products [56], may have the anti-inflammatory effects of other members of this class of compounds found in fruits, vegetables, and some spices. Katske et al. [57] administered 500 mg twice daily to 22 BPS patients for 4 weeks. All but one patient had some improvement in the O'Leary/Sant symptom and problem scores as well as in a global assessment score. Further studies are necessary to determine efficacy.

Antibiotics

Warren et al. [58] randomized 50 patients to receive 18 weeks of placebo or antibiotics including rifampin plus a sequence of doxycycline, erythromycin, metronidazole, clindamycin, amoxicillin, and ciprofloxacin for 3 weeks each. Intent to treat analysis demonstrated that 12 of 25 patients in the antibiotic and 6 of 25 patients in the placebo group reported overall improvement while 10 and 5, respectively, noticed improvement in pain and urgency. The study was complicated by the fact that 16 of the patients in the antibiotic group underwent new BPS therapy during the study as did 13 of the placebo patients. There was no statistical significance. What was statistically significant were adverse events in 80% of participants who received antibiotic compared to 40% in the placebo group. Nausea and/or vomiting and diarrhea were the predominant side effects. Most patients on antibiotics correctly guessed what treatment arm they were in, and those that guessed correctly were significantly more likely to note improvement after the study. No duration in improvement after completion of the trial of antibiotics was reported.

Burkhard et al. [59] recorded a 71% success in 103 women presenting with a history of urinary urgency and frequency and chronic urethral and/or pelvic pain often associated with dyspareunia and/or a history of recurrent urinary tract infection. This was a large, inclusive group and one that is probably broader than the bladder pain syndrome we are focusing on. Nevertheless, she recommended empiric doxycycline in this group. The overwhelming majority of BPS patients have been treated with empiric antibiotics prior to diagnosis.

At this time there is no evidence to suggest that antibiotics have a place in the therapy of BPS in the absence of a culture-documented infection [60]. Nevertheless, it would not be unreasonable to treat patients with *one* empiric course of antibiotic, if they have never been on an antibiotic for their urinary symptoms.

Methotrexate

Low-dose oral methotrexate significantly improved bladder pain in four of nine women with BPS, but did not change urinary frequency, maximum voided volume, or mean voided volume [61]. No placebo-controlled RCT has been done with this agent.

Montelukast

Mast cell triggering releases two types of proinflammatory mediators, including granule-stored preformed types such as heparin and histamine, and newly synthesized prostaglandins, and leukotriene B_4 and C_4. Classic antagonists, such as montelukast, zafirlukast, and pranlukast, block cysteinyl leukotriene 1 receptors. In a pilot study [62], ten women with BPS and detrusor mastocytosis received 10 mg of montelukast daily for 3 months. Frequency, nocturia, and pain improved dramatically in eight of the patients. Further study would seem to be warranted, especially in patients with detrusor mastocytosis, defined as >28 per mm^2.

Nifedipine

The calcium channel antagonist nifedipine inhibits smooth muscle contraction and cell-mediated immunity. In a pilot study [63], 30 mg of an extended-release preparation was administered to ten female patients and titrated to 60 mg daily in four of the patients who did not get symptom relief. Within 4 months five patients had at least a 50% decrease in symptom scores, and three of the five were asymptomatic. No further studies have been reported.

Misoprostol

The oral prostaglandin analogue misoprostol was studied in 25 patients at a dose of 600 μg daily [64]. At 3 months 14 patients were significantly improved, and at 6 months 12 patients still had a response. A cytoprotective action in the urinary bladder was postulated.

Guidelines from the American Urological Association suggest that frontline treatment options for oral medication for BPS can include amitriptyline, cimetidine, hydroxyzine, and/or PPS sodium. Cyclosporine should be reserved for use by experienced clinicians after less potentially morbid alternatives have been exhausted [65].

References

1. Barrington JW, Stephenson TP. Pentosanpolysulphate for interstitial cystitis. Int Urogynecol J Pelvic Floor Dysfunct. 1997;8(5):293–5.
2. Fritjofsson A, Fall M, Juhlin R, Persson BE, Ruutu M. Treatment of ulcer and nonulcer interstitial cystitis with sodium pentosanpolysulfate: a multicenter trial. J Urol. 1987;138(3):508–12.
3. Holm-Bentzen M, Jacobsen F, Nerstrom B, Lose G, Kristensen JK, Pedersen RH, et al. A prospective double-blind clinically controlled multicenter trial of sodium pentosanpolysulfate in the treatment of interstitial cystitis and related painful bladder disease. J Urol. 1987;138(3):503–7.
4. Parsons CL, Schmidt JD, Pollen JJ. Successful treatment of interstitial cystitis with sodium pentosanpolysulfate. J Urol. 1983;130(1):51–3.
5. Mulholland SG, Hanno P, Parsons CL, Sant GR, Staskin DR. Pentosan polysulfate sodium for therapy of interstitial cystitis. A double-blind placebo-controlled clinical study. Urology. 1990;35(6):552–8.
6. Parsons CL, Benson G, Childs SJ, Hanno P, Sant GR, Webster G. A quantitatively controlled method to study prospectively interstitial cystitis and demonstrate the efficacy of pentosanpolysulfate. J Urol. 1993;150(3):845–8.
7. Sairanen J, Hotakainen K, Tammela TL, Stenman UH, Ruutu M. Urinary epidermal growth factor and interleukin-6 levels in patients with painful bladder syndrome/interstitial cystitis treated with cyclosporine or pentosan polysulfate sodium. Urology. 2008;71(4):630–3.
8. Sant GR, Propert KJ, Hanno PM, Burks D, Culkin D, Diokno AC, et al. A pilot clinical trial of oral pentosan polysulfate and oral hydroxyzine in patients with interstitial cystitis. J Urol. 2003;170(3):810–5.
9. Nickel J, Barkin J, Forrest J, Mosbaugh P, Payne C, Hernandez-Graulau J, et al. k. Urology. 2001;165(5 (suppliment)):67A.
10. Jepsen JV, Sall M, Rhodes PR, Schmidt D, Messing E, Bruskewitz RC. Long-term experience with pentosanpolysulfate in interstitial cystitis. Urology. 1998;51(3):381–7.
11. Hanno PM. Analysis of long-term Elmiron therapy for interstitial cystitis. Urology. 1997;49(5A Suppl):93–9.
12. Rice L, Kennedy D, Veach A. Pentosan induced cerebral sagittal sinus thrombosis: a variant of heparin induced thrombocytopenia J Urol. 1998;160:2148.
13. Zaslau S, Riggs DR, Jackson BJ, Adkins FC, John CC, Kandzari SJ, et al. In vitro effects of pentosan polysulfate against malignant breast cells. Am J Surg. 2004;188(5):589–92.
14. Bade JJ, Laseur M, Nieuwenburg A, van der Weele LT, Mensink HJ. A placebo-controlled study of intravesical pentosanpolysulphate for the treatment of interstitial cystitis. Br J Urol. 1997;79(2):168–71.
15. Hampson SJ, Woodhouse CRJ. Sodium pentosanpolysulphate in the management of haemorrhagic cystitis: experience with 14 patients. Eur Urol. 1994;25:40–2.
16. Parsons CL. Successful management of radiation cystitis with sodium pentosanpolysulfate. J Urol. 1986;136:813–4.
17. Toren P, Norman R. Cyclophosphamide induced hemorrhagic cystitis successfully treated with pentosanpolysulfate. J Urol. 2005;173:103.

18. Baldessarini RJ. Drugs and the treatment of psychiatric disorders. In: Gilman AG, Goodman SS, Rall TW, et al., editors. The Pharmacological basis of therapeutics. 7th ed. New York: Macmillan Publishing Company; 1985. p. 387–445.
19. Barrett DM, Wein AJ. Voiding dysfunction: diagnosis, classification, and management. In: Gillenwater JY, Grayhack JT, Howards SS, et al., editors. Adult and pediatric urology. Chicago: Year Book Medical Publishers; 1987. p. 863–92.
20. Hanno PM, Wein AJ. Medical treatment of interstitial cystitis (other than Rimso-50/Elmiron). Urology. 1987;29(4 Suppl):22–6.
21. Renshaw DC. Desipramine for interstitial cystitis. JAMA. 1988;260(3):341.
22. Hanno PM, Buehler J, Wein AJ. Use of amitriptyline in the treatment of interstitial cystitis. J Urol. 1989;141(4):846–8.
23. Hanno PM. Amitriptyline in the treatment of interstitial cystitis. Urol Clin North Am. 1994;21(1):89–91.
24. Kirkemo AK, Miles BJ, Peters JM. Use of amitriptyline in the treatment of interstitial cystitis. J Urol. 1990;143:279A.
25. Pranikoff K, Constantino G. The use of amitriptyline in patients with urinary frequency and pain. Urology. 1998;51(5A Suppl):179–81.
26. van Ophoven A, Pokupic S, Heinecke A, Hertle L. A prospective, randomized, placebo controlled, double-blind study of amitriptyline for the treatment of interstitial cystitis. J Urol. 2004;172(2):533–6.
27. van Ophoven A, Hertle L. Long term results of amitriptyline treatment for interstitial cystitis. J Urol. 2005;173(4):86.
28. Hertle L, Van OA. Long-term results of amitriptyline treatment for interstitial cystitis. Aktuelle Urol. 2010;41 Suppl 1:S61–5.
29. Foster Jr HE, Hanno PM, Nickel JC, Payne CK, Mayer RD, Burks DA, et al. Effect of amitriptyline on symptoms in treatment naive patients with interstitial cystitis/painful bladder syndrome. J Urol. 2010;183(5):1853–8.
30. McQuay HJ, Moore RA. Antidepressants and chronic pain. BMJ. 1997;314(7083):763–4.
31. Low PA, Dotson RM. Symptomatic treatment of painful neuropathy. JAMA. 1998;280:1863–4.
32. Ray W, Meredith S, Thapa P, Hall K, Murray K. Cyclic antidepressants and the risk of sudden cardiac death. Clin Pharmacol Ther. 2004;75:234–41.
33. Wammack R, Remzi M, Seitz C, Djavan B, Marberger M. Efficacy of oral doxepin and piroxicam treatment for interstitial cystitis. Eur Urol. 2002;41(6):596–600.
34. van Ophoven A, Hertle L. The dual serotonin and noradrenaline reuptake inhibitor duloxetine for the treatment of interstitial cystitis: results of an observational study. J Urol. 2007;177(2):552–5.
35. Simmons JL. Interstitial cystitis: an explanation for the beneficial effect of an antihistamine. J Urol. 1961;85:149–55.
36. Theoharides TC. Hydroxyzine in the treatment of interstitial cystitis. Urol Clin North Am. 1994;21(1):113–9.
37. Simons F. Advances in H1-antihistamines. N Engl J Med. 2004;351(21):2203–17.
38. Minogiannis P, El Mansoury M, Betances JA, Sant GR, Theoharides TC. Hydroxyzine inhibits neurogenic bladder mast cell activation. Int J Immunopharmacol. 1998;20(10):553–63.
39. Theoharides TC, Sant GR. Hydroxyzine for symptomatic relief of interstitial cystitis symptoms. In: Sant GR, editor. Interstitial cystitis. Philadelphia: Lippincott-Raven; 1997. p. 241–6.
40. Theoharides TC, Sant GR. Hydroxyzine therapy for interstitial cystitis. Urology. 1997;49(5A Suppl):108–10.
41. Lewi HJ. Cimetidine in the treatment of interstitial cystitis. Br J Urol. 1996;77(suppliment 1):28.
42. Seshadri P, Emerson L, Morales A. Cimetidine in the treatment of interstitial cystitis. Urology. 1994;44(4):614–6.

43. Thilagarajah R, Witherow RO, Walker MM. Oral cimetidine gives effective symptom relief in painful bladder disease: a prospective, randomized, double-blind placebo-controlled trial. BJU Int. 2001;87:207–12.
44. Dasgupta P, Sharma SD, Womack C, Blackford HN, Dennis P. Cimetidine in painful bladder syndrome: a histopathological study. BJU Int. 2001;88(3):183–6.
45. Tincello DG, Walker AC. Interstitial cystitis in the UK: results of a questionnaire survey of members of the Interstitial Cystitis Support Group. Eur J Obstet Gynecol Reprod Biol. 2005;118(1):91–5.
46. Forsell TRMIH. Cyclosporine in severe interstitial cystitis. J Urol. 1996;155:1591.
47. Sairanen J, Forsell T, Ruutu M. Long-term outcome of patients with interstitial cystitis treated with low dose cyclosporine A. J Urol. 2004;171(6 Pt 1):2138–41.
48. Sairanen J, Tammela TL, Leppilahti M, Multanen M, Paananen I, Lehtoranta K, et al. Cyclosporine A and pentosan polysulfate sodium for the treatment of interstitial cystitis: a randomized comparative study. J Urol. 2005;174(6):2235–8.
49. Ueda T, Tamaki M, Ogawa O, Yamauchi T, Yoshimura N. Improvement of interstitial cystitis symptoms and problems that developed during treatment with oral IPD-1151T. J Urol. 2000;164(6):1917–20.
50. Oravisto KJ, Alfthan OS. Treatment of interstitial cystitis with immunosuppression and chloroquine derivatives. Eur Urol. 1976;2(2):82–4.
51. Foster HESSWM. Nitric oxide and interstitial cystitis. Advances in Urology. 1997;10:1.
52. Smith SD, Wheeler MA, Foster Jr HE, Weiss RM. Improvement in interstitial cystitis symptom scores during treatment with oral L-arginine. J Urol. 1997;158(3 Pt 1):703–8.
53. Ehren I, Lundberg JO, Adolfsson J, Wiklund NP. Effects of L-arginine treatment on symptoms and bladder nitric oxide levels in patients with interstitial cystitis. Urology. 1998;52(6):1026–9.
54. Korting GE, Smith SD, Wheeler MA, Weiss RM, Foster Jr HE. A randomized double-blind trial of oral l-arginine for treatment of interstitial cystitis. J Urol. 1999;161(2):558–65.
55. Cartledge JJ, Davies AM, Eardley I. A randomized double-blind placebo-controlled crossover trial of the efficacy of L-arginine in the treatment of interstitial cystitis. BJU Int. 2000;85(4):421–6.
56. Theoharides TC, Kempuraj D, Vakali S, Sant GR. Treatment of refractory interstitial cystitis/painful bladder syndrome with CystoProtek—an oral multi-agent natural supplement. Can J Urol. 2008;15(6):4410–4.
57. Katske F, Shoskes DA, Sender M, Poliakin R, Gagliano K, Rajfer J. Treatment of interstitial cystitis with a quercetin supplement. Tech Urol. 2001;7(1):44–6.
58. Warren JW, Horne LM, Hebel JR, Marvel RP, Keay SK, Chai TC. Pilot study of sequential oral antibiotics for the treatment of interstitial cystitis. J Urol. 2000;163(6):1685–8.
59. Burkhard FC, Blick N, Hochreiter WW, Studer UE. Urinary urgency and frequency, and chronic urethral and/or pelvic pain in females. Can doxycycline help? J Urol. 2004;172(1):232–5.
60. Maskell R. Broadening the concept of urinary tract infection. Br J Urol. 1995;76:2–8.
61. Moran PA, Dwyer PL, Carey MP, Maher CF, Radford NJ. Oral methotrexate in the management of refractory interstitial cystitis. Aust N Z J Obstet Gynaecol. 1999;39(4):468–71.
62. Bouchelouche K, Nordling J, Hald T, Bouchelouche P. Treatment of interstitial cystitis with montelukast, a leukotriene D(4) receptor antagonist. Urology. 2001;57(6 Suppl 1):118.
63. Fleischmann J. Calcium channel antagonists in the treatment of interstitial cystitis. Urol Clin North Am. 1994;21(1):107–11.
64. Kelly JD, Young MR, Johnston SR, Keane PF. Clinical response to an oral prostaglandin analogue in patients with interstitial cystitis. Eur Urol. 1998;34(1):53–6.
65. Hanno PM, Burks D, Clemens JQ, Dmochowski R, Erickson D, FitzGerald MP, et al. AUA guideline for the diagnosis and treatment of interstitial cystitis/bladder pain syndrome. J Urol. 2011;185(6):2162–70.

Chapter 22
Pain Treatment in Bladder Pain Syndrome

John Hughes and Salma Mohammed

Medical Treatment

The term bladder pain syndrome (BPS) implies that there is nociception at the level of the bladder. Current understanding of the pathophysiology, pain pathways involved and the psychological components is less than complete. Evidence suggests that BPS involves changes in neural processing resulting in chronic pain of visceral origin [1, 2]. These pains are therefore considered as neuropathic. The innervation of the pelvis includes somatic, visceral and autonomic components. With insufficient research into the specific management of BPS the medical management tends to be that used for other visceral and neuropathic pains. Consideration also has to be given to the possibility of a somatic contribution.

Patients present with ill-defined symptoms involving biological, psychological and social domains. By definition clearly defined conditions have been excluded before the diagnosis of BPS is made. Further research is required into both the pathophysiology of this type of pain as well as the treatment.

The management of BPS warrants a multidisciplinary approach with contributions from various specialties including urology, gynaecology, gastroenterology, psychology, physiotherapy, genitourinary medicine and pain medicine [3].

Since BPS has somatic, visceral and neuropathic components general recommendations for its management are derived from the management of chronic pain (Table 22.1) [4].

J. Hughes, M.B.B.S., F.R.C.A., F.F.P.M.R.C.A. (✉)
Pain Management Unit, The James Cook University Hospital,
Marton Road, Middlesbrough TS4 3BW, UK
e-mail: john@hughesj.demon.co.uk

S. Mohammed, M.B.B.S., F.R.C.A.
Anaesthesia, Intensive Care and Pain Medicine, Pain Management Unit,
The James Cook University Hospital, Middlesbrough, UK

J. Nordling et al. (eds.), *Bladder Pain Syndrome: A Guide for Clinicians*,
DOI 10.1007/978-1-4419-6929-3_22, © Springer Science+Business Media New York 2013

Table 22.1 Pharmacological treatment of chronic pelvic pain [4]

Drug	Type of pain	Level of evidence	Grade of recommendation	Comment
Paracetamol	Somatic pain	1b	A	Benefit is limited and based on arthritic pain.
COX 2 antagonists	–	1b	A	Avoid in patients with cardiovascular risk factors.
NSAIDs	Dysmenorrhoea	1a	B	Better than placebo but unable to distinguish between different NSAIDs.
Tricyclic antidepressants	Neuropathic pain	1a	A	–
	Pelvic pain	3	C	Evidence suggests that pelvic pain is similar to neuropathic pain.
Anticonvulsants, e.g. Gabapentin	Neuropathic pain	1a	A	–
Opioids	Chronic nonmalignant pain	1a	A	Limited long-term data, should only be used by clinicians experienced in their use.
	Neuropathic pain	1a	A	Benefit is probably clinically significant, caution with use, as above.

COX cyclooxygenase-2, *NSAID* nonsteroidal anti-inflammatory drug
From Fall M, Baranowski A, Elneil S, Engeler D, Hughes J, et al. EAU guidelines on Chronic Pelvic Pain. European Urology. 2010; 57:35–48. Reprinted with permission from the European Association of Urology

Medications

Simple Analgesics

Paracetamol (Acetaminophen)

Paracetamol is usually a well-tolerated synthetic nonopiod analgesic with very few side effects [5]. It has analgesic and antipyretic properties and has been used in somatic pain including arthritic pain [6, 7].

Paracetamol acts centrally by inhibiting brain cyclo-oxygenase (COX) and nitric oxide synthase. Brain COX seems to reduce the production of prostaglandins and therefore the central sensitisation that results from inflammation [8, 9].

When used with a traditional nonsteroidal anti-inflammatory drug (NSAID), it enhances the analgesic effect of the NSAID and allows the use of a lower dose of the NSAID [5].

NSAIDs

NSAIDs can be classified into the nonspecific COX inhibitors and the specific COX-2 inhibitors.

- Nonspecific COX inhibitors (e.g. aspirin, diclofenac, ibuprofen).
- Specific COX-2 inhibitors (e.g. celecoxib, parecoxib, etoricoxib).

NSAIDs inhibit the enzyme COX which thereby prevents the production of prostaglandins and thromboxanes from membrane phospholipids. COX exists as two isoenzymes, COX-1 and COX-2. COX-1 (the constitutive form) is responsible for the protective prostaglandins that maintain renal blood flow, haemostatic function and the protective gastric mucosal barrier. COX-2 (the inducible form) occurs at the site of tissue damage and facilitates the inflammatory response. Therefore, inhibition of COX-1 seems to produce the adverse effects of NSAIDs while inhibition of COX-2 seems to result in the anti-inflammatory, analgesic and antipyretic effects of NSAIDs. Even though the COX-2 inhibitors have been designed to minimise gastrointestinal complications compared to the non-specific COX inhibitors, they are associated with a small but definite risk of myocardial and cerebrovascular events [10].

There is, however, very little evidence to support the use of NSAIDs in the management of BPS. NSAIDs have been found to be superior to placebo and maybe superior to paracetamol in studies investigating different types of analgesia for dysmenorrhoea [11].

Neuropathic Analgesics

These are groups of drugs that are used for neuropathic pain and have little analgesic effect if used for acute somatic pain.

Tricyclic Antidepressants

Tricyclic antidepressants (TCAs) predominantly have their pain-modulating effect by inhibiting the reuptake of norepinephrine and serotonin at the presynaptic membrane. They also have anticholinergic effects that account for many of the side effects. A recent Cochrane review concluded that TCAs and venlafaxine are effective for neuropathic pain with a number needed to treat of three. There is however limited evidence supporting the use of the newer selective serotonin reuptake inhibitors. The preemptive use of antidepressants to prevent the development of neuropathic pain remains unclear [12].

To date, there is very little strong evidence supporting the use of TCAs in humans in the treatment of BPS. These drugs are options of treatment from whatever data is available [13, 14]. An animal study suggests that it may have a role in cystitis [15]. The algorithm (Fig. 22.1) can be considered where there is suggestion of nerve injury or central sensitisation.

TCAs tend to be used in lower dosages than those used for the treatment of depression. Amitriptyline and nortriptyline are used in a dose of up to 150 mg daily. Duloxetine at a dose of 60–120 mg has been found to decrease the intensity of pain in diabetic neuropathy and fibromyalgia and has been used as an alternative in the treatment of neuropathic pain in some countries [16–18].

Anticonvulsants

Anticonvulsants have been used for many years in pain management. Gabapentin and pregabalin have fewer side effects compared to the older anticonvulsants and are suggested as the preferred anticonvulsants for neuropathic pain [18]. The exact mechanism of action of gabapentin and pregabalin in chronic pain is unknown but they appear to be calcium channel blockers.

There is little evidence supporting the use of anticonvulsants in genitourinary pain [19]. However, where there is a suggestion of neuropathic pain or central sensitisation they should be considered. Anticonvulsants have no role in the management of acute pain [19]. In a Cochrane review, pregabalin at dosages of 600 mg daily had a number needed to treat of 3–5 for neuropathic pain and 11 in fibromyalgia [20].

NMDA Antagonists (e.g. Ketamine)

This NMDA channel is known to play an important role in the development and maintenance of chronic pain. It is thought to be most important when there is evidence of central sensitisation and opioid tolerance [21–25].

Ketamine is a noncompetitive NMDA receptor antagonist and also exhibits action at sodium channels and opioid receptors (kappa and mu) [26]. Ketamine has been used in many chronic pain conditions such as peripheral neuropathies with allodynia, stump and phantom limb pain, central pain and cancer-related pain. In BPS ketamine may be of potential benefit if there is evidence of nerve injury or central sensitisation.

At low doses, ketamine has anti-hyperalgesia, anti-allodynic and tolerance protective effects [26]. It may therefore be useful in opioid-resistant pain. There are few papers to support its use and safety profile in long-term use [27]. There is some suggestion that ketamine may be incriminated in causing BPS [28, 29]. Oral ketamine should only be started by a physician familiar with its use.

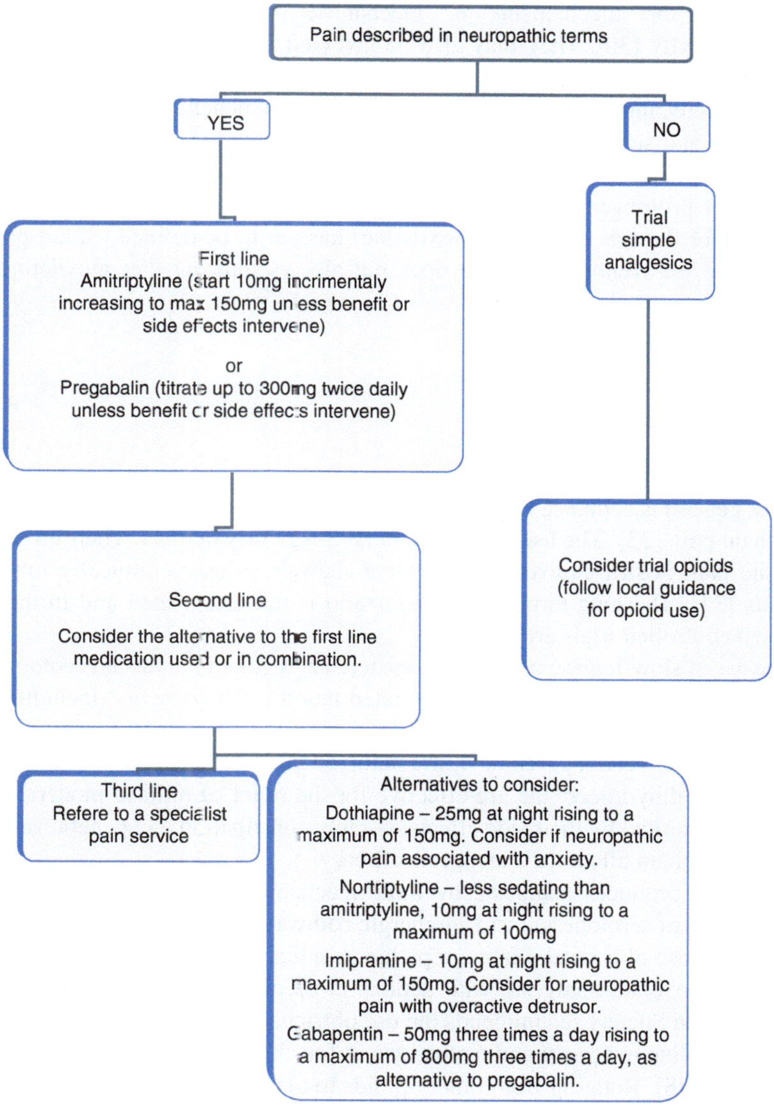

Fig. 22.1 Guidelines for the use of neuropathic analgesics. Modified from EAU guidelines [4] and NICE [18] with permission from the European Association of Urology

Na Channel Blockers

It is thought that changes in certain sodium channel isoforms may be involved in neuropathic pain processing. As a result, injured afferent nerves become susceptible to generating more prolonged and higher frequency discharges, with a reduced refractory period. These changes associated with the sodium channels are thought to underlie the mechanisms of mechanosensitivity, thermosensitivity and chemosensitivity [30]. They may also be involved in the development of visceral hyperalgesia.

In one study, intravenous lidocaine was found to be beneficial in reducing neuropathic pain and sensory phenomenon such as allodynia [31]. A positive lidocaine infusion may be followed by repeated infusions and the benefit from a single infusion may be prolonged.

A role for the oral analogue (Mexiletine) has yet to be defined [32]; a positive response to intravenous lidocaine does not always indicate that mexiletine will work.

Opioids

It is the general acceptance that opioids have a role in the treatment of chronic nonmalignant pain [33]. The use of opioids in BPS is poorly defined. Their use in neuropathic pain is still equivocal but a meta-analysis suggests clinically important benefits [34]. The long-term risk–benefit ratio is not established and further randomised controlled trials are needed.

The use of slow-release opioids administered at regular intervals is recommended for chronic pain. The dose should be titrated based on the benefits (including pain and function) and side effects.

Morphine, oxycodone, fentanyl, tramadol, codeine and methadone can be used. Codeine and dihydrocodeine are effective for the relief of mild to moderate pain. Their use is limited by their side effects; notably constipation and genetic variances in the metabolism affect their analgesic efficacy.

Tramadol produces analgesia by three mechanisms, an opioid effect and an enhancement of serotonergic and adrenergic pathways [35, 36]. A Cochrane review supports the use of tramadol in neuropathic pain management [37].

Methadone is an analgesic with actions at opioid and NMDA receptors. The Canadian Pain Society recommends the use of tramadol and controlled-release opioids as third-line treatment and methadone as fourth-line treatment for moderate to severe pain [38]. Rotating from other opioids to methadone is not an exact science due to its pharmacokinetics [39].

Buprenorphine and pentazocine both have agonist and antagonist actions at opioid receptors and can induce withdrawal symptoms in opioid-tolerant patients. Topical buprenorphine patches may offer similar advantages to topical fentanyl.

The decision to start long-term opioids should be made by a trained specialist only after all other reasonable treatment strategies have failed and in conjunction with the patient's primary care physician. General guidelines for the use of opioids in chronic pain should be followed [40, 41].

Nonpharmacological Treatments

Interventional Treatments

(a) Nerve blocks.
These blocks should be performed by pain physicians trained in performing them, with appropriate monitoring and resuscitation facilities. Procedures may be undertaken for either diagnostic and or therapeutic reasons. The details of specific blocks fall outside the scope of this chapter.

(b) Suprapubic transcutaneous electrical nerve stimulation (TENS) in BPS.
Current experience is limited to open studies. In one study 54 % of patients were helped by TENS. Less favourable results were obtained in non-Hunner lesion BPS (type 3C) [42]. It is difficult to assess the efficacy of TENS in the treatment of BPS with accuracy. This mode of treatment involves the application of high-intensity stimuli at specific sites over a prolonged period of time and so designing controlled studies is quite difficult.

(c) Sacral neuromodulation in BPS.
Patients with Chronic reflex sympathetic dystrophy treated with neurostimulation have reported a reduction in pain intensity as well as an improved quality of life [43]. There may be a role in BPS.
This procedure is invasive and expensive and as such it is reserved for patients unresponsive to conservative treatment. It usually involves the application of electrodes through the sacral foramina three or four. The mechanism of action remains unclear.

(d) Botulinum toxin.
Recent studies have shown that botulinum toxin might be a safe and effective treatment for BPS [44].

Conclusion

The diagnosis of BPS is one of exclusion after all clearly defined causes have been ruled out. Further research is warranted into the mechanisms and medical management of BPS.

Current understanding is that it is possibly a pain of visceral origin and this type of pain is considered to be neuropathic. General recommendations are therefore derived from the management of chronic pain. As with most types of neuropathic pain, a multidisciplinary approach is used with contributions from various specialties.

The medical management involves targeting various aspects of the pain pathway with the different groups of drugs available. When the traditional conservative management fails, then the use of interventional procedures is considered.

The use of medications should be part of a biopsychosocial model of pain management and include input from other disciplines as part of an individualised management plan for the patient.

References

1. Buffington CAT. Comorbidity of interstitial cystitis with other unexplained clinical conditions. J Urol. 2004;172(4 Pt 1):1242–8.
2. Buffington CAT. Bladder pain syndrome/interstitial cystitis—etiology and animal research. In: Baranowski AP, Abrams P, Fall M, editors. Urogenital pain in clinical practice. Informa healthcare, 2008, New York, ISBN-10:0-8493-9932-7 p. 169–83.
3. Baranowski AP, Abrams P, Berger RE, et al. Urogenital pain–time to accept a new approach to phenotyping and, as a consequence, management. Eur Urol. 2008;53(1):60–7.
4. Fall M, Baranowski A, Elneil S, Engeler D, Hughes J, et al. EAU guidelines on chronic pelvic pain. Eur Urol. 2010;57:35–48.
5. Bannworth B, Pehourq F. Pharmacologic basis for using paracetemol: pharmacokinetic and pharmacodynamic issues. Drugs. 2003;63: Spec No 2:5–13.
6. Bradley JD, Brandt KD, Katz BP, Kalasinski LA, Ryan SI. Treatment of knee osteoarthritis: relationship of clinical features of joint inflammation to the response to a nonsteroidal anti-inflammatory drug or pure analgesic. J Rheumatol. 1992;19(12):1950–4.
7. Temple AR, Benson GD, Zinsenheim JR, Schweinle JE. Multicenter, randomized, double-blind, active-controlled, parallel-group trial of the long-term (6–12 months) safety of acetaminophen in adult patients with osteoarthritis. Clin Ther. 2006;28(2):222–35.
8. Bianchi M, Panerai AE. The dose-related effects of paracetamol on hyperalgesia and nociception in the rat. Br J Pharmacol. 1996;117:130–2.
9. Koppert W, Wehrfritz A, Körber N, Sittl R, et al. The cyclooxygenase isozyme inhibitors parecoxib and paracetamol reduce central hyperalgesia in humans. Pain. 2004;108(1–2):148–53.
10. Fitzgerald G. Coxibs and cardiovascular disease. N Engl J Med. 2004;351(17):1709–11.
11. Marjoribanks J, Proctor ML, Farquhar C. Nonsteroidal anti-inflammatory drugs for primary dysmenorrhoea. Cochrane Database Syst Rev. 2003;(4):CD001751.
12. Saarto T, Wiffen P. Antidepressants for neuropathic pain: a Cochrane review. J Neurol Neurosurg Psychiatry. 2010;81:1372–3.
13. Phatak S, Foster Jr HE. The management of interstitial cystitis: an update. Nat Clin Pract Urol. 2006;3:45–53.
14. Pontari MA. Chronic prostatitis/chronic pelvic pain syndrome in elderly men: toward better understanding and treatment. Drugs Aging. 2003;20(15):1111–25.
15. Chew DJ, Buffington CA, Kendall MS, DiBartola SP, Woodworth BE. Amitriptyline treatment for severe recurrent idiopathic cystitis in cats. J Am Vet Med Assoc. 1998;213(9):1282–6.
16. Raskin J, Pritchett YL, Wang F, et al. A double-blind, randomized multicenter trial comparing duloxetine with placebo in the management of diabetic peripheral neuropathic pain. Pain Med. 2005;6(5):346–56.
17. Lunn MP, Hughes RA, Wiffen PJ. Duloxetine for treating painful neuropathy or chronic pain. Cochrane Database Syst Rev. 2009;(4):CD007115.
18. Neuropathic pain. National Institute of Health and Clinical Excellence. Clinical Guideline 96. http://www.nice.org.uk/nicemedia/live/12948/58253/58253.pdf. Published March 2010.
19. Wiffen P, Collins S, McQuay H, et al. Anticonvulsant drugs for acute and chronic pain. Cochrane Database Syst Rev. 2005;(3):CD001133.
20. Moore RA, Straube S, Wiffen PJ, et al. Pregabalin for acute and chronic pain in adults. Cochrane Database Syst Rev. 2009;(3):CD007076.
21. Price DD, Mayer DJ, Mao J, Caruso FS. NMDA-receptor antagonists and opioid receptor interactions as related to analgesia and tolerance. J Pain Symptom Manage. 2000;19(1 Suppl):S7–S11.
22. Eide PK, Jørum E, Stubhaug A, Bremnes J, Breivik H. Relief of post-herpetic neuralgia with the N-methyl-D-aspartic acid receptor antagonist ketamine: a double-blind, cross-over comparison with morphine and placebo. Pain. 1994;58(3):347–54.
23. Guirimand F, Dupont X, Brasseur L, Chauvin M, et al. The effects of ketamine on the temporal summation (wind-up) of the RIII nociceptive flexion reflex and pain in humans. Anesth Analg. 2000;90:408–14.

24. Laurido C, Pelissier T, Pérez H, Flores F, et al. Effect of ketamine on spinal cord nociceptive transmission in normal and monoarthritic rats. Neuroreport. 2001;12(8):1551–4.
25. Mikkelsen S, Ilkjaer S, Brennum J, Borgbjerg F, et al. The effect of naloxone on ketamine-induced effects on hyperalgesia and ketamine-induced side effects in humans. Anesthesiology. 1999;90(6):1539–45.
26. Visser E, Schug SA. The role of ketamine in pain management. Biomed Pharmacother. 2006;60(7):341–8.
27. Blonk MI, Koder BG, van den Bemt PM, Huygen FJ. Use of oral ketamine in chronic pain management: a review. Eur J Pain. 2010;14(5):466–72.
28. Middela S, Pearce I. Ketamine-induced vesicopathy: a literature review. Int J Clin Pract. 2011;65(1):27–30.
29. Wood D, Cottrell A, Baker SC, et al. Recreational ketamine: from pleasure to pain. BJU Int. 2011;107:1881–4.
30. Cummins T, Sheets P, Waxman S. The roles of sodium channels in nociception: implications for mechanisms of pain. Pain. 2007;131(3):243–57.
31. Baranowski AP, De Courcey J, Bonello E. A trial of intravenous lidocaine on the pain and allodynia of postherpetic neuralgia. J Pain Symptom Manage. 1999;17(6):429–33.
32. Galer BS, Harle J, Rowbotham MC. Response to intravenous lidocaine infusion predicts subsequent response to oral mexiletine: a prospective study. J Pain Symptom Manage. 1996;12(3):161–7.
33. McQuay H. Opioids in pain management. Lancet. 1999;353(9171):2229–32.
34. Eisenberg E, McNicol E, Carr DB. Opioids for neuropathic pain. Cochrane Database Syst Rev. 2006;3:CD006146.
35. Sagata K, Minami K, Yanagihara N, Shiraishi M, et al. Tramadol inhibits norepinephrine transporter function at desipramine-binding sites in cultured bovine adrenal medullary cells. Anesth Analg. 2002;94(4):901–6.
36. Desmeules JA, Piguet V, Collart L, Dayer P. Contribution of monoaminergic modulation to the analgesic effect of tramadol. Br J Clin Pharmacol. 1996;41(1):7–12.
37. Hollingshead J, Dühmke RM, Cornblath DR. Tramadol for neuropathic pain. Cochrane Database Syst Rev. 2006;3:CD003726.
38. Moulin DE, Clark AJ, Gilron I, et al. Pharmacological management of chronic neuropathic pain: consensus statement and guidelines from the Canadian Pain Society. Pain Res Manag. 2007;12(1):13–21.
39. Fredheim OM, Borchgrevink PC, Klepstad P, Kaasa S, Dale O. Long term methadone for chronic pain: a pilot study of pharmacokinetic aspects. Eur J Pain. 2007;11(6):599–604.
40. Kalso E, Allan L, Dellemijn PL, Faura CC, et al. Recommendations for using opioids in chronic non-cancer pain. Eur J Pain. 2003;7(5):381–6.
41. The British Pain Society. Opioids for persistent pain: Good practice. London: The British Pain Society; 2010. http://www.britishpainsociety.org/book_opioid_main.pdf.
42. Fall M, Lindström S. Transcutaneous electrical nerve stimulation in classic and nonulcer interstitial cystitis. Urol Clin North Am. 1994;21(1):131–9.
43. Kemler MA, Barendse GAM, et al. Spinal cord stimulation in patients with chronic reflex sympathetic dystrophy. N Engl J Med. 2000;343:618–24.
44. Pinto R, Lopes T, Frias B, Silva A, et al. Trigonal injection of botulinum toxin A in patients with refractory bladder pain syndrome/interstitial cystitis. Eur Urol. 2010;58(3):360–5.

Chapter 23
Intravesical Therapy

Mauro Cervigni and Arndt van Ophoven

Introduction and Overview

Because of the absence of definitive diagnostic tests and generally accepted standard clinical criteria, bladder pain syndrome (BPS) is a diagnosis of exclusion; as a result, the design of randomized controlled trials (RCTs) for its management is extremely difficult. Therefore, data regarding the efficacy of therapies are limited and often based on uncontrolled studies or case series. Although more than 180 different treatments have been tried in BPS, data are still inconclusive.

Intravesical treatments for BPS were recently analyzed in a Cochrane review: only bacillus Calmette–Guerin (BCG) and oxybutin seemed to be relatively well tolerated and gave the most promising results. However, it was repeatedly noted by the authors that the available evidence is extremely limited.

Nevertheless, instillation therapy continues to remain an important therapeutic approach to BPS for ameliorating or delaying recurrence of symptoms. It appears to be wise to apply the lessons learned from intravesical treatment of superficial bladder cancer to improve the treatment of BPS and lower urinary tract symptoms (LUTS) in general.

Instillations of drugs into the bladder create a high concentration of drugs locally at the disease site without increasing systemic levels, which can explain the low risk of systemic side effects.

M. Cervigni, M.D. (✉)
Department of Urogynecology, S. Carlo-IDI, Catholic University,
Viale Glorioso 13, Rome 00153, Italy

Department Obstetrics and Gynecology, Catholic University,
Rome, Italy
e-mail: m.cervigni@idi.it

A. van Ophoven, M.D., Ph.D.
Division of Neuro-Urology, Marienhospital Herne, University Hospital of Bochum,
Widumerstr. 8, Herne 44627, Germany

J. Nordling et al. (eds.), *Bladder Pain Syndrome: A Guide for Clinicians*,
DOI 10.1007/978-1-4419-6929-3_23, © Springer Science+Business Media New York 2013

Table 23.1 Intravesical medications for treatment of PBS/IC: Results[a]

Drug	RCT	Success
DMSO	Yes	70%
BCG	Yes	Conflicting RCT data as to efficacy
RTX	Yes	No proven efficacy
Hyaluronic acid	Yes	No proven efficacy
Heparin	No	60%
Chondroitin sulfate	No	33%
Lidocaine	No	65%
PPS	Yes	Suggestion of possible efficacy 40%

[a]Adapted by Hanno P. Painful bladder syndrome. In Abrams P, Cardozo L, Khoury S, Wein A, editors. Incontinence. Paris; 2009, pp. 1455–1520

A large body of evidence supports the notion that symptoms of BPS emanate from underlying inflammation in the bladder. Animal studies have reported infiltration of neutrophils, enhanced activation of several inflammatory cytokines in the bladder, and increase in inflammatory gene expression. It is believed that activation of mast cells and disruptions in the bladder permeability barrier are the other key events in the bladder inflammation associated with BPS. The intravesical route offers reasonable adjunctive therapies for immediate symptom relief during symptom flare up.

Given the multifactorial nature of the disease, therapy is often tailored to improve therapeutic outcomes with multimodal treatment through pharmacological and non-pharmacological approaches such as hydrodistention acting via different and often synergistic mechanisms of action.

Disadvantages include the need for intermittent catheterization, which can be painful in BPS patients, and furthermore the cost and the general risk of iatrogenic infection.

Finally regulatory approvals and availability for the various instillations throughout the world differ from nation to nation. What follows are treatments that have been reported in the recent literature, some of which are commonly used (Table 23.1).

Dimethyl Sulfoxide

Dimethyl sulfoxide (DMSO) is believed to reduce inflammation, relax muscles, eliminate pain, dissolve collagen, and degranulate mast cells. It has long been used as a therapeutic agent for BPS. Its mechanism of action, however, has not been clarified. In a randomized study Peeker et al. reported that frequency and pain were improved in ulcer-type BPS patients, although no improvement was observed in maximum bladder capacity [1]. In a non-randomized controlled study Perez-Marrero et al. reported that 53% of the patients showed remarkable improvement in subjective evaluation (placebo 18%) and 93% in objective evaluation (placebo 35%) [2]. Around an

80% improvement rate has been reported in case series and retrospective studies. With regard to side effects after instillation of DMSO, most patients recognize a garlic-like odor, which disappears within a day, and about 10% of patients report bladder irritative symptoms which resolve with or without symptomatic treatment [3]. It is hypothesized that these transient exacerbations occur as the result of mast cell degranulation. The number of significant side effects is considered to be small [4]. DMSO may accelerate the absorption of other drugs instilled simultaneously, including hydrocortisone, heparin, and sodium bicarbonate [5].

Resiniferatoxin

Resiniferatoxin (RTX) is produced from *Euphorbia resinifera*, a cactus-like plant of Morocco. Its homovanilling ring is a natural ligand of the capsaicin receptor in a subpopulation of primary afferent sensory neurons involved in the transmission of pain [6, 7]. When it is administered intravesically, it binds to Transient Receptor Potential Vanilloid 1 (TRPV 1) receptors located in C fibers in suburothelium and in urothelial cells [8].

Till now, RTX has been used for neurogenic and idiopathic overactive detrusor and overactive bladder [9, 10]. During the last years this drug has also been used for the treatment of BPS.

A pretreatment analgesia must be performed using an intravesical instillation of 20–100 ml of 2–4% lidocaine solution, held in the bladder for 10–30 min to increase tolerability. RTX was prepared at a dose of 30–100 ml of a 10–100 nM solution in ethanol. The drug was retained in the bladder for 30 min. The different treatment schemes included single, multiple instillation or prolonged infusion of 10 nM of RTX for 10 days by a pump connected to suprapubic catheter.

Recently, a systematic review was conducted by Mourtzoukou et al. on the use of RTX in BPS and concluded that data regarding clinical effectiveness of RTX are contradictory [11]. Payne et al. conducted the largest randomized placebo-controlled study that showed that single administration of RTX at doses of 0.01 to 0.10 mM did not improve overall symptoms, pain, urgency, frequency, nocturia, or average void volume during 12-week follow-up. RTX resulted in a dose-dependent increase in the incidence of instillation pain but was otherwise generally well tolerated [12]. Other two studies, that used a single dose of RTX in BPS patients, had more encouraging results although they included small samples [13, 14]. Both studies showed an improvement of symptoms, either statistically significant or not, and this improvement was present even 3 months after treatment.

Apostolidis et al. investigated the effects of a single intravesical instillation of 100 ml 50 nM RTX solution in 15 patients with frequency and urgency, four of whom had a clinical and histopathological diagnosis of BPS. The overall results showed a statistically significant improvement of maximum cystometric capacity urodynamic volume at the first desire to void, and 24-h frequency at all follow-up points (at 1, 3, and 6 months after treatment) [15].

Peng et al. reported the effect of intravesical instillation of low-dose RTX (10 nM) once weekly for 4 weeks: 7 (54%) out of 13 patients that received instillations reported excellent (2/7) or improved (5/7) therapeutic results [16]. Three patients had a significant increase in functional bladder capacity; pain and quality of life significantly improved 12 weeks after initial infusion.

Lazzeri et al. reported the effect of a prolonged infusion of RTX in five patients with BPS and showed a reduction in frequency, nocturia, and pain 4 weeks after the end of infusion ($p<0.01$), while pain remained significantly lower at 12-week follow-up ($p<0.05$) [17].

The treatment with RTX is generally well tolerated, and only a small number of patients report important side effects: pain during instillation is the most frequent complaint (0–87.5%). The pain is of 1-h duration and is accompanied with increase in systolic blood pressure during instillation. Increase in urgency and burning sensation at the suprapubic or urethral level during infusion is less frequently reported.

A critical evaluation of the available literature regarding the role of RTX in the treatment of patients with BPS suggests that its effectiveness is still questionable.

Substitution Therapy

Glycosaminoglycans (GAGs) are long, linear polysaccharide compounds synthesized by urothelial cells and associated to the urothelial cell membrane, where they reinforce the surface and form an additional permeability barrier; in this way GAGs reduce the direct contact of urine with the urothelium [18]. GAG deficiency has been suggested as a primary cause of BPS and GAG substitution concepts have obtained a predominant position in BPS therapy [19].

At present, three GAG substituents (heparin, hyaluronan, and chondroitin sulfate) and one heparinoid [pentosanpolysulfate (PPS)] are used for substitution therapy.

Pentosanpolysulfate

PPS is a semisynthetic mucopolysaccharide available for oral and intravesical treatment. Its structure is similar to heparin, with a similar postulated mode of action when used locally. Oral administration of PPS is a well-established first-choice treatment. There is still poor evidence concerning the results of the intravesical instillation therapy. In a randomized controlled trial, Bade et al. found benefit in 4 patients out of 10 on PPS versus 2 of 10 on placebo [20]. They noted a significant decrease in nocturia and an increase in bladder capacity. In a prospective, uncontrolled, open-label study, 29 BPS patients received 300 mg PPS intravesically twice a week for 10 weeks and thereafter a voluntary maintenance therapy once a month [21]. Complete response was observed 3, 6, and 12 months after treatment in 16, 27, and 14% of patients, respectively. In most patients, benefits lasted for a short time and required sustainment therapy or a renewed treatment. A recent placebo-controlled study of 41 patients found that the addition of a 6-week course of intravesical PPS to a regimen of oral PPS significantly improved results [22]. No significant side effects are considered to be present using PPS intravesically.

Heparin

Heparin has similarities to the GAG layer of the bladder. When instilled into the bladder, theoretically it might replace the damaged GAG layer. Kuo reported that the International Prostate Symptom Score, as well as bladder capacity at initial desire to void and maximum bladder capacity, improved significantly [23]. According to the report by Parsons et al. symptoms were reduced in 56% of patients treated 3 times weekly for 12 weeks [24]. These reports suggest the efficacy of heparin; however, there is no randomized comparative study to give conclusive evidence. One study indicated that intravesical heparin instillations may prolong the response to DMSO treatment [25]. No significant side effects have been reported, as it does not affect systemic coagulation parameters. In the case of patients with hematuria, however, it may exacerbate local hemorrhage. The instillation method has not been standardized. Generally, 10,000–40,000 units of heparin are instilled. It is unusual to have pain or irritation as a result of instillation, and retention times can be 30 min or more. Instillation frequency can be up to every other day and is often administered at home by the patient. Parsons et al. reported that when 40,000 units of heparin combined with 1–2% lidocaine was instilled 3 times a week for 2 weeks, about 80% efficacy was obtained [26]. There is no upper limit for the duration of the treatment, but a long-term effect is unknown. Welk and Teichman treated 23 IC patients with a solution of lidocaine, heparin, and sodium bicarbonate [27]. The results of this study demonstrated that this solution provides relief not only of voiding symptoms and pain but also of dyspareunia.

Hyaluronic Acid

Hyaluronic acid (HA), a GAG present in the bladder mucosa, plays an important protective role on the underlying urothelium. HA inhibits adherence of immune complexes to polymorphonuclear cells, leukocyte migration, and aggregation. It also binds to lymphocytes and endothelial cells, blocking the ICAM-1 receptors and alleviating the inflammatory process. A few studies on HA in PBS/IC are available in the literature: Morales et al. reported a 71% partial or complete response to treatment with HA after 12 weeks, with a subsequent relapse after 24 weeks [28]. A lower response rate of only 30% was demonstrated by another author on a small group of PBS/IC patients, achieving improvement in both pain and frequency [29].

Kallenstrup et al. reported a positive response to treatment in 65% of patients, with a follow-up of 3 years. A significant reduction in pain score was noted (2.2-fold decrease in pain score after 3 months and 5.2-fold decrease after 3 years), while reduction in urinary frequency was not observed [30]. Similar results on pain emerge from the study by Daha et al. [31]. The greatest symptomatic improvement observed in this study was achieved in a selected group of patients, whose bladder showed a 30% reduction in maximum bladder capacity following cystometry done with KCl as compared to NaCl ($p = 0.003$). Two other groups reported the use of HA intravesical instillation combined with hydrodistension under general anesthesia. Leppilahti et al. reported complete or partial response in 8 patients out of 12 with this technique [32]. Ahmad et al. recently reported their experience on 23 patients: they obtained a response rate of 74% with an average follow-up of 15.8 months [33].

Chondroitin Sulfate

Chondroitin sulfate (CS), which is less expensive and more inert than heparinoids, hyaluronan, or PPS, has been introduced to restore the barrier function lost due to epithelial dysfunction in BPS. In an open-label study, Steinhoff et al. used chondroitin sulfate in patients with BPS and positive potassium test. Thirteen patients were followed for the entire 13-month study. A total of 6/13 (46.2%) showed a good response, 2/13 (15.4%) had a fair response, 4/13 (30.8%) had a partial response, and 1/13 (7.7%) showed no response [34].

In a multicenter, community-based open-label study Nickel et al. showed that 47% of the 53 enrolled patients were responders at week 10. At 24 weeks, 60% were responders. There was a statistically and clinically significant decrease in the mean symptom and bother scores from baseline at 10 weeks and 24 weeks ($p < 0.001$). There were no significant safety issues during the study [35].

In a multicenter, randomized, double-blind study 65 patients were randomized. At week 7, 22.6% of the vehicle control group were responders compared with 39.4% of the active therapy group ($p = 0.15$). Overall, 76.9% of the patients in the study reported at least 1 adverse event; most were mild or moderate, the majority associated with the vehicle control treatment. The difference in treatment effect in this small underpowered study was not statistically significant, although twice as many patients reported a clinically significant benefit with intravesical chondroitin sulfate treatment compared with vehicle control treatment [36].

Hyaluronic Acid Plus Chondroitin Sulfate

To maximize the potential for urothelial restoration, and to elucidate the optimal dose and schedule, HA 1.6% and CS 2.0% were combined for intravesical instillation therapy in the course of two independent preliminary, open-label, uncontrolled studies, each in 23 patients with BPS. There was significant symptomatic improvement for patients in both studies. In one study, weekly bladder instillations of the combination of agents were administered for 20 weeks, then monthly for 3 months, with a mean follow-up for another 5 months [37]. In the other study, the same combination of agents was administered intravesically weekly for 12 weeks and, if there was a response, biweekly for 6 months [38].

Bacillus Calmette–Guerin

The efficacy of intravesical BCG for the treatment of BPS was evaluated in three RCTs. Peters et al. conducted a randomized double-blind study showing a 60% improvement compared to 27% [39] placebo response with good long-term results at 27 months [40]. The most recent NIDDK-sponsored RCT supports these findings demonstrating benefit in 21% of the BCG group compared to 12% in the placebo group ($p=0.062$) [41]. In a crossover trial BCG versus DMSO, none of the patients improved on BCG at first treatment, whereas seven improved using DMSO, two when DMSO was the first-line treatment, and five when DMSO followed BCG [1].

Conclusion

Different therapeutic strategies are possible for intravesical treatment. Agents like hyaluronic acid, heparin, and BTX-A show promising tendencies in recent research, and combination with other therapeutic modalities. On the contrary, BCG and RTX do not seem to have any improving effect on symptoms in BPS. Adverse or side effects are seen with DMSO and RTX. Generally, it is necessary to do more research in this field. Controlled studies with larger populations, possibly divided in well-defined subgroups (classic and non-ulcer BPS), are strongly needed.

References

1. Peeker R, Haghsheno MA, Holmang S, Fall M. Intravesical bacillus Calmette-Guerin and dimethyl sulfoxide for treatment of classic and nonulcer BPS: a prospective, randomized double-blind study. J Urol. 2000;164:1912.
2. Perez-Marrero R, Emerson LE, Feltis JT. A controlled study of dimethyl sulfoxide in BPS. J Urol. 1988;140:36.
3. Sant GR. Intravesical 50% dimethyl sulfoxide (Rimso-50) in treatment of BPS. Urology. 1987;29:17.

4. Rossberger J, Fall M, Peeker R. Critical appraisal of dimethyl sulfoxide treatment for BPS: discomfort, side-effects and treatment outcome. Scand J Urol Nephrol. 2005;39:73.
5. Hanno P. BPS and related disorders. In: Walsh PC, editor. Campbell's urology. Philadelphia: Elsevier; 2002. p. 631–68.
6. Szallasi A, Blumberg PM. Resiniferatoxin, a phorbol-related diterpene, acts as an ultrapotent analog of capsaicin, the irritant constituent in red pepper. Neuroscience. 1989;30:515–20.
7. Szallasi A, Blumberg PM. Resiniferatoxin and its analogs provide novel insights into the pharmacology of the vanilloid (capsaicin) receptor. Life Sci. 1990;47:1399–408.
8. Avelino A, Cruz F. TRPV 1 (vanilloid receptors) in the urinary tract: expression, function and clinical applications. Naunyn Schmiedebergs Arch Pharmacol. 2006;373:289–99.
9. Silva C, Rio ME, Criz F. Desensitization of bladder sensory fibers by intravesical resiniferatoxin, a capsaicin analog: long-term results for the treatment of detrusor hyeprreflexia. Eur Urol. 2000;38:444–52.
10. Silva C, Ribeiro MJ, Cruz F. The effect of intrevesical resiniferatoxin in patients with idiopathic detrusor instability suggests that involuntary detrusor contraction are triggered by C-fiber input. J Urol. 2002;168:575–9.
11. Mourtoukou EG, Iavazzo C, Falagas ME. Resiniferatoxin in the treatment of BPS: a systematic review. Int Urogynecol J Pelvic Floor Dysfunct. 2008;19:1571–6.
12. Payne CK, Mosbaugh PG, Forrest JB, et al. Intravesical resiniferatoxin for the treatment of BPS: a randomized, double blind, placebo controlled trial. J Urol. 2005;173:1590–4.
13. Lazzeri M, Beneforti P, Spinelli M, Zanollo A, Barbagli F, Turini D. Intravesical resiniferatoxin for the treatment of hypersensitive disorder: a randomized placebo controlled study. J Urol. 2000;164:676–9.
14. Chen TY, Corcos J, Camel M, et al. Prospective, randomized, double-blind study of safety and tolerability of intravesical resiniferatoxin (RTX) in BPS (IC). Int Urogynecol J Pelvic Floor Dysfunct. 2005;16:293–7.
15. Apostolidis A, Gonzales GE, Fowler CJ. Effect of intravesical resiniferatoxin (RTX) on lower urinary tract symptoms, urodynamic parameters, and quality of life of patients with urodynamic increased bladder sensation. Eur Urol. 2006;50:1299–305.
16. Peng CH, Kuo HC. Multiple intravesical instillationof low-dose resiniferatoxin in the treatment of refractory BPS. J Urol. 2007;78:78–81.
17. Lazzeri M, Spinelli M, Beneforti P, et al. Intravesical infusion of resiniferatoxin by a temporary in situ drug delivery system to treat interstitiasl cystitis. Eur Urol. 2000;164:676–9.
18. Hurst RE. Structure, function, and pathology of proteoglycans and glycosaminoglycans in the urinary tract. World J Urol. 1994;12:3–10.
19. Toft BR, Nordling J. Recent developments of intravesical therapy of painful bladder syndrome/BPS: a review. Curr Opin Urol. 2006;16:268–72.
20. Bade JJ, Laseur M, Nieuwenburg A, et al. A placebo controlled study of intravesical pentosanpolysulphate for the treatment of BPS. Br J Urol. 1997;79:168–71.
21. Daha LK, Lazar D, Simak R, Pfuger H. The effects of intravesical pentosanpolysulphate treatment on the symptoms of patients with bladder pain syndrome/BPS: preliminary results. Int Urogynecol J Pelvic Floor Dysfunct. 2008;19:987–90.
22. Davis EL, El Khoundary SR, Talbott EO, et al. Safety and efficacy of the use of intravesical and oral pentosan polysulphate sodium for BPS: a randomized double-blind clinical trial. J Urol. 2008;179:177–85.
23. Kuo HC. Urodynamic results of intravesical heparin therapy for women with frequency urgency syndrome and BPS. J Formos Med Assoc. 2001;100:309.
24. Parsons CL, Housley T, Schmidt JD, Lebow D. Treatment of BPS with intravesical heparin. Br J Urol. 1994;73:504.
25. Perez-Marrero R, Emerson LE, Maharajh DO, et al. Prolongation of response to DMSO by heparin maintenance. Urology. 1993;41(Suppl):64.
26. Parsons CL. Successful downregulation of bladder sensory nerves with combination of heparin and alkalinized lidocaine in patients with BPS. Urology. 2005;65:45.

27. Welk BK, Teichman JM. Dyspareunia response in patients with BPS treated with intravesical lidocaine, bicarbonate, and heparin. Urology. 2008;71:67–70.
28. Morales A, Emerson L, Nickel JC. Intravesical hyaluronic acid in the treatment of refractory BPS. J Urol. 1996;156:45–8.
29. Porru D, Campus G, Tudino D, Valdes E, Vespa A, Scarpa RM, Usai E. Results of treatment of refractory BPS with intravesical hyaluronic acid. Urol Int. 1997;59(1):26–9.
30. Kallenstrup EB, Joregensen S, Nordling J, Hald T. Treatment of BPS with Cystistat®: a hyaluronic acid product. Scand J Urol Nephrol. 2005;39:143–7.
31. Daha LK, Riedl CR, Lazar D, Hohlbrugger G, Pfluger H. Do cystometric findings predict the results of intravesical hyaluronic acid in women with BPS? Eur Urol. 2005;47:393–7.
32. Leppilahti M, Hellstrom P, Tammela TL. Effect of diagnostic hydrodistension and four intravesical hyaluronic acid instillations on bladder ICAM-1 intensity and association of ICAM-1 intensity with clinical response in patients with interstitialcystitis. Urology. 2002;60(1):46–51.
33. Ahmad I, Sarath Krishna N, Meddings RM. Sequential hydrodistension and intravesical instillation of hyaluronic acid under general anaesthesia for treatment of refractory BPS: a pilot study. Int Urogynecol J Pelvic Floor Dysfunct. 2008;19:543–6.
34. Steinhoff G, Ittah B, Rowan S. The efficacy of chondroitin sulfate 0.2% in treating BPS. Can J Urol. 2002;9(1):1454–8.
35. Nickel JC, Egerdie B, Downey J, Singh R, Skehan A, Carr L, Irvine-Bird K. A real-life multicentre clinical practice study to evaluate the efficacy and safety of intravesical chondroitin sulphate for the treatment of BPS. BJU Int. 2009;103(1):56–60. Epub 2008 Sep 3.
36. Nickel JC, Egerdie RB, Steinhoff G, Palmer B, Hanno P. A multicenter, randomized, double-blind, parallel group pilot evaluation of the efficacy and safety of intravesical sodium chondroitin sulfate versus vehicle control in patients with BPS/painful bladder syndrome. Urology. 2010;76:804–9.
37. Cervigni M, Natale F, Nasta L, Padoa A. A combined intravesical therapy with hyaluronic acid and chondroitin for refractory painful bladder syndrome/BPS. Int Urogynecol J Pelvic Floor Dysfunct. 2008;19:943–7.
38. Porru D, Cervigni M, et al. Results of endovesical hyaluronic acid/chondroitin sulfate in the treatment of BPS/painful bladder syndrome. Rev Recent Clin Trials. 2008;3:126–9.
39. Peters K, Diokno A, Steinert B, et al. The efficacy on intravesical Tice strain bacillus Calmette-Guerin in the treatment of BPS: a double-blind, prospective, placebo controlled trial. J Urol. 1997;157:2090–4.
40. Peters KM, Diokno AC, Steinert BW, Gonzalez JA. The efficacy of intravesical bacillus Calmette-Guerin in the treatment of BPS: long-term followup. J Urol. 1998;159:1483.
41. Mayer R, Propert KJ, Peters KM, et al. A randomized controlled trial of intravesical bacillus calmette-guerin for treatment of refractory BPS. J Urol. 2005;173:1186–91.

Chapter 24
Hydrodistention, Transurethral Resection and Other Ablative Techniques in the Treatment of Bladder Pain Syndrome

Magnus Fall, Jørgen Nordling, and Ralph Peeker

Hydrodistension

Bumpus [1] was the first one to describe hydrodistension as a therapy for interstitial cystitis. He found in patients subjected to distension of the bladder under anaesthesia that there was a considerable, although temporary, relief of pain. Subsequently, the method was established as a standard therapeutic measure. As late as 40 years ago hydrodistension was a standard procedure, little else to be offered to patients with intolerable bladder pain. As is not uncommon, the scientific foundation of this method in the treatment of bladder pain syndrome (BPS)/interstitial cystitis is still not more than empirical. Explanations of the effect are speculative, the most favoured hypotheses ranging from disruption of the intramural sensory neural network to decrease of the blood supply to the detrusor.

When used as a therapeutic measure, distension during general anaesthesia has to be administered at regular intervals. The common interval between treatments used to be 3 months, providing temporary relief of pain although mostly short-lived and seldom sustained to the next treatment. Compared to ablation of lesions by transurethral resection, hydrodistension is inferior [2]. In exceptional cases, hydrodistension may be adequate to maintain pain relief for half a year or more, and in such cases it may be a realistic option although such cases are extremely rare.

M. Fall, M.D., Ph.D. (✉)
Department of Urology, Institute of Clinical Sciences, Sahlgrens University Hospital, Bruna straket 11B, Gothenburg 41345, Sweden
e-mail: magnus.fall@urology.gu.se

J. Nordling, M.D., Dr. Med. Sci., F.E.B.U.
Department of Urology, University of Copenhagen, Herlev Hospital, Herlev, Denmark

R. Peeker
Department of Urology, Sahlgrenska University Hospital, Bruna Straket 11, Gothenburg 41345, Sweden

J. Nordling et al. (eds.), *Bladder Pain Syndrome: A Guide for Clinicians*, 317
DOI 10.1007/978-1-4419-6929-3_24, © Springer Science+Business Media New York 2013

Prolonged Distension

In 1972, Helmstein presented a method to treat superficial tumours of the urinary bladder [3]. He used a catheter furnished with a large balloon, transurethrally inserted into the bladder and expanded with fluid until an intravesical pressure above the arterial pressure was reached. The objective of this treatment was to reach a manifest pressure reducing the blood flow to the bladder and maintaining this pressure during periods of 30 min. Since the procedure is very painful, treatment had to be administered during regional or general anaesthesia. This modality was tested in severe urgency and also tried in interstitial cystitis. Dunn et al. [4] found this method useful but longer follow-up has been unfavourable and because of the complicated procedure the method has almost been abandoned.

Ablative Techniques

Transurethral Resection and Coagulation

The idea of resecting inflamed bladder tissue in BPS is not new; rather it dates back some one hundred years when Guy Hunner reported on open resection of ulcers [5]. Later, when transurethral techniques became available, transurethral resection and fulguration were on trial in limited investigations, also resulting in favourable but variable symptomatic outcome [6, 7]. In the 1980s, a more systematic application of the transurethral technique, with careful and radical electro-resection of all lesions, was described [2]. This technique yielded quite favourable results, also long-term, and implies complete resection of all lesions, including a peripheral oedema zone and the underlying superficial detrusor muscle, using a minimum of coagulation. Thus, broad coagulation of the resected surfaces is avoided, using solely pinpoint treatment of bleeding vessels. The reason for this mode of procedure is to avoid promotion or enhancement of bladder contracture, a well-known complication to the classic Hunner type, ESSIC BPS type 3C disease. Some 10 years ago the hitherto largest series on this technique was published. In this study, the long-term outcome in 103 patients with classic IC and their response to complete TUR of visible lesions were retrospectively evaluated [8]. In that series, an initial satisfactory symptomatic effect in nine of ten patients with BPS type 3C was registered. Interestingly, the included patients could be divided into four relatively distinct groups: long-term good responders (long-term remission for 3 years or more with a maximum of three resections), short-term good responders (need for repeated resections to stay symptomatically relieved and follow up less than 3 years), patients with bladder contracture (developed over more than 2 years) and end-stage disease (within 2 years after diagnosis). The excellent symptomatic effect in many patients with ESSIC 3C disease makes TURB a first-line treatment, with few comparable alternatives.

TUR has been suggested to result in symptom improvement by removal of intramural nerve endings engaged by the inflammatory process. Surgical complications are most commonly retroperitoneal bladder perforation and persistent hematuria. Such complications are rare and typically just require prolonged catheter drainage [8].

Laser

Neodymium (Nd): YAG laser has been used in urology since the 1960s. Shanberg et al. were the first to use it for treatment of BPS [9]. Laser ablation penetrates approximately 5 mm, heating tissue to 60–70 degree C, thought to be leaving elastic fibres undamaged. Laser is among some considered advantageous over TURB, since repeated resections are supposed to cause bladder contracture. The opposite argument can be inflicted on laser, since the depth of the laser effect is difficult to determine, bladder perforation occurring also with laser. Careful performance of TURB allows a reasonably good control of the extent of surgical damage. Which one of the two techniques might induce less reparative activity in the bladder wall remains an open question.

Essentially, the transurethral methods are only applicable in ESSIC type 3C disease with circumscript inflammatory lesions. Diffuse widespread glomerulations are not accessible to endoscopic ablation; in fact they are not necessarily an expression of a disease confined to the urinary bladder. The disease mechanisms and the response to various treatments are so far speculative. Ablation implies removal of intramural sensory nerves and inflammatory aggregates having an effect on nerves engaged by the inflammatory process. Traditionally, mast cells have been thought to reflect intensity and grade of 3C disease. Therefore, it has been hypothesised that patients with a high mast cell density respond more favourably to TUR-B; however a recent report could not demonstrate that the mast cell density in the lamina propria predicted outcome after TUR [10]. Hypotheses do not always turn out positive and many enigmas in BPS remain to be solved.

References

1. Bumpus HC. Interstitial cystitis: its treatment by over-distension of the bladder. Med Clin North Am. 1930;13:1495–8.
2. Fall M. Conservative management of chronic interstitial cystitis: transcutaneous electrical nerve stimulation and transurethral resection. J Urol. 1985;133:774–8.
3. Helmstein K. Treatment of bladder carcinoma by a hydrostatic pressure technique. Report on 43 cases. Br J Urol. 1972;44:434–50.
4. Dunn M, Ramsden PD, Roberts JBM, et al. Interstitial cystitis, treated by prolonged bladder distension. Br J Urol. 1977;49:641–5.
5. Hunner GL. A rare type of bladder ulcer: further notes, with a report of eighteen cases. JAMA. 1918;70:203–12.

6. Kerr Jr W. Interstitial cystitis: treatment by transurethral resection. J Urol. 1971;105:664–6.
7. Greenberg E, Barnes R, Stewart S, et al. Transurethral resection of Hunner's ulcers. J Urol. 1974;111:764–6.
8. Peeker R, Aldenborg F, Fall M. Complete transurethral resection of ulcers in classic interstitial cystitis. Int Urogynecol J PelvicFloor Dysfunct. 2000;11:290–5.
9. Shanberg AM, Malloy T. Treatment of interstitial cystitis with neodymium: YAG laser. Urology. 1987;29(4 Suppl):31–3.
10. Rössberger J, Fall M, Gustafsson-Kåbjörn C, et al. Does mast cell density predict the outcome after transurethral resection of Hunner's lesions in patients with type 3C bladder pain syndrome/interstitial cystitis? Scand J Urol Nephrol. 2010;44(6):433–7.

Chapter 25
Botulinum Toxin Treatment in Bladder Pain Syndrome

Paul P. Irwin and Paulo Dinis Oliveria

Botulinum toxin (BTX) has become a widely used treatment for refractory overactive bladder (OAB) symptoms due to both neurogenic [1] and idiopathic [2] detrusor overactivity. Several reports of its use in bladder pain syndrome (BPS) suggest that it may have a role to play in the management of this condition also.

BTX is a protein that is produced naturally by *Clostridium botulinum*. The toxin is taken up by endocytosis at nerve terminals where it stops the vesicular release of neurotransmitters at the synapse. It does this by cleaving the SNAP-25 protein, which is required for normal vesicle fusion with the plasma membrane of the axon synapse. Depending on the nerves affected, the synaptic release of not only acetylcholine but also all neurotransmitters from the nerve terminal is prevented.

Neurobiology and Possible Modes of Action

The precise mechanism of action of BTX in BPS is speculative. The little we know about it may be extrapolated through our evolving understanding of the neurobiology of the OAB, in particular the concept of the urothelium as a syncytium or "sensory web". The urothelium appears to function as a transducer of mechanical and chemical stimuli and communicates with the underlying nerve plexus, detrusor smooth muscle and myofibroblasts. Urothelial cells express several receptors/ion channels that are also found on suburothelial afferent nerves. These include, among many others, the ion channel TRPV1 and the ATP-gated

P.P. Irwin, M.Ch., F.R.C.S.I. (Urol) (✉)
Michael Heal Department of Urology, Leighton Hospital, Mid Cheshire Hospitals NHS Trust, Middlewich Road, Crewe, Cheshire CW1 4QJ, UK
e-mail: paul.irwin@mcht.nhs.uk

P.D. Oliveria, M.D., Ph.D.
Department of Urology, Hospital de São João,
Porto, Portugal

J. Nordling et al. (eds.), *Bladder Pain Syndrome: A Guide for Clinicians*,
DOI 10.1007/978-1-4419-6929-3_25, © Springer Science+Business Media New York 2013

purinergic receptor $P2X_3$. There are also many neurotransmitters involved in afferent signalling in the urothelium, including ATP, substance P (SP), nitric oxide (NO), calcitonin gene-related peptide (CGRP), tachykinins and acetylcholine [3–5]. These neurotransmitters are released not only from the afferent nerve fibres; many are released from the urothelium itself. In this way, through the release of its neurotransmitters, the urothelium may control the firing thresholds and activity of the underlying afferent nerves and detrusor muscle.

The suburothelial plexus of afferent nerves consists of myelinated Aδ and unmyelinated C fibres. Afferent signals from these fibres are relayed centrally to the periaqueductal grey area of the midbrain. Normal bladder stretch activates Aδ fibre discharge, while C fibres are normally silent, becoming active in inflammatory conditions. In neurogenic detrusor overactivity (NDO) suburothelial C-fibres become more prominent and active. They begin to discharge in response to mechanical stimuli which leads to increased parasympathetic stimulation of the bladder and therefore DO. Evidence is growing that a similar mechanism applies in idiopathic detrusor overactivity (IDO) in which an increased density of nerve fibres that are immunoreactive to TRPV1, $P2X_3$, SP and CGRP has been observed. Following successful treatment of OAB with BTX injection, the proportion of suburothelial afferent nerve fibres expressing $P2X_3$ and TRPV1 is reduced significantly, while the overall nerve fibre density is unaltered [4]. These changes are seen only in the nerve fibres; receptor expression in the urothelium is unaltered. It therefore appears that at least part of the therapeutic effect of BTX in DO may be due to reduced expression of sensory receptors in otherwise intact afferent nerves. It is postulated that the reduction in the density of $P2X_3$ and TRPV1 receptor levels may reduce the sensitivity of aberrant C-fibres to stretch and thereby reduce overactivity in the detrusor.

Many of the mechanisms involved in the pathophysiology of DO are known to apply also in BPS. Aberrant C-fibre activity is certainly present as is the increased expression of TRPV1 and P2X3 receptors. It is also known that urothelial stretch, as occurs in bladder filling, causes the urothelium to release ATP. This release is amplified in patients with NDO and it is also a prominent finding in tissue from patients with BPS [6]. ATP has the effect of lowering the threshold for activating the ion currents through TRPV1 receptors. This is a possible mechanism by which large amounts of ATP, released from damaged or sensitised urothelial cells in response to injury or inflammation, may trigger the sensation of pain [7]. BTX abolishes the stretch-induced release of ATP from the urothelial side of the bladder but not that from the basal/serosal side. This suggests that ATP release from the urothelium occurs by exocytotic release [8]. However urothelium, in contrast to sensory nerves, does not express SV2 or SNAP-25, which would preclude a direct action of BTX-A.

Recent work by Portuguese researchers has identified a further effect of BTX treatment in BPS, namely, a reduction in urinary levels of the neurotrophins NGF and brain-derived growth factor (BDNF). NGF is produced by urothelial cells and detrusor muscle fibres, while BDNF arises from urothelial cells and sensory nerve fibres. The mechanism for this reduction in urinary neurotrophin levels is unknown, but it may reflect a reduction in sensory nerve density in the trigone [9].

There are thus four probable mechanisms by which BTX might have a therapeutic impact in BPS:

1. Prevention of Ach release from presynaptic nerve terminals.
2. Reduced expression of P2X3 and TRPV1 receptors on afferent nerves.
3. Prevention of stretch-induced ATP release from the urothelium.
4. Reduced production of neurotrophins NGF and BDNF.

Botulinum Toxin Treatment in BPS

Table 25.1 summarises those studies that have looked at BTX in BPS. With three exceptions all were small open-label trials [9–18]. Most treatments are done under general anaesthetic, although local anaesthesia using intravesical lignocaine and sodium bicarbonate is a useful alternative. The authors have found that BTX injection in BPS patients is considerably more challenging than when done for OAB. The BPS bladder is generally of smaller capacity and has an inflamed urothelium that bleeds readily at each injection site. This necessitates the use of continuous irrigation, for which general anaesthesia is ideal.

Most urologists inject the toxin into the trigone, on the basis that this is where sensory afferent nerve concentration is greatest. This may also minimise the risk of post-operative urinary retention. One group who injected the trigone alone reported no problems with urinary retention [9] whereas those groups who injected the trigone and other areas reported an incidence of urinary retention of between 3 and 18% [11–13].

Patient improvement rates are variable between studies, as are the means of patient selection and the instruments used to measure outcomes. However, all non-randomised studies showed improvement in symptoms in between 69 and 100% of patients [9–15].

Although patient numbers are limited in published randomised controlled trials, two of them show significantly better improvement rates for BTX-A when compared to either hydrodistension or pentosan polysulphate.

Kou and Chancellor performed an excellent randomised controlled trial of intravesical BTX-A plus hydrodistension versus hydrodistension alone in 67 patients who satisfied the NIDDK criteria and who had persistent symptoms despite being on pentosan polysulphate treatment. The patients were randomly assigned to one of the three treatments: BTX-A (100 units) followed 2 weeks later by hydrodistension, BTX-A (200 units) followed 2 weeks later by hydrodistension or hydrodistension alone. While patients in all three treatment groups experienced a significant decrease in their symptom scores, those who received BTX-A plus hydrodistension experienced superior and longer lasting symptomatic relief than those who had hydrodistension alone. The effect of BTX injection treatment was also durable as 55% remained asymptomatic at 12 months. There was no difference in the degree of pain control and bladder capacity increase between the

Table 25.1 Summary of trials of botulinum toxin A in the management of Bladder Pain Syndrome

Authors	Number and trial description	Anaesthetic GA/LA	Sites injected	BTX-A dose	Outcome	CISC
Smith et al. [10]	13 NIDDK Non-randomised	GA/sedation	20–30 Trigone + post wall	200 units Dysport® 7 cases Botox® 6 cases	9/13 (69%) improved symptoms lasted mean of 3.7 months	0
Giannantoni et al. [11]	14 "ESSIC equivalent" Pilot	GA	20 Trigone + post wall	200 units Botox®	12/14 (85.7%) improved symptoms and C_{max} at 3 months	2
Carl et al. [12]	29 NIDDK Non-randomised	GA/sedation	20–25 Trigone + post wall	500 units	Significant improvement in all symptoms in 24/35 (83%) as well as improved CMG parameters. By 6 months seven required repeat treatment	1
Ramsay et al. [13]	11 NIDDK Non-randomised	GA	20–30 Suburothelium Dome + trigone	200–300 units Brand not stated	Significant improvements in BFLUTS and KHQ scores lasting 10–14 weeks	2
Liu [14]	19 (+HD 2 weeks later) Non-randomised	GA	Suburothelium	100–200 units Brand not stated	Significant reduction in pain and frequency at 3 months. Response seen in 10/14 (74%) who received 100 units and 4/5 (80%) who received 200 units	0
Giannantoni et al. [15]	15 ESSIC Non-randomised	GA	20 Trigone + post wall	200 units Botox®	13/15 (86.6%) improved at 3 months. Pain recurred in 11 by 5 months and in all cases at 12 months	2
Kuo et al. [16]	44 NIDDK RCT: BTX + HD versus HD alone	GA	40 Posterior + lateral walls	100–200 units Botox®	31/44 (71%) success at 6 months and significantly better results versus HD alone. Higher rate of voiding dysfunction in those receiving 200 units	0

Gottsch et al. [17]	20 RCT versus saline	Not stated	2 Periurethral	50 units	No improvement at 3 months in any symptom compared to placebo	0
Rasheed et al. [18]	28 RCT versus PPS	LA	30 Bladder+trigone	300 units	Significant improvement in all parameters at 20 weeks compared to PPS instillations	Not stated
Pinto [9]	26 ESSIC Non-randomised	Sedation	10 Trigone	100 units Botox®	Significant improvements in all parameters, including CMG, for 10 months. 16 requested repeat treatment	0

NIDDK National Institute of Diabetes and Diseases of the Kidney criteria, *CMG* cystometrography (urodynamics), *BFLUTS* bristol female lower urinary tract symptoms, *KHQ* Kings Health Questionnaire, *RCT* randomised controlled trial, *HD* hydrodistension, *PPS* pentosan polysulphate

two doses of BTX-A. However, vthose who received the larger dose experienced a higher rate of voiding dysfunction and, although none appear to have required self-catheterisation, three patients did need "temporary catheterisation" [16].

A study from Egypt randomised 28 female patients to intravesical BTX-A injection treatment or instillations of pentosan polysulphate. These women satisfied the NIDDK criteria. At 21 weeks post treatment the improvements in pain, frequency, nocturia and urgency were significantly greater for the BTX group than for those who received PPS instillations [18]. However, another trial showed no difference between the injection of BTX and saline injections. Gottsch et al. randomised 20 patients to receive periurethral injections of either BTX-A (50 units) or saline. No significant improvement in symptoms was found in either group at 3 months and there was no difference between the two study groups [17]. However, in this study BTX was injected transperineally under ultrasound guidance, a technique not used by others. Furthermore, the injected volume was small (two injections of 1 ml per injection). Since BTX is taken up only by nerve terminals, and since these are located mainly between the detrusor and urothelial layers, such an approach might not hit the desired target.

Despite these variations in technique, mode of injection and patient selection, virtually all non-randomised and two randomised trials have shown a clear benefit of BTX injection treatment for BPS. It is indeed a promising treatment option and one that deserves further study.

References

1. Duthie J, Wilson DI, Herbison GP, Wilson D. Botulinum toxin injections for adults with overactive bladder syndrome. Cochrane Database Syst Rev. 2007;18(3):CD005493.
2. Anger J, Weinberg A, Suttorp MJ, Letwin MS, Shekelle PG. Outcomes of intravesical botulinum toxin for idiopathic overactive bladder symptoms: a systematic review of the literature. J Urol. 2010;183:2258–64.
3. Apostolidis A, Haferkamp A, Aoki KR. Understanding the role of botulinum toxin A in the treatment of the overactive bladder: more than just muscle relaxation. Eur Urol. 2006;5(11): 670–78 suppl.
4. Apostolidis A, Popat R, Yiangou Y, Cockayne D, Ford APD, Davis JB, Dasgupta P, Fowler CJ, Anand P. Decreassed sensory receptors P2X3 and TRPV1 in suburothelial nerve fibres following intradetrusor injections of botulinum toxin for human detrusor overactivity. J Urol. 2005;174:977–83.
5. Birder LA, Kanai AJ, Cruz F, Moore K, Fry CH. Is the urothelium intelligent? Neurourol Urodyn. 2010;29(4):598–602.
6. Sun Y, Keay S, DeDeyne PG, Chai TC. Augmented stretch-activated adenosine triphosphate release from bladder uroepithelial cells in patients with interstitial cystitis. J Urol. 2001;166:1951–6.
7. Birder L, de Groat W, Mills I, Morrison J, Thor K, Drake M. Neural control of the lower urinary tract: peripheral and spinal mechanisms. Neurourol Urodyn. 2010;29(1):128–39.
8. Khera M, Somogyi GT, Kiss S, Boone TB, Smith CP. Botulinum toxin A inhibits ATP release from bladder urothelium after chronic spinal cord injury. Neurochem Int. 2004;45(7):987–93.
9. Pinto R, Lopes T, Frias B, Silva A, Silva JA, Silva CM, Cruz C, Cruz F, Dinis P. Trigonal injection of botulinum toxin A in patients with refractory bladder pain syndrome/interstitial cystitis. Eur Urol. 2010;58(3):366–8.

10. Smith CP, Radziszewski P, Borkowski A, Somogyi GT, Boone TB, Chancellor MB. Botulinum toxin A has antinocceptive effects in treating interstitial cystitis. Urology. 2004;64:871–5.
11. Giannantoni A, Costantini E, Di Stasi SM, Tascini MC, Bini V, Porena M. Botulinum A toxin intravesical injections in the treatment of painful bladder syndrome: a pilot study. Eur Urol. 2006;49:704.
12. Carl S, Grosse J, Laschke S. Treatment of interstitial cystitis with botulinum toxin type A. Eur Urol. 2007;6:248.
13. Ramsay AK, Small DR, Conn IG. Intravesical botulinum toxin type A in chronic interstitial cystitis: results of a pilot study. Surgeon. 2007;5(6):331–3.
14. Liu HT, Kuo HC. Intravesical botulinum toxin A injections plus hydrodistension can reduce nerve growth factor production and control bladder pain in interstitial cystitis. Urology. 2007;70(3):463–8.
15. Giannantoni A, Porena M, Costantini E, Zucchi A, Mearini L. Botulinum A toxin intravesical injection in patients with painful bladder syndrome: 1-year follow-up. J Urol. 2008;179(3):1031–4.
16. Kuo HC, Chancellor MB. Comparison of intravesical botulinum toxin type A injections plus hydrodistension with hydrodistension alone for the treatment of refractory interstitial cystitis/painful bladder syndrome. BJU Int. 2009;104:657–61.
17. Gottsch HP, Miller JL, Yang CC, Berger RE. A pilot study of botulinum toxin for interstitial cystitis/painful bladder syndrome. Neurourol Urodyn. 2011;30:93–6.
18. Rasheed T, Farahat A, Bahnasy M, Bindary A, Tatawy H. A prospective randomized study of intravesical pentosan polysulfate and botulinum toxin-A for the treatment of painful bladder syndrome/interstitial cystitis. Eur Urol Suppl. 2010;9(2):641.

Chapter 26
Neurostimulation for Bladder Pain Syndrome

Dominique El-Khawand and Kristene E. Whitmore

Introduction

Neurostimulation, also known as neuromodulation, is an innovative and minimally invasive surgical treatment for various refractory conditions including lower urinary tract (LUT) dysfunctions, chronic pain, Parkinson's disease, and gastroparesis. It involves extrinsic stimulation of nerves, the spine, or the brain in order to obtain the desired therapeutic effect. For the LUT, neuromodulation is primarily achieved via sacral nerve stimulation (SNS), although pudendal and posterior tibial nerve stimulations have been described.

Tanagho and Schmidt initially described SNS for the treatment of voiding dysfunction in 1988 [1]. Since then, The US Food and Drug Administration has approved SNS for four indications: urinary urge incontinence (1997), urgency–frequency syndrome, nonobstructive urinary retention (1999) and chronic fecal incontinence (2011). Currently, InterStim (Medtronic Inc., Minneapolis, MN) is the only available device for SNS in the United States. Although not officially approved for the treatment of Bladder Pain Syndrome (BPS), multiple recent clinical studies have emerged showing its benefit for patients with this chronic debilitating condition, improving the pain and the urgency–frequency symptoms, as well as the quality of life.

D. El-Khawand, M.D. (✉) • K.E. Whitmore
Division of Female Pelvic Medicine and Reconstructive Surgery,
Department of Obstetrics and Gynecology, Drexel University College of Medicine,
207 N. Broad St., 4th Floor, Philadelphia, PA 19107, USA
e-mail: dominique_Khawand@yahoo.com

J. Nordling et al. (eds.), *Bladder Pain Syndrome: A Guide for Clinicians*,
DOI 10.1007/978-1-4419-6929-3_26,

Mechanism of Action

The bladder wall contains visceral parasympathetic afferents in the form of lightly myelinated Aδ (delta) fibers and unmyelinated C fibers, possessing predominantly mechanosensitive (tension) and chemosensitive (nociception) properties, respectively [2]. Upon bladder filling, Aδ (delta) fibers respond to physiologic low-threshold intravesical pressure, whereas C fibers are typically silent. In animal models, unmyelinated bladder afferents exhibit impulse transmission following chemical irritation, and in the presence of significant epithelial inflammation may exhibit both spontaneous activity and novel mechanosensitivity [3, 4]. Such C fiber plasticity may play a role in the evolution of BPS symptoms. Physiologic bladder filling in the presence of chronic inflammation could produce an afferent barrage resulting in frequency, urgency, and pain [5].

Sacral neuromodulation (SNM) is thought to function in part through the inhibition of C fiber impulse transmission to the central nervous system. This theory is supported by experimental evidence provided by Shaker et al., who administered SNS to spinalized animals with (C fiber-mediated) bladder hyperreflexia [6]. Thirty-nine female Sprague–Dawley rats were divided equally into three groups: normal controls; spinally transected at T10; and spinally transected and electrically stimulated. Three weeks after transection, bladder hyperreflexia and C fiber activity were confirmed by urodynamics and increased L6 dorsal root ganglia levels of neuropeptide (substance P, neurokinin A, and calcitonin gene-related peptide), respectively. Electrostimulation of S1 in group 3 resulted in the absence of appreciable detrusor activity upon filling, in addition to significantly less neuropeptide within the L6 dorsal root ganglia than in group 2, consistent with decreased C fiber impulse delivery.

Inhibition of C fiber transmission by SNM may occur as a result of primary somatic afferent activation, as typically employed SNS impulse parameters exhibit an affinity for somatic (versus visceral) and afferent (versus efferent) nerve fibers [7, 8]. Somatic afferent inhibition of C fiber transmission may be explained by the "gate theory" introduced by Melzack and Wall in 1965, in which well-myelinated large-diameter (somatic) fibers impair impulse delivery by poorly myelinated small-diameter (visceral) fibers to higher centers [9].

Visceral and somatic afferent pathways converge at the level of sacral cord; thus, by stimulating somatic afferents as in posterior tibial nerve stimulation, bladder activity is inhibited by blocking bladder afferent input to the sacral cord [10]. Similar findings have been demonstrated with stimulation of the pudendal nerve in spinalized cats. Further examination of the afferent branches of the pudendal nerve has identified two distinct branches (cranial urethral sensory and dorsal nerve of the penis) that can mediate electrically evoked bladder contractions and presented evidence for two distinct micturition pathways (spino-bulbo-spinal vs. spinal reflexes) activated by selective afferent pudendal nerve stimulation [11]. Furthermore, effects of SNM may occur at the spinal and supraspinal levels by inhibiting the spinal neurons involved in the micturition reflexes, interneurons involved in spinal segmental reflexes, and postganglionic neurons [12].

Patient Selection

Neuromodulation's minimally invasive nature, safety profile, and staged reversible technique make it an appealing option for patients with intractable, debilitating BPS symptoms who have failed conventional conservative interventions (e.g., dietary modifications, behavioral and physical therapy, medical treatment) and before having more invasive surgical therapies. However, patients should be extensively counseled about the off-label use of the device and the potential complications, and an informed consent is obtained.

To determine the eligibility for the chronic pulse generator implantation, each patient should undergo an initial screening test. Two tests are available: the percutaneous nerve evaluation (PNE) and the first stage lead placement (FSLP) using tined leads. If the patient demonstrates adequate improvement of urinary symptoms during this trial period (as documented by ≥50% improvement of parameters based on pre- and post-procedure voiding diaries and pain scores), the second stage with the implantation of a programmable pulse generator is performed [13]. Because of the decreased risk of lead migration and the longer test duration, the FSLP test has a higher response rate [14]. Borawski et al. found that FSLP better predicted progression to implantation when compared to PNE in a prospective randomized trial of patients with urge incontinence (88% versus 46%, $n=30$) [15]. In another retrospective study, 42 patients received bilateral PNE and 11 received bilateral FSLP. Eighty-two percent of FSLP progressed to implantable pulse generator (IPG) placement, while only 47% of patients receiving PNE progressed to chronic implantation [16].

Patients are contraindicated for implant of the InterStim System if they have not demonstrated an appropriate response to test stimulation or are unable to operate the neurostimulator. Also, diathermy (e.g., shortwave diathermy, microwave diathermy, or therapeutic ultrasound diathermy) is contraindicated because diathermy's energy can be transferred through the implanted system (or any of the separate implanted components), which can cause tissue damage. Similarly, magnetic resonance imaging is not recommended in patients who have any implanted components of the neurostimulation system.

Overview of the Procedure

The procedure for SNM is divided into two parts: the initial screening test and the implantation of the chronic IPG. In the initial description of SNM for voiding dysfunction, the screening test consisted of a bilateral PNE, which was essentially a "blind" placement of a temporary electrode through the S3 foramen using anatomical/bony landmarks without the aid of fluoroscopy. The screening trial would last for several days. Patients who had a successful screening evaluation underwent placement of a chronic lead under general anesthesia, where the appropriate sacral foramen was identified without fluoroscopy, and the lead was attached through a deep presacral incision directly to the posterior sacral periosteum.

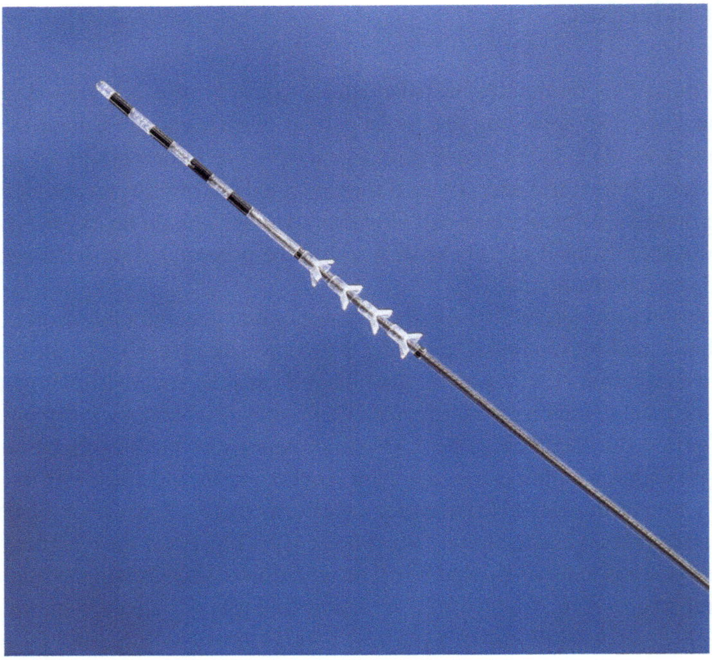

Fig. 26.1 The tined lead eliminated the need for deep anchoring and decreased the rate of lead migration. Reprinted with permission of Medtronic, Inc. ©2012. Please note that the information addresses InterStim Therapy for interstitial cystitis, a use which the FDA has not approved. Medtronic does not market its products for unapproved indications and makes no representations regarding the safety and/or efficacy for unapproved uses

In 2002, the FDA approved of the tined lead (Fig. 26.1), which eliminated the need for a deep incision and anchoring. This modification revolutionized the procedure, allowing for a minimally invasive approach under a combination of intravenous sedation and local anesthesia. This procedure was first described by Spinelli et al. in 2003 and uses a combination of intraoperative fluoroscopy to improve the accuracy of lead placement and the tined lead device to minimize migration during the screening trial. Previously, the rigid, non-coiled test lead used in the PNE was easily dislodged during the screening trial after a brief period, resulting in a higher rate of false negative screening tests. In the staged trial, the tined lead may be left in place for several weeks to allow for a longer screening period. Those with a successful tined lead-staged trial can then proceed with the second-stage implantation of the programmable pulse generator and expect to experience the same benefit derived from the trial.

Because of the expense and degree of invasiveness, most of the time, a staged trial is conducted using only a single lead. Some investigators have suggested that stimulating only one side limits the ability of the screening trial to fully assess for symptomatic improvement. A bilateral PNE allows for two sides to be tested in a more economical and less invasive fashion. In contrast to previous trials, anterior–posterior (AP) and lateral fluoroscopy can be employed during the PNE procedure to improve lead placement within the foramen. Both the stage I lead placement and the bilateral PNE under fluoroscopic guidance, as described below, are used in current practice as formal screening trials prior to generator implantation [13].

Surgical Technique

Percutaneous Nerve Evaluation

This procedure may be performed in the office under local anesthesia or in the operating room under local anesthesia with intravenous sedation. The patient is placed in a prone position with a 30° flexion in the hips to position the sacrum horizontally. Two or three pillows may be placed under the abdomen to minimize lumbar lordosis. The patient is draped to allow visualization of the anus as well as the feet in order to check for appropriate motor responses. The nonsterile ground pad is affixed to the patient's heel or calf. Strict antiseptic techniques should be used throughout the procedure. If fluoroscopy is not available, bony landmarks can be used to identify the S3 level by palpation. At the level of the upper border of the greater sciatic notch, the S3 sacral foramen is located 2 cm from the midline. The S2 and S4 foramina are located 2 cm cephalad and caudal to S3, respectively. Also S3 foramen can be found 9 cm cephalad from the drop-off of the sacrum and 2 cm from the midline.

If fluoroscopy is available, the sacral foramina can be located 2 cm from the midline at the level of the line connecting the inferior borders of the sacroiliac (SI) joints. The foramen needle is typically inserted 1–2 cm cephalad from the spot identified as the S3 level, piercing the skin at an angle of approximately 60°, and traverses a certain distance of skin and adipose tissue before it reaches the foramen (Fig. 26.2). Insertion at this angle ensures that the needle is aligned perpendicular to the bony surface. If the patient is overweight, the insertion point may be above the mark. Because the sacrum is curved, the angle of insertion varies for each foramen. The margins of the foramen should be identified with the tip of the needle before it is inserted into the foramen. The nerve and vascular bundle is usually located on the upper medial side of the foramen. For most patients, the 3.5 in. (9 cm) needle is appropriate. For larger patients the 5 in. (12 cm) foramen needle may be needed.

To test the nerve responses, the mini-hook (J-hook) on the patient cable is connected to the uninsulated portion of the foramen needle (a black band below the hub). The test stimulator is turned "ON" and the amplitude intensity is increased gradually to obtain sensory or motor responses (Table 26.1). Slight adjustments in the depth and angle of the needle can produce marked changes in response. To locate the optimal S3 response and increase the likelihood of success, the test should be repeated contralaterally or at the S2 or S4 sites. If no site produces the desired response, the nerve may have been anesthetized by the local anesthetic, or the patient may not be responding to stimulation. It is critical to accurately document the responses to stimulation.

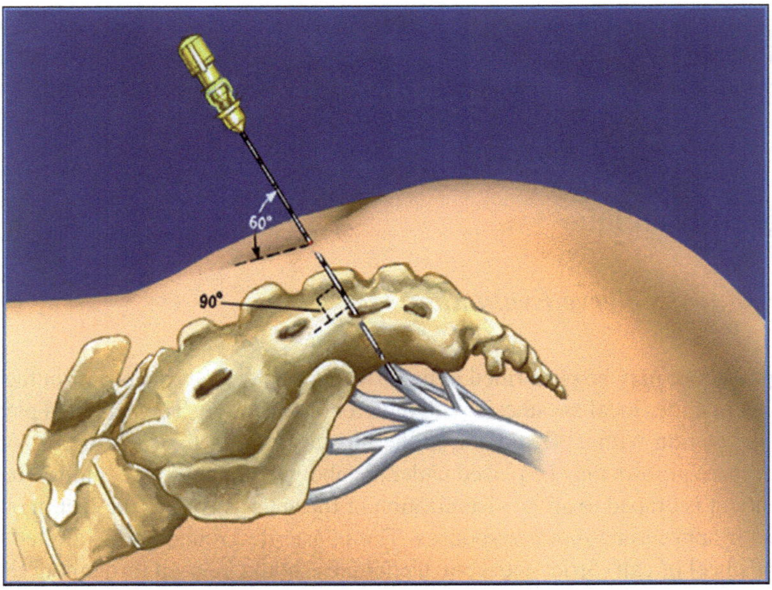

Fig. 26.2 The needle is inserted at a 60° angle to the skin into the upper medial aspect of the S3 foramen. Reprinted with permission of Medtronic, Inc. ©2012. Please note that the information addresses InterStim Therapy for interstitial cystitis, a use which the FDA has not approved. Medtronic does not market its products for unapproved indications and makes no representations regarding the safety and/or efficacy for unapproved uses

The temporary test stimulation lead is a coiled, insulated, multistranded wire, which elongates when stretched or stressed. A stainless steel connector pin is located at the proximal end of the lead and the exposed electrode is located at the distal end. The lead is gently threaded with the fingers through the needle cannula. When the lead passes the needle tip, a slight resistance is felt. To avoid shearing the tip of the lead, the needle should not be advanced once the lead has exited the tip.

Lateral fluoroscopy may help to assess the depth and position of the lead. When properly positioned, the electrode should lie approximately 2.5 cm beyond the periosteum, and 0.5–1 cm anterior to the sacral surface. Once the lead is positioned, nerve response is confirmed by connecting the J-hook to the connector pin of the lead and turning the test stimulator amplitude "ON." The foramen needle and lead stylet are removed carefully. The appropriate response is reconfirmed. The lead is fixed to the skin with tape to avoid displacement and appropriate dressing is applied.

Stage 1: Test Stimulation with a Chronic Lead

This is usually performed in the operating room under intravenous sedation and local anesthesia. Fluoroscopy should be available. The procedure starts similarly

Table 26.1 Sacral nerves motor and sensory responses to test stimulation

Nerve root	Motor		Sensory
	Pelvic floor	Lower extremity	
S2	Clamp of the anal sphincter (anterior/posterior shortening of perineal structures)	Plantar flexion of the entire foot with lateral rotation	Contraction of the base of the penis or vagina
S3	Bellow's reflex (lifting and dropping of the pelvic floor; look for deepening and flattening of the buttock groove)	Plantar flexion of the great toe	Paresthesia or pulling sensation in the rectum, scrotum, labia, or vagina
S4	Bellow's reflex only	None	Pulling in rectum only

to what was described above for the PNE. Once the foramen needle is in position, the stylet is removed and a guidewire is inserted as a place holder prior to removing the foramen needle. A small stab incision (5 mm) is made to accommodate the lead introducer. It must be wide and deep enough to prevent trapping the lead in the skin. The two-part lead introducer (dilator and sheath) slides over the guidewire, and is advanced into the foramen, until the radiodense marker is at the anterior surface of the sacrum. The dilator is then removed. The tined lead (with stylet inserted) is advanced through the sheath until the second white marker on the lead body aligns with the introducer sheath handle. At this point the four electrodes are exposed, but not the tines (this is clearly visible under fluoroscopy). The position of the electrodes is confirmed by stimulating each electrode separately and checking for motor and sensory responses (see Table 26.1). The position can be adjusted accordingly. The optimal position for the lead is in the upper medial aspect of the foramen, parallel to the sacral nerve, with electrodes "2" and "3" straddling the anterior margin of the sacrum (Fig. 26.3). With the electrodes in the optimal position, the lead body (proximal to the sheath) is held steady while the sheath is backed out of the incision. Best practices indicate that many surgeons perform this step under live fluoroscopy to verify that the electrodes maintain their position. As the sheath is removed, the tines deploy and anchor the lead in place. The incision used for the lead introducer is also used for tunneling the lead to the future neurostimulator site. This site should be below the belt line, and is usually located lateral to the outer edge of the sacrum and about 3–5 cm below the posterior superior iliac crest. The percutaneous lead extension is then placed by making a small stab wound lateral or contralateral to the future neurostimulator pocket site where the extension will exit the skin. A tunnel is made between the two sites and the extension is fed through the tube. After cleaning body fluids from the lead and the percutaneous extension connector, the protective boot is slipped over the end of the lead. The lead and percutaneous extension are connected, the screws

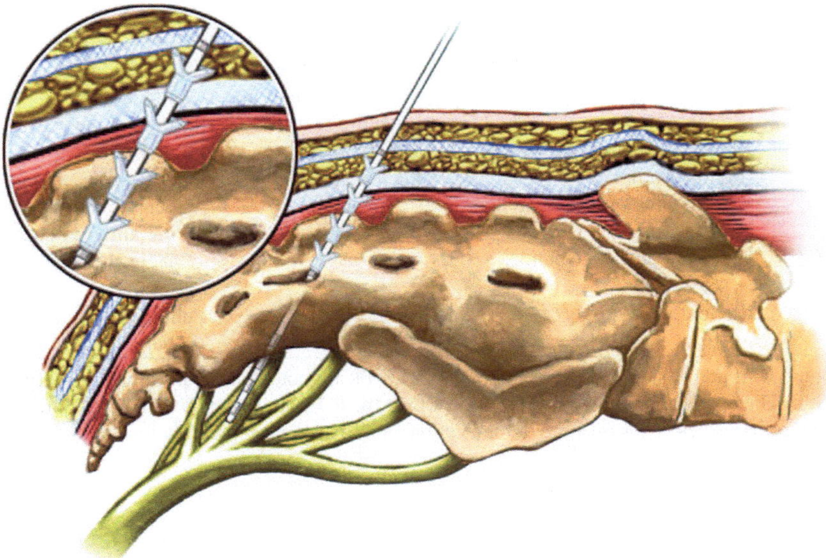

Fig. 26.3 Illustration of the correct position of the electrodes of a chronic lead. Note how the tines anchor the lead to the surrounding tissue and prevent displacement. Reprinted with permission of Medtronic, Inc. ©2012. Please note that the information addresses InterStim Therapy for interstitial cystitis, a use which the FDA has not approved. Medtronic does not market its products for unapproved indications and makes no representations regarding the safety and/or efficacy for unapproved uses

are tightened, and the protective boot is pushed over the connection. Sutures are used to secure the boot at the end of the connection closest to the percutaneous extension. The externalized part of the percutaneous lead extension is secured with a transparent dressing. The percutaneous lead extension pin connector is locked into the twist-lock connector on the screening cable which is later connected to an external generator for the duration of the trial period (Fig. 26.4).

Stage 2: Chronic Implant Placement

The site of the lead connection to the percutaneous extension is opened, the boot is removed, and the extension wire is disconnected. A subcutaneous pocket is created bluntly or with electrocautery at a depth of 1–1.5 in (2.5–4 cm). The lead is then securely connected to the IPG which is then placed in the pocket (Fig. 26.5). Before closing the pocket, the system integrity should be checked using the physician's programmer. Liberal irrigation throughout the procedure may help prevent infection (we use a gentamicin/saline solution).

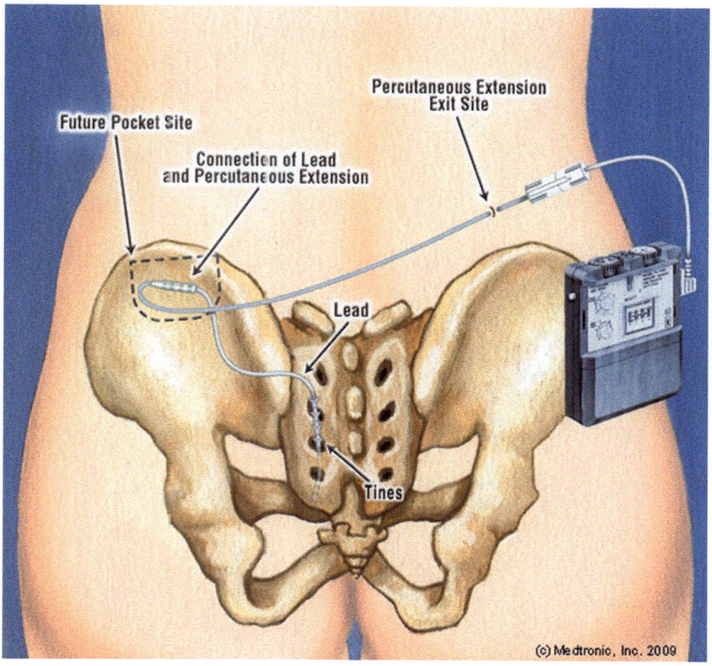

Fig. 26.4 Test stimulation using a chronic lead (stage 1). Reprinted with permission of Medtronic, Inc. ©2012. Please note that the information addresses InterStim Therapy for interstitial cystitis, a use which the FDA has not approved Medtronic does not market its products for unapproved indications and makes no representations regarding the safety and/or efficacy for unapproved uses

Clinical Results

The use of SNM in patients with BPS has been the subject of multiple research studies since its FDA approval for urgency and frequency. Maher et al. prospectively followed 15 women with refractory BPS who received S3 SNM. Seventy-three percent of the participants reported improvement in pelvic pain, daytime frequency, nocturia, and urgency. Eighty-seven percent of the participants reported a 50% decrease in bladder pain. Forty-seven percent of the patients had a 50% decrease in 24-h voiding frequency. Mean bladder pain decreased from 8.9 to 2.4 on a scale of 0 to 10. Additionally, the quality of life parameters of social functioning, bodily pain, and general health significantly improved during the stimulation period [17].

Whitmore et al. conducted a multicenter prospective observational study on women with refractory BPS ($n = 33$) who had failed other forms of treatment. They found that there was a statistically significant improvement in bladder pain, urinary frequency, and both average and maximum voided volumes, as well as the interstitial cystitis symptom and problem indices after the FSLP. Seventy-seven percent of patients had subjective improvement and 52% underwent IPG placement (stage 2) [5].

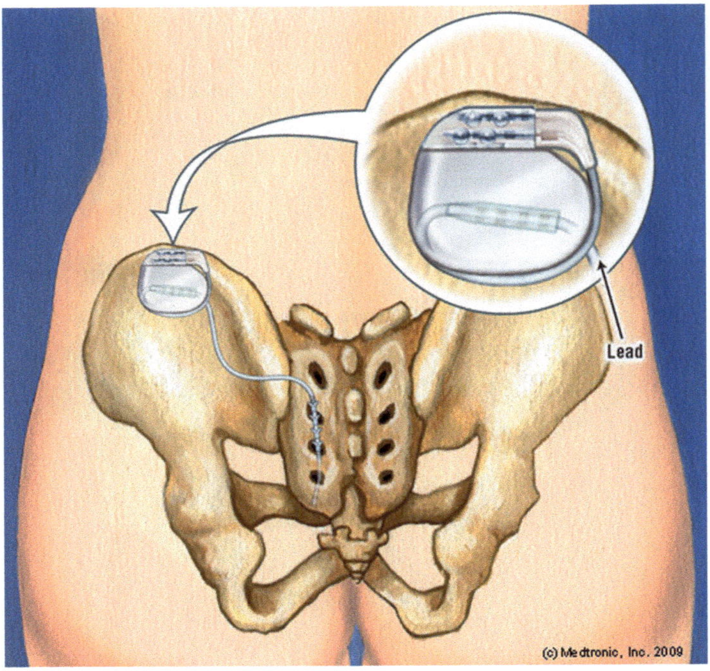

Fig. 26.5 Implantation of a chronic pulse generator (stage 2). Reprinted with permission of Medtronic, Inc. ©2012. Please note that the information addresses InterStim Therapy for interstitial cystitis, a use which the FDA has not approved. Medtronic does not market its products for unapproved indications and makes no representations regarding the safety and/or efficacy for unapproved uses

Comiter, in 2003, prospectively examined the efficacy of SNS on 25 patients with refractory BPS. Of those, 17 (68%) had a successful trial test and qualified for chronic IPG placement. When evaluated at a mean of 14-month follow-up, their mean daytime frequency and nocturia improved, mean voided volume increased, and average pain decreased from 5.8 to 1.6 on a 0–10 point visual analog pain scale (VAS; $P<0.01$). By the last postoperative visit, 94% of the implanted patients reported sustained improvement [18].

The direct effect of SNM on pain secondary to BPS was studied by Peters and Konstandt. Twenty-one patients (17 females and 4 males) who had failed a mean of six prior treatments were examined retrospectively with a mean follow-up of 15.4 months after having a chronic IPG. Overall, 95% of participants reported a moderate to marked improvement of their pain. The mean narcotic use, measured in intramuscular morphine dose equivalents (MDEs), significantly decreased by 36%, from 81.6 to 52 mg/day. Of the 18 patients who were using narcotics before SNS, four remained narcotic-free [19].

Along with alleviating BPS symptoms, more objectively, SNS has been shown to alter hypothesized urinary markers for BPS. Chai et al. reported normalization of epidermal growth factor-like growth factor (HB-EGF) and antiproliferative factor (APF) after S3 neurostimulation [20].

The reports on long-term success of SNS in patients with BPS have been encouraging. Recently Powell and Kreder reported only 9% (2 out of 22) loss of efficacy at a mean follow-up of 60 months [21]. Of 39 patients who had the screening test, 22 underwent chronic generator implantation after documenting 50% improvement in the presenting complaint. Long-term success rate was 86% (19/22). Half of the devices had to be explanted for various reasons (e.g., depleted batteries, malfunction, infection, ...) and most of those patients had reimplantation with continued benefit. Loss of efficacy was responsible for only three (14%) of the explants and one device was replaced with return of benefit. Gajewski and Al-Zahrani reported good long-term success of the SNM in 72% of the patients at a median follow-up of 61 months. In their study, the presence of urgency was a positive predictor of the long-term success of the implant [22].

Complications

Complication rates of SNM for the specific indication of BPS have not been separately reported. A review by Leong et al. extracted the adverse events from several published reports on the use of SNS for other urinary indications [23]. They concluded that adverse events are usually related to the implant procedure and the presence of the implant or of undesirable stimulation. The most common adverse event reported was pain at the implant site, which occurred between 3% and 42%. Other adverse events reported were lead migration (1–21%), bowel dysfunction (4–7%), and infection (4–10%) (Table 26.2). Another review by Brazzelli et al. looking at published studies before 2004 reported a reoperation rate of 33%, mainly secondary to pain and infection, and chronic lead removal in 9% of patients [24].

Technical improvements throughout the years have decreased the incidence of adverse events significantly. Two important improvements were the introduction of tined leads and the gluteal placement of the IPG instead of abdominal. In the advent of these changes, both the incidence of adverse events and the reoperation rate per implanted patient have decreased. The majority of adverse events do not require surgical intervention. Decreased efficacy due to electrode migration and undesirable stimulation can easily be solved by reprogramming the IPG [23]. A retrospective analysis among 83 implanted patients with a reduced response or complications, such as pain at the IPG site, showed that 18% of the cases could be helped conservatively. Furthermore, the incidence of adverse events is lower with the new tined leads in comparison with non-tined leads (28 and 73%, respectively) [25]. A study among 235 patients confirmed that tined leads migrated less often, which occurred among five patients (2.1%) [26]. The available data indicate that the further development and optimization of SNM limit the risk of adverse events [23].

Table 26.2 Most common adverse events with sacral neuromodulation

Adverse event	Rate (%)
Pain at implant site	3–42
Lead migration	1–21
Infection	4–10
Bowel dysfunction	4–7

Data from Leong RK, De Wachter SG, van Kerrebroeck PE. Current information on sacral neuromodulation and botulinum toxin treatment for refractory idiopathic overactive bladder syndrome: a review. Urol Int. 2010;84(3):245–253

Other Neuromodulation Techniques

Pudendal Nerve Stimulation

The pudendal nerve innervates the pelvic floor muscles, external urethral and anal sphincters, and pelvic organs, and many sacral nerve sensory afferent fibers originate from it. Therefore, chronic pudendal nerve stimulation (CPNS) may be a viable alternative for people with BPS who fail SNS. Although no pudendal nerve-specific device is commercially available, recent data regarding its efficacy is starting to emerge. The technique is performed by advancing a foramen needle medial to the ischial tuberosity towards the ischial spine. Proper placement is verified by electromyography of the anal sphincter and typical motor (anal contraction) and sensory (pulsation in the vaginal or scrotal area) responses. Once the pudendal nerve is identified, a quadripolar lead electrode is positioned and correct responses are again verified. The lead is then tunneled to a mid-buttock incision, where it is connected to an external generator during the screening period and then to an implantable generator if indicated [27].

In a prospective, single blinded, randomized crossover trial, by Peters, 30 patients with voiding dysfunction received a sacral and pudendal lead to test independently [27]. Pudendal stimulation was rated as superior to sacral for improving pelvic pain ($P=0.024$), urinary urgency ($P=0.005$), frequency ($P=0.007$), and bowel function ($P=0.049$). In a subset analysis of only those with BPS ($n=22$), 77% of subjects also chose CPNS as the superior lead after 6 months of follow-up [28]. The same author later reported on 55 patients (of whom 26 had BPS) who received CPNS with a median follow-up of 24 months. Significant improvements in frequency, voided volume, incontinence, and urgency were found. Pain and incontinence severity did not change. ICPI and ICSI scores significantly improved over 12 months; however, the mean scores for the BPS subgroup were approaching baseline values after 1 year [29].

Posterior Tibial Nerve Stimulation

Posterior tibial nerve stimulation technique consists of inserting a 0.22 mm needle about 5–6 cm above the medial tibial malleolus. The needle is connected to an external electric generator and correct placement is verified by flexion of the great toe. The stimulation is usually applied 30 min weekly for 10 weeks. Data regarding its efficacy for patients with BPS is conflicting [30–32].

Caudal Epidural Sacral Nerve Stimulation

Zabihi et al. reported the benefit of bilateral caudal epidural SNM in 30 patients (21 females, 9 males) with refractory BPS and chronic pelvic pain followed over a mean of 16 months. Twenty-three (77%) patients had successful trial stimulation and were chronically implanted. ICSI and ICPI significantly improved by 35 and 38%, respectively. The pain score improved by 40% ($P=0.04$). The procedure is performed by advancing the foramen needle into the epidural space through the sacral hiatus, under fluoroscopic guidance. Once correct placement is confirmed, the quadripolar tined lead is properly positioned and deployed over the S2–S4 sacral nerve roots. The leads are stimulated intraoperatively to achieve sacral S2–S4 motor and sensory responses [33].

References

1. Tanagho EA, Schmidt RA. Electrical stimulation in the clinical management of the neurogenic bladder. J Urol. 1988;140(6):1331–9.
2. de Groat WC. A neurologic basis for the overactive bladder. Urology. 1997;50(6A Suppl):36–52. discussion 53–36.
3. Habler HJ, Janig W, Koltzenburg M. Activation of unmyelinated afferent fibres by mechanical stimuli and inflammation of the urinary bladder in the cat. J Physiol. 1990;425:545–62.
4. McMahon SB. Neuronal and behavioural consequences of chemical inflammation of rat urinary bladder. Agents Actions. 1988;25(3–4):231–3.
5. Whitmore KE, Payne CK, Diokno AC, Lukban JC. Sacral neuromodulation in patients with interstitial cystitis: a multicenter clinical trial. Int Urogynecol J Pelvic Floor Dysfunct. 2003;14(5):305–8. discussion 308–309.
6. Shaker H, Wang Y, Loung D, Balbaa L, Fehlings MG, Hassouna MM. Role of C-afferent fibres in the mechanism of action of sacral nerve root neuromodulation in chronic spinal cord injury. BJU Int. 2000;85(7):905–10.
7. Hohenfellner M, Dahms SE, Matzel K, Thuroff JW. Sacral neuromodulation for treatment of lower urinary tract dysfunction. BJU Int. May 2000;85 Suppl 3:10–9. discussion 22–13.
8. Fowler CJ, Swinn MJ, Goodwin RJ, Oliver S, Craggs M. Studies of the latency of pelvic floor contraction during peripheral nerve evaluation show that the muscle response is reflexly mediated. J Urol. 2000;163(3):881–3.
9. Melzack R, Wall PD. Pain mechanisms: a new theory. Science. 1965;150(699):971–9.
10. Elkelini MS, Abuzgaya A, Hassouna MM. Mechanisms of action of sacral neuromodulation. Int Urogynecol J Pelvic Floor Dysfunct. 2010;21 Suppl 2:S439–46.
11. Yoo PB, Woock JP, Grill WM. Bladder activation by selective stimulation of pudendal nerve afferents in the cat. Exp Neurol. 2008;212(1):218–25.
12. Leng WW, Chancellor MB. How sacral nerve stimulation neuromodulation works. Urol Clin North Am. 2005;32(1):11–8.

13. Williams ER, Siegel SW. Procedural techniques in sacral nerve modulation. Int Urogynecol J Pelvic Floor Dysfunct. 2010;21 Suppl 2:453–60.
14. Baxter C, Kim JH. Contrasting the percutaneous nerve evaluation versus staged implantation in sacral neuromodulation. Curr Urol Rep. 2010;11(5):310–4.
15. Borawski KM, Foster RT, Webster GD, Amundsen CL. Predicting implantation with a neuromodulator using two different test stimulation techniques: a prospective randomized study in urge incontinent women. Neurourol Urodyn. 2007;26(1):14–8.
16. Bannowsky A, Wefer B, Braun PM, Junemann KP. Urodynamic changes and response rates in patients treated with permanent electrodes compared to conventional wire electrodes in the peripheral nerve evaluation test. World J Urol. 2008;26(6):623–6.
17. Maher CF, Carey MP, Dwyer PL, Schluter PL. Percutaneous sacral nerve root neuromodulation for intractable interstitial cystitis. J Urol. 2001;165(3):884–6.
18. Comiter CV. Sacral neuromodulation for the symptomatic treatment of refractory interstitial cystitis: a prospective study. J Urol. 2003;169(4):1369–73.
19. Peters KM, Konstandt D. Sacral neuromodulation decreases narcotic requirements in refractory interstitial cystitis. BJU Int. 2004;93(6):777–9.
20. Chai TC, Zhang C, Warren JW, Keay S. Percutaneous sacral third nerve root neurostimulation improves symptoms and normalizes urinary HB-EGF levels and antiproliferative activity in patients with interstitial cystitis. Urology. 2000;55(5):643–6.
21. Powell CR, Kreder KJ. Long-term outcomes of urgency-frequency syndrome due to painful bladder syndrome treated with sacral neuromodulation and analysis of failures. J Urol. 2010;183(1):173–6.
22. Gajewski JB, Al-Zahrani AA. The long-term efficacy of sacral neuromodulation in the management of intractable cases of bladder pain syndrome: 14 years of experience in one centre. BJU Int. 2010;107(8):1258–64.
23. Leong RK, De Wachter SG, van Kerrebroeck PE. Current information on sacral neuromodulation and botulinum toxin treatment for refractory idiopathic overactive bladder syndrome: a review. Urol Int. 2010;84(3):245–53.
24. Brazzelli M, Murray A, Fraser C. Efficacy and safety of sacral nerve stimulation for urinary urge incontinence: a systematic review. J Urol. 2006;175(3 Pt 1):835–41.
25. Sutherland SE, Lavers A, Carlson A, Holtz C, Kesha J, Siegel SW. Sacral nerve stimulation for voiding dysfunction: one institution's 11-year experience. Neurourol Urodyn. 2007;26(1):19–28. discussion 36.
26. Deng DY, Gulati M, Rutman M, Raz S, Rodriguez LV. Failure of sacral nerve stimulation due to migration of tined lead. J Urol. 2006;175(6):2182–5.
27. Peters KM, Feber KM, Bennett RC. Sacral versus pudendal nerve stimulation for voiding dysfunction: a prospective, single-blinded, randomized, crossover trial. Neurourol Urodyn. 2005;24(7):643–7.
28. Peters KM, Feber KM, Bennett RC. A prospective, single-blind, randomized crossover trial of sacral vs pudendal nerve stimulation for interstitial cystitis. BJU Int. 2007;100(4):835–9.
29. Peters KM, Killinger KA, Boguslawski BM, Boura JA. Chronic pudendal neuromodulation: expanding available treatment options for refractory urologic symptoms. Neurourol Urodyn. 2010;29(7):1267–71.
30. Congregado Ruiz B, Pena Outeirino XM, Campoy Martinez P, Leon Duenas E, Leal Lopez A. Peripheral afferent nerve stimulation for treatment of lower urinary tract irritative symptoms. Eur Urol. 2004;45(1):65–9.
31. Zhao J, Nordling J. Posterior tibial nerve stimulation in patients with intractable interstitial cystitis. BJU Int. 2004;94(1):101–4.
32. Zhao J, Bai J, Zhou Y, Qi G, Du L. Posterior tibial nerve stimulation twice a week in patients with interstitial cystitis. Urology. 2008;71(6):1080–4.
33. Zabihi N, Mourtzinos A, Maher MG, Raz S, Rodriguez LV. Short-term results of bilateral S2-S4 sacral neuromodulation for the treatment of refractory interstitial cystitis, painful bladder syndrome, and chronic pelvic pain. Int Urogynecol J Pelvic Floor Dysfunct. 2008;19(4):553–7.

Chapter 27
Bladder Augmentation, Urinary Diversion and Cystectomy in Patients with Bladder Pain Syndrome

Jørgen Nordling, Magnus Fall, and Ralph Peeker

Introduction

Bladder Pain Syndrome (BPS) is a disease characterised by pain perceived in the bladder often leading to frequent voiding day and night. Some patients have to void up to 50 times per day and night. It is easily understandable that voiding this often has a major impact on the quality of life for the unfortunate patient suffering from this disease. It differs however between patients to which degree frequent voiding or pain, or both, are the most bothersome symptoms.

Diagnostic criteria for BPS have been under heated debate during the last 8 years. From this discussion it has become evident, that it is not today possible to define any useful diagnostic test for making the diagnosis of BPS. The diagnosis is therefore clinical, based on symptoms, cystoscopy and biopsy also being helpful, and exclusion of confusable diseases by specific investigations.

The influence of BPS on quality of life has been evaluated by Koziol et al. [1] demonstrating a significant negative effect on the ability to travel, employment, leisure activities and sleep. Michael et al. [2] found that the quality of life in females with "interstitial cystitis" was especially affected in the psychosocial dimensions like vitality and mental health.

To find and document effective treatments of a relatively rare disease, with no clear clinical definition, is a difficult task. Many treatments are anecdotal or based

J. Nordling (✉)
Department of Urology, Herlev Hospital, University of Copenhagen, Copenhagen, Denmark
e-mail: jnordling@dadlnet.dk

M. Fall
Department of Urology, Institute of Clinical Sciences, Sahlgrens Academy at University of Gothenburg, Göteborg, Sweden

R. Peeker
Department of Urology, Sahlgrenska University Hospital, Gothenburg, Sweden

J. Nordling et al. (eds.), *Bladder Pain Syndrome: A Guide for Clinicians*,
DOI 10.1007/978-1-4419-6929-3_27,

on empiric data and proper prospective, randomised, controlled studies are rather the exception than the rule. Treatment includes behavioural treatments, diets, oral medications, bladder distention and bladder irrigation directed against the frequent voiding and/or the pain. Only when all these treatments have failed is surgery considered.

Surgery includes surgery on the nervous system and surgery on the bladder.

Surgery on the Nervous System

Old methods like sympathetic denervation [3], parasympathetic denervation [4] and cystolysis [5, 6] are now abandoned since positive effects were found to be short-lived while side effects persisted.

In recent years, neuromodulation and especially sacral neuromodulation have gained some interest.

Cystoplasty and Urinary Diversion

If all other treatments have failed major surgery may be necessary to relieve patients from their disabling symptoms. This includes bladder augmentation, urinary diversion and partial or total cystectomy.

It is essential that a patient has been through an extensive workup and trials of treatment before irreversible surgery is undertaken—all reasonable conservative measures should be tried first. It must be remembered that major reconstructive surgery includes extensive and, in principle, irreversible procedures for conditions that otherwise imply a modest risk of death or life-threatening complications. Apart from the more immediate problems intra- and postoperatively, there are less obvious ones like metabolic consequences [11] and the late development of cancer after incorporation of ileum into the urinary tract [7, 8]. Reconstructive procedures therefore have to be regarded as last resorts when there are no other treatments with reasonable efficacy to be offered.

The decision of which type of reconstruction to choose in BPS can sometimes be difficult. Therefore, decision-making should invariably be preceded by a thorough and appropriate patient counselling, to communicate possible risks with the procedure and to give the patient realistic expectations on the result of operation. Of course, every patient considered for a complicated reconstruction must be fitted to cope with the consequences of operation, to benefit from treatment. Continent urinary diversion, or cystoplasty, requires a patient with an unspoiled cognitive ability and a good manual dexterity. In a younger patient, meeting the abovementioned prerequisites, a continent diversion might be preferable whereas an older patient probably is better served with a Bricker conduit. A fact to communicate is a high risk of re-operation for patients with a continent cutaneous stoma. In this context, an important notion is that a recent report revealed that although some 90% of the patients had a well-functioning reservoir at the time of follow-up, patients with benign functional or inflammatory diseases were experiencing comparatively more problems with their reservoirs than patients with, e.g., spinal cord injury or malignant disease [9].

When selecting the appropriate procedure, a careful preoperative assessment of renal and bowel function is important. The amount of bowel surface to be allowed to be incorporated into the urinary tract must be decided [10]. In contrast to the urothelium, the bowel mucosa has a significant permeability to ammonium chloride, the resorption of which may bring about hyperchloremic metabolic acidosis. A patient with compromised kidney function can have difficulties in compensating for this uptake and as a consequence, continent urinary diversion can only be recommended to patients with a glomerular filtration rate in excess of 40 ml/min/1.73m^2 body surface. Furthermore, the isolation of an ileal segment may compromise bile acid reabsorption which in turn may result in diarrhoea and even, particularly in patients with preoperatively compromised anal sphincter function, anal incontinence [11]. Uptake of folic acid/cobolamin may likewise be compromised.

Bladder Augmentation

In a smaller proportion of patients the inflammatory process within the bladder wall results in severe fibrosis and a contracted bladder with sometimes a very small capacity even in general anaesthesia. These patients do often have a most severe frequency, while bladder pain becomes less important. These are the patients best suited for bladder augmentation with or without resection of the patients' own bladder [12, 13]. The use of different bowel segments for bladder augmentation has been reported in numerous articles, including ileum [12, 14–21], ileocoecum [12, 22–26], coecum [14, 26], right colon [12, 15, 27], sigmoid colon [16, 24, 28] and gastric segments [29, 30]. In the chapter on BPS from the 4th International Consultation on Incontinence it was concluded: *There is no significant difference between bowel segments with regard to outcome except for gastric tissue substitution which is associated with dysuria and persistent pain due to production of acids* [31].

Cystoplasty might be performed supratrigonally (trigone sparing) or infratrigonally. Good results were reported for the supratrigonal approach [14, 16, 24, 32, 33], although the report from Nielsen et al. in 1990 was less favourable with two failures in eight patients [23]. Van Ophoven reported 5 years results of orthotopic substitution enteroplasty in 18 patients with only two failures. Three patients needed self-catheterisation and one a suprapubic catheter [34]. In 1998 Peeker et al. [13] reported excellent results in patients with end-stage ulcerative or classic BPS (ESSIC 3C) but not so in patients with non-ulcer disease (ESSIC 2X). A follow-up on an extended series was published in 2007 further emphasising this conclusion [35].

More favourable results have been reported in patients with small cystoscopic bladder capacity (<200 ml) [23, 36–39]. Cystoscopic low bladder capacity might be due to fibrosis as an end-stage result of long-lasting inflammation. However, cystoscopic low bladder capacity might also be due to existing inflammation with oedema and thickening of the bladder wall and as a consequence be reversible. Sairanen et al. described the long-term effect of cyclosporine treatment in BPS patients [40], and in many of these patients functional bladder capacity after treatment by far exceeded cystoscopic bladder capacity before treatment. Three patients with *cystoscopic bladder capacity of 200 ml*, and an average functional bladder capacity of 70 ml, had a *functional capacity of 290, 220 and 350 ml* after treatment. Two patients with a maximal cystoscopic capacity of 300 ml and a functional capacity of 92 and 100 ml increased the functional capacity to 490 and 350 ml. In all patients a substantial increase in bladder capacity was registered. This phenomenon has also been noted in a subgroup of patients with classic Hunner disease treated with long-term suprapubic TENS [41]. Cystoscopic bladder capacity therefore cannot be taken as the only and ultimate sign of end-stage disease. Obviously, treatments with a capability to subside the disease process can also influence anaesthetic bladder capacity. It still remains to be shown if biopsy findings of characteristics and grade of inflammation and/or grade of fibrosis in the detrusor might increase the prognostic significance of a low cystoscopic capacity.

Example of Technique: Supratrigonal Cystectomy and Ileocystoplasty

Access to the abdominal cavity is obtained via a midline laparotomy incision. After cystotomy, the ureters are intubated with two baby-feeding catheters anchored to the ureteral ridge with 4-0 Catgut sutures. Subtotal resection of the bladder is performed, leaving only the internal urethral meatus and both ureteral orifices (Fig. 27.1). A 40 cm segment of the ileum is isolated, taking care to preserve the vascular supply, and with the distal transection margin located 30–40 cm proximal to the ileocaecal valve. The segment is detubularised antimesenterically (Fig. 27.2), double-folded to a spherical shape (Figs. 27.3 and 27.4) and anastomosed to the trigone remnant using an uninterrupted resorbable 3-0 suture. Postoperatively, an external drain tube should be left in situ for 1–3 days, depending on the amount of discharge. The baby-feeding tubes are extracted after 1 week. An indwelling evacuation catheter should be left open, inside the cystoplasty, for at least 10 days, after which clamping of the catheter may begin with the emptying intervals initially being 1 hour, gradually increasing. The catheter is usually removed after 2–3 weeks.

Bladder augmentation with infratrigonal bladder resection sparing the bladder neck is reported less frequently [42–45]. Ureteral re-implantation is needed and complications like urine leakage, urethral stricture and reflux might occur [44]. Linn et al. compared supratrigonal and infratrigonal bladder resection in patients with BPS and found 3 failures in 17 patients with infratrigonal resection and half of the patients with good outcome required self-catheterisation [33]. The need for intermit-

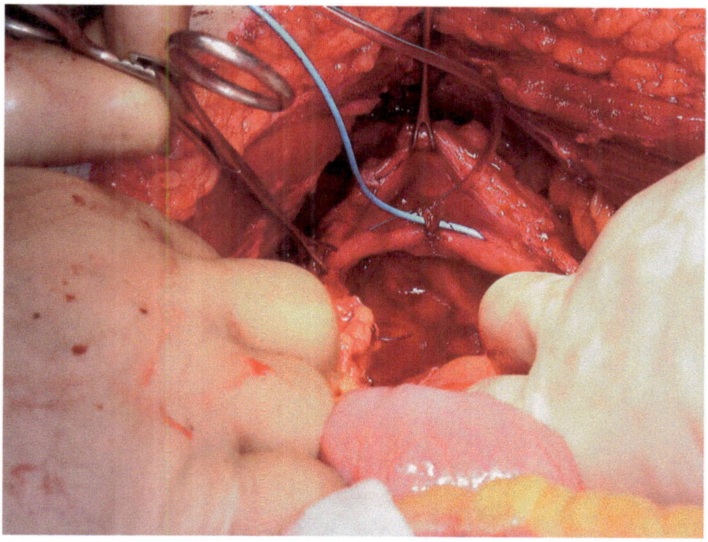

Fig. 27.1 Supratrigonal portion of the bladder resected, leaving just the trigone

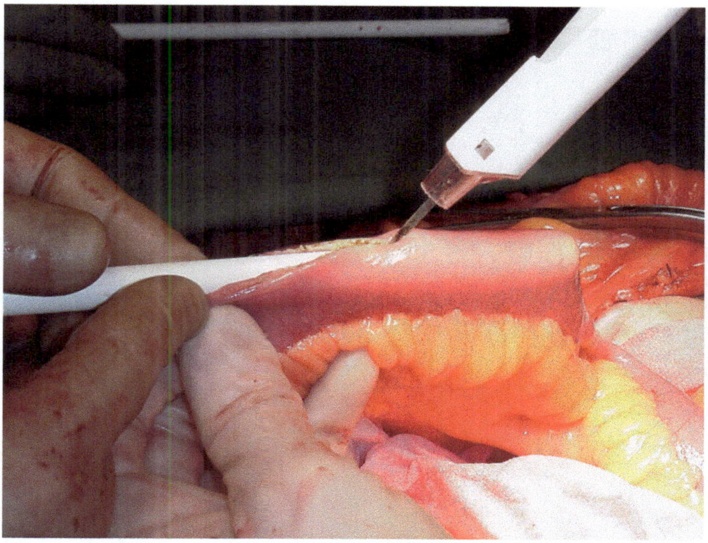

Fig. 27.2 Ileum segment isolated and opened antimesenterically

tent catheterisation is in many cases not an acceptable outcome due to the hypersensitivity of the bladder base and urethra making the procedure much too painful.

In the chapter on BPS from the 4th International Consultation on Incontinence it was concluded: *There is some weak evidence that cystoplasty with supratrigonal resection may benefit some selected patients with end stage ESSIC type 3C BPS.*

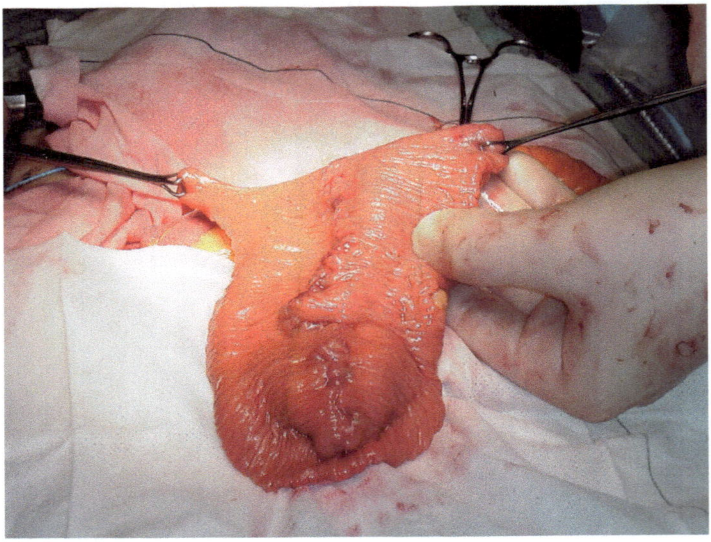

Fig. 27.3 U-shape folding of the opened ileum

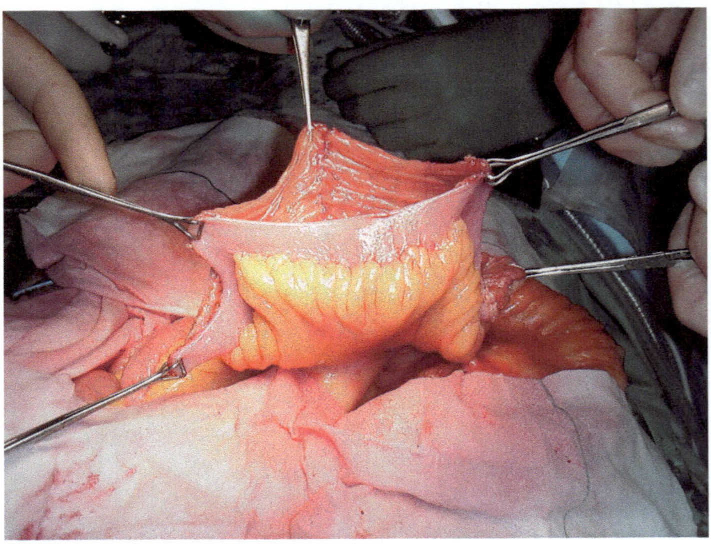

Fig. 27.4 Once again folding the ileum plate creates the cystoplasty, with a triangular opening adjusted to the size of the trigone

There is no compelling evidence that infratrigonal cystectomy with cystoplasty has any outcome advantage over supratrigonal cystectomy but it tends to be associated with more complications and poorer functional bladder rehabilitation [31].

Urinary Diversion

In a questionnaire to urologists in the USA Gershbaum and Moldwin [46] found urinary diversion to be the most common surgical treatment for BPS. It is therefore a little surprising that the literature on the subject is extremely sparse. It is often just mentioned in the text that this is the ultimate treatment to relieve patients from their symptoms and diversion with or without cystectomy is often successful [15, 36, 37, 47, 48]. It has been a subject of discussion whether urinary diversion should be accompanied by simultaneous cystectomy, or if cystectomy should be reserved for those patients having persistent pain or intolerable infectious problems from their bladder.

We have recently scrutinised our own experiences and from the essential aspects there is agreement. Nordling reviewed the Copenhagen experiences from the last 10 years. Of 16 patients with BPS 15 became pain free and 1 had persistent unchanged pain. All patients had detrusor mastocytosis [49]. One had a Hunner lesion. Cystoscopic bladder capacity was median 490 ml with a range from 100 ml to 4,000 ml. The patient with persistent pain later had a cystectomy without any effect on the pain. One patient had a cystectomy because of pyocystos with good result.

Rössberger [35] reviewed the Gothenburg results. During a 25-year period 47 subjects were treated with major surgery. In 28 out of 34 patients with Type 3C BPS the initial surgical procedure did result in complete symptom resolution. Of the remaining six patients, four could successfully be managed by a supplementary surgery: diversion, cystectomy or transurethral resection of lesions in the trigonal remnant, respectively. Only 3 of the 13 patients with non-ulcer disease experienced symptom resolution after reconstructive surgery and two out of these required supravesical diversion. Eight patients had a supplementary secondary simplex cystectomy in an attempt to treat persistent suprapubic pain, without relief of pain. Early intra- and post-operative complications were few. However, the need for re-operations in patients with non-ulcer BPS having undergone continent urinary diversion was high, mainly related to nipple valve problems. In this series, a very marked difference in outcome was found in patients with end-stage classic Hunner type of disease vs. non-ulcer BPS.

Continent urinary diversion using an intestinal reservoir has become the treatment of choice in patients having a cystectomy due to bladder cancer. This has therefore been suggested for patients with BPS due to the better quality of life with an internal urinary reservoir. Experience has however shown unexpected complications such as reoccurrence of pain in the intestinal reservoir. Again the literature on the subject is sparse, although chronic inflammatory changes have been seen in the cystoplasty pouch [50, 51]. The persistent pain after major irreversible surgery is an enigma and often causes patients to defer surgery for many years. In this discussion it must however be remembered that two major symptoms cause the poor quality of life seen in these patients: PAIN and FREQUENCY. At least it can be promised that frequency is alleviated by a urinary diversion making daily life much easier and making it possible to have a full night's sleep. These results also seem to demonstrate a very good chance of pain relief.

In the chapter on BPS from the 4th International Consultation on Incontinence it was concluded: *Urinary diversion with or without cystectomy may be the ultimate option for refractory patients. Continent diversion may have better cosmetic and life style outcome but recurrence of pain in the pouch is a real possibility* [31].

Conclusion

Urinary bladder augmentation should be reserved for the end-stage BPS patient with a contracted bladder and with urinary frequency as the main problem, when pain is not any more a significant symptom. Urinary diversion is to be reserved for the patient, whose quality of life is more or less destroyed because of pain and urinary frequency and who has demonstrated an unsatisfactory response to less invasive treatments. Continent urinary diversion might be an alternative but risks of pain in the pouch and nipple valve problems are real limitations.

References

1. Koziol JA, Clark DC, Gittes RF, Tan EM. The natural history of interstitial cystitis: a survey of 374 patients. J Urol. 1993;149(3):465–9.
2. Michael YL, Kawachi I, Stampfer MJ, Colditz GA, Curhan GC. Quality of life among women with interstitial cystitis. J Urol. 2000;164(2):423–7.
3. Douglass H. Excision of the superior hypogastric plexus in the treatment of intractable interstitial cystitis. Am J Surg. 1934;25:249–57.
4. Moulder MK, Meirowsky AM. The management of Hunner's ulcer by differential sacral neurotomy: preliminary report. J Urol. 1956;75:261–2.
5. Hunner GL. A rare type of bladder ulcer in women: report of cases. Boston Med Surg J. 1915;172:660–4.
6. Worth PH. The treatment of interstitial cystitis by cystolysis with observations on cystoplasty. A review after 7 years. Br J Urol. 1980;52(3):232.
7. Ali-el-Dein B, Gomha M, Ghoneim MA. Critical evaluation of the problem of chronic urinary retention after orthotopic bladder substitution in women. J Urol. 2002;168(2):587–92.
8. Lane T, Shah J. Carcinoma following augmentation ileocystoplasty. Urol Int. 2000;64(1):31–2.
9. Jonsson O, Olofsson G, Lindholm E, Tornqvist H. Long-time experience with the Kock ileal reservoir for continent urinary diversion. Eur Urol. 2001;40(6):632–40.
10. Mills RD, Studer UE. Metabolic consequences of continent urinary diversion. J Urol. 1999;161(4):1057–66.
11. Olofsson G, Fjalling M, Kilander A, Ung KA, Jonsson O. Bile acid malabsorption after continent urinary diversion with an ileal reservoir. J Urol. 1998;160(3 Pt 1):724–7.
12. Webster GD, Maggio MI. The management of chronic interstitial cystitis by substitution cystoplasty. J Urol. 1989;141(2):287–91.
13. Peeker R, Aldenborg F, Fall M. The treatment of interstitial cystitis with supratrigonal cystectomy and ileocystoplasty: difference in outcome between classic and nonulcer disease. J Urol. 1998;159(5):1479–82.

14. von Garrelts B. Interstitial cystitis: thirteen patients treated operatively with intestinal bladder substitutes. Acta Chir Scand. 1966;132(4):436–43.
15. Badenoch AW. Chronic interstitial cystitis. Br J Urol. 1971;43(6):718–21.
16. Bruce PT, Buckham GJ, Carden AB, Salvaris M. The surgical treatment of chronic interstitial cystitis. Med J Aust. 1977;1(16):581–2.
17. Awad SA, Al Zahrani HM, Gajewski JB, Bourque-Kehoe AA. Long-term results and complications of augmentation ileocystoplasty for idiopathic urge incontinence in women. Br J Urol. 1998;81(4):569–73.
18. Guillonneau B, Toussaint B, Bouchot O, Buzelin JM. Treatment of interstitial cystitis with sub-trigonal cystectomy and enterocystoplasty. Prog Urol. 1993;3(1):27–31.
19. Christmas TJ, Holmes SA, Hendry WF. Bladder replacement by ileocystoplasty: the final treatment for interstitial cystitis. Br J Urol. 1996;78(1):69–73.
20. Shirley SW, Mirelman S. Experiences with colocystoplasties, cecocystoplasties and ileocystoplasties in urologic surgery: 40 patients. J Urol. 1978;120(2):165–8.
21. Koskela E, Kontturi M. Function of the intestinal substituted bladder. Scand J Urol Nephrol. 1982;16:129–33.
22. DeJuana CP, Everett Jr JC. Interstitial cystitis: experience and review of recent literature. Urology. 1977;10(4):325–9.
23. Nielsen KK, Kromann-Andersen B, Steven K, Hald T. Failure of combined supratrigonal cystectomy and Mainz ileocecocystoplasty in intractable interstitial cystitis: is histology and mast cell count a reliable predictor for the outcome of surgery? J Urol. 1990;144(2 Pt 1):255–8.
24. Kontturi MJ, Hellstrom PA, Tammela TL, Lukkarinen OA. Colocystoplasty for the treatment of severe interstitial cystitis. Urol Int. 1991;46(1):50–4.
25. Whitmore WF, Gittes RF. Reconstruction of the urinary tract by cecal and ileocecal cystoplasty: review of a 15-year experience. J Urol. 1983;129:494–8.
26. Holm-Bentzen M, Klarskov P, Opsomer R, Hald T. Cecocystoplasty: an evaluation of operative results. Urol Int. 1986;41:21–5.
27. Seddon JM, Best L, Bruce AW. Intestinocystoplasty in treatment of interstitial cystitis. Urology. 1977;10(5):431–5.
28. Hradec H. Bladder substitution indications and results in 114 operations. J Urol. 1965;94:406–17.
29. Singla A, Galloway N. Early experience with the use of gastric segment in lower urinary tract reconstruction in adult patient population. Urology. 1997;50:630–5.
30. Leong CH. Use of stomach for bladder replacement and urinary diversion. Ann R Coll Surg Engl. 1978;60:282–9.
31. Hanno P, Lin A, Nordling J, Nyberg L, van Ophoven A, Ueda T. Bladder pain Syndrome. In: Abrams P, Cardozo L, Khoury S, Wein A, editors. Incontinence. Paris: Health Publications Ltd.; 2009. p. 1459–520.
32. Dounis A, Gow JG. Bladder augmentation–a long-term review. Br J Urol. 1979;51(4):264–8.
33. Linn JF, Hohenfellner M, Roth S, Dahms SE, Stein R, Hertle L, et al. Treatment of interstitial cystitis: comparison of subtrigonal and supratrigonal cystectomy combined with orthotopic bladder substitution. J Urol. 1998;159(3):774–8.
34. van Ophoven A, Oberpenning F, Hertle L. Long-term results of trigone-preserving orthotopic substitution enterocystoplasty for interstitial cystitis. J Urol. 2002;167(2 Pt 1):603–7.
35. Rössberger J, Fall M, Jonsson O, Peeker R. Long-term results of reconstructive surgery in patients with bladder pain syndrome/interstitial cystitis: subtyping is imperative. Urology. 2007;70(4):638–42.
36. Counseller VS. Bilateral transplantation of the ureters of the female. Am J Obstet Gynecol. 1937;33:234–48.
37. Hand JR. Interstitial cystitis: report of 223 cases (204 women and 19 men). J Urol. 1949;61:291–310.
38. Messing EM, Stamey TA. Interstitial cystitis: early diagnosis, pathology, and treatment. Urology. 1978;12(4):381–92.

39. Hohenfellner M, Black P, Linn JF, Dahms SE, Thuroff JW. Surgical treatment of interstitial cystitis in women. Int Urogynecol J Pelvic Floor Dysfunct. 2000;11(2):113–9.
40. Sairanen J, Forsell T, Ruutu M. Long-term outcome of patients with interstitial cystitis treated with low dose cyclosporine A. J Urol. 2004;171(6 Pt 1):2138–41.
41. Fall M. Conservative management of chronic interstitial cystitis: transcutaneous electrical nerve stimulation and transurethral resection. J Urol. 1985;133(5):774–8.
42. Lotenfoe RR, Christie J, Parsons A, Burkett P, Helal M, Lockhart JL. Absence of neuropathic pelvic pain and favorable psychological profile in the surgical selection of patients with disabling interstitial cystitis. J Urol. 1995;154(6):2039–42.
43. Bejany DE, Politano VA. Ileocolic neobladder in the woman with interstitial cystitis and a small contracted bladder. J Urol. 1995;153(1):42–3.
44. Nurse DE, McCrae P, Stephenson TP, Mundy AR. The problems of substitution cystoplasty. Br J Urol. 1988;61(5):423–6.
45. Hughes OD, Kynaston HG, Jenkins BJ, Stephenson TP, Vaughton KC. Substitution cystoplasty for intractable interstitial cystitis. Br J Urol. 1995;76(2):172–4.
46. Gershbaum D, Moldwin R. Practice trends for the management of interstitial cystitis. Urology. 2001;57(6 Suppl 1):119.
47. Freiha FS, Faysal MH, Stamey TA. The surgical treatment of intractable interstitial cystitis. J Urol. 1980;123(5):632–4.
48. Webster GD, Galloway N. Surgical treatment of interstitial cystitis. Indications, techniques, and results. Urology. 1987;29(4 Suppl):34–9.
49. Nordling J, Anjum FH, Bade JJ, Bouchelouche K, Bouchelouche P, Cervigni M, et al. Primary evaluation of patients suspected of having interstitial cystitis (IC). Eur Urol. 2004;45(5):662–9.
50. Kisman OK, Niejeholt AA, van Krieken JH. Mast cell infiltration in intestine used for bladder augmentation in interstitial cystitis. J Urol. 1991;146:1113–4.
51. Baskin LS, Tanagho EA. Pelvic pain without pelvic organs. J Urol. 1992;147(3):683–6.

Part V
Patient Perspective

Chapter 28
A Patient Perspective

Jane M. Meijlink, BA Hons

Bladder Pain Syndrome (BPS) has a deep impact on the life of both the patient and the patient's family. Understanding the patient perspective and the physical, psycho-emotional and social impact of BPS on the patient is an important step towards successful treatment by the health professional.

Despite the fact that today's health consumer in the developed world has a much greater knowledge of medical issues than ever before due to better health education and use of the Internet, genitourinary disorders are still stigmatised and considered taboo throughout both the developed and developing world. A bladder disorder is an intimate matter which patients feel embarrassed and uncomfortable to discuss, while their friends and relatives certainly do not want to hear about it. Consequently, many patients in different countries and cultures around the world are reluctant to seek professional help for their bladder disorder, let alone any related sexual dysfunction.

While increased awareness of this bladder syndrome in recent decades has led to quicker referral and diagnosis in some parts of the world, a patient with BPS symptoms may nevertheless still spend years without the right diagnosis. The first hurdle is the primary care health provider who may assume that the patient has an infection, even when urine tests appear to be negative. Furthermore, with nothing visible in the urine, many patients have either been told that there is nothing physically wrong and that it is all in the mind or have been referred to the wrong specialist and undergone unnecessary surgery including hysterectomy and even appendectomy. Since the primary care level is still the big stumbling block for BPS patients, it is vital to increase awareness of BPS at this level to ensure recognition of the symptoms at an early stage and referral to the right specialist. But this is not the end of the story, since although many more urologists and urogynaecologists than previously can today diagnose BPS, they are not always willing to take on these time-consuming patients who often require a complex, multidisciplinary approach.

J.M. Meijlink, BA Hons (✉)
International Painful Bladder Foundation (IPBF),
Burgemeester Le Fevre De Montignylaan 73, 3055 NA Rotterdam, The Netherlands
e-mail: jane-m@dds.nl

J. Nordling et al. (eds.), *Bladder Pain Syndrome: A Guide for Clinicians*,
DOI 10.1007/978-1-4419-6929-3_28,

Diagnosis a Relief

It can come as an immense relief to patients who may have been suffering from their bladder for years to be given the diagnosis of a disease with a name. On the other hand, however, patients who may have suddenly developed a severe form of BPS, and received a relatively quick diagnosis, may be shocked to learn that they have an incurable disorder. The prospect of suffering from these symptoms for the rest of their life is terrifying. They may be angry that this has happened to them and look round for someone or something to blame, or they may become panic-stricken and depressed. Living with a debilitating, painful disease of unknown cause, for which there is no cure, no single effective treatment for all patients and, worst of all, which the doctors themselves do not seem to understand or even agree on, is indeed an alarming prospect. However, if a patient has chronic bladder symptoms with no diagnosis and doctors have been suggesting that it is psychosomatic, the patient's family and friends are likely to think that the doctor knows best and to take the same approach. After all, the patient looks perfectly well. However, this can lead to devastating depression, loss of confidence, self-doubt and even suicide.

Importance of Official Recognition by Authorities

There are other reasons in today's world of officialdom why a diagnosis is important. Without a doctor's diagnosis of an officially recognised condition with a registered name, it may be impossible to obtain any kind of social security benefit, disability pension, reimbursement of medical costs or recognition of the illness by an employer or an authority. This importance of an officially recognised condition is one of the many reasons why the interstitial cystitis patient organisations have been so concerned at the many different names in circulation (painful bladder syndrome, BPS, etc.), since the name now registered everywhere with authorities is "interstitial cystitis" or translations of this in other languages. If the diagnosed name does not match the name registered with authorities, the patient runs the risk of receiving no reimbursement or social benefit and being faced with accusations of malingering by an employer.

Treatment

The ultimate aim of treatment is to alleviate the symptoms and improve the patient's quality of life. Not all patients experience the key symptoms of pain, urgency and frequency in equal degrees. There are as many variations as there are patients. While some patients suffer severe pain, others may say that they have no perception of pain as such, but have extreme problems with urgency and/or frequency with perhaps a persistent feeling of pressure, heaviness or discomfort. Treatment should be focused on whatever causes the patient the most bother and detriment to quality of life.

Treatment of BPS requires a great deal of time and patience on the part of the doctor in collaboration with the patient who will be required to play an active role, particularly in the field of behavioural and dietary modification. Since patients differ greatly, treatment has to be individualised and, until patients have been categorised into phenotypes or treatment sub-types, it may still largely be a question of trial and error, particularly if it is the non-Hunner's lesion type.

A BPS patient may need to use a combination of drugs, all of which may have side effects, and many BPS patients seem to have a bigger problem with drug intolerance than normal people. If the pain is severe and intractable, referral to a pain clinic is an option. However, care should be taken to find a pain consultant who has good knowledge of BPS and is willing to work in collaboration with the urologist; otherwise the patient may once again end up being diagnosed as psychosomatic.

If patients feel that their regular medication is having little or no effect, or the side effects are intolerable, they are more likely to resort to self-medication in the form of herbal or homeopathic remedies or any of the wide array of alternative therapies on offer. There is nothing worse than feeling that you have no control over your symptoms and consequently no control over your life. Desperate BPS patients are therefore wide open to suggestion and will try anything and this makes them potential victims of Internet advertising for the so-called cures for IC. If the doctor does not provide an office "climate" in which the patient feels able to openly discuss complementary and alternative treatment, the patient will simply go ahead without mentioning it. This can lead to potentially dangerous situations if certain herbal treatments are combined with conventional medicine. An ideal method is to create a treatment plan for each patient that can include complementary and alternative therapies in an open, safe way and in which the patient can play an active rather than a purely passive role. These could include for example trigger-point therapy, hypnotherapy, myofascial pain therapy, pelvic floor re-education, acupuncture and herbal supplements. Relaxation techniques can help reduce physical or psychological stress and include yoga, Tai chi, guided imagery and meditation. There are many complementary and alternative therapies that may help to alleviate symptoms, relax the patient and help to achieve a better quality of life. Any therapy that can help the patient to relax and de-stress is likely to improve his/her quality of life.

Impact on the Life of the Patient

BPS can have a deep impact on the social, psychological, occupational, domestic, physical and sexual life of the patient and affect the very structure of his/her life.

The frequent and often urgent need to urinate can form an obstacle to work, travel, visiting friends or even just popping out to the shop round the corner. When outside the safety of their own home, IC patients' life is dominated by the question: "Where am I going to find the next toilet?" Before every outing, the patient will carefully plan a network of toilets. This kind of situation can make patients afraid to leave the safety of their home. There are many patients who almost never go out and are literally prisoners of their BPS. If they think that there will be no toilet, they stay at home. In addition, the sheer embarrassment and shame they feel at having to urinate so frequently make many patients avoid associating with their friends and colleagues. So the disabling social consequences of BPS should not be underestimated either, since they may lead to isolation from friends, relatives, former activities, employment and life in general.

Impact on Work

The frequent and/or urgent need to urinate may make it difficult for some patients to continue working or they may be forced to change to a different type of job where they do have the possibility of frequent access to toilets. Work in some jobs becomes impossible when you have to keep running to the toilet, whether you are a bus driver, a teacher or a ballet dancer. If you work in an office or shop and keep going to the toilet, you risk getting fired because the boss thinks you are slacking. Fatigue due to lack of proper sleep or other causes can also be a hazard in some professions involving driving or operating machinery. A positive aspect is that today's computerised world means that there are many more opportunities of working from home than in the past, even setting up your own home-based business. There is nothing to stop BPS patients from becoming entrepreneurs!

Financial Impact

The impact of BPS on their work and career may cause patients considerable financial loss. They either cannot work or they lose their job and then have to fight tooth and nail for disability benefit because in some countries BPS is not registered as an official disease. In countries where many patients have no access to social security benefits, being unable to work may mean total dependence on relatives or even starvation. Many patients around the world have no medical insurance and no money to pay for treatment. And even in Western Europe, many of the treatments for BPS are not reimbursed. A chronic disease like BPS may therefore be a major long-term financial headache for patients and their families. It is consequently essential to ensure that doctors worldwide are made aware of affordable, low-price, generic drugs for BPS, including cheap anaesthetic cocktails to provide quick relief from intense pain.

Impact on the Whole Family

BPS has an impact on the entire family from many points of view. It affects relationships with partners and children because you cannot act like a normal parent or a normal partner. A BPS patient may be tired, irritable and unable to cope, to look after the family and to do normal everyday things with the partner and children. The financial impact may also affect the whole family by leading to a reduction in the family's standard of living. Members of the family may become resentful at this impact on their lives.

Sexual Impact

BPS can have a big impact on intimate relationships since sexual intercourse may be painful for both male and female BPS patients, either because the urethra, bladder and vagina are too painful or in the case of men because of the pain of ejaculation. This aspect of the impact of BPS on the patient's life should never be underestimated. Sex is a normal part of the lives of most human beings. If this form of intimacy is taken away, relationships may start to show cracks about which the patient may be deeply concerned or it may lead to divorce. Since some patients may find it difficult or impossible to broach this intimate subject with their doctor, it is an aspect that the doctor should raise and if necessary offer the patient the possibility of sex counselling. Every endeavour should be made to find ways of overcoming sexual dysfunction and the distress it causes and there are indeed many possible solutions. The important first step is "communicating" that a problem exists. If the health provider can speak to the patient clearly and directly about these sexual issues, this will create a climate that may help the patient to open up.

Psychological and Emotional Impact

Suffering from a chronic disorder for which there is no known cure is in itself likely to lead to depression, anxiety and panic attacks. Patients are continually anxious about the future: will the bladder symptoms get worse, will they be able to cope, will surgery be necessary and will their partner support them or abandon them? They may be disillusioned with the medical professionals who failed to diagnose their bladder disorder for years and who now appear to be unable to provide adequate treatment and have little or no time for them. Consequently they may feel isolated and abandoned and feel rightly or wrongly that nobody cares what happens to them. There may also be a sense of anger that this has happened to them and they may keep wishing that they could turn the clock back to their life without BPS, looking backwards rather than trying to cope with the situation and looking forwards.

Physical and Psychological Impact of Lack of Sleep and Fatigue

The physical and psychological impact of lack of sleep due to night-time frequency and the impact of daytime fatigue from other causes should also be taken into account and every endeavour made to find solutions. This means enrolling the help of the patient to make a careful analysis of all the possible causes of the tiredness. Causes of fatigue and lethargy may include sleep disruption and consequent lack of proper deep sleep, insomnia, medication, various physical disorders, psychological disorders, autoimmune diseases and even excessive activity or over-exercising. Fatigue in an individual patient may be caused by a combination of several of these factors.

Without proper sleep, people deteriorate both physically and psychologically. Even night-time frequency of just two or three times a night can cause considerable tiredness because some people have difficulty falling asleep again, once they have been out of bed to the bathroom. BPS patients in a flare or the most severe BPS patients may be out of bed continually throughout the night. This means that they get no chance to achieve the deep sleep that refreshes the mind and body. This leads to daytime fatigue and lack of energy, irritability, lack of motivation and concentration, memory lapses and depression. However, if a patient is very tired all day but is getting a reasonable amount of sleep, it is essential to check out other causes for the fatigue such as anaemia, hypothyroidism, heart failure, low blood pressure, infectious diseases including glandular fever or simply the impact of chronic pain. All kinds of medication can also cause daytime drowsiness and lethargy.

Chronic fatigue of autoimmune origin (e.g. Systemic Lupus Erythematosus and particularly Sjögren's syndrome) can be very debilitating and also occurs in fibromyalgia. When no identifiable cause of this kind of fatigue can be found, it is called chronic fatigue syndrome. This type of chronic fatigue, which may have both physical and mental effects, has no bearing on whether you feel you have slept well or not.

Quite apart from the problems in leading a normal home life, fatigue or daytime drowsiness can make it difficult or impossible for the patient to work, while driving a vehicle or using machinery can be dangerous in such a situation.

Patients with chronic fatigue need to learn to pace themselves, not feel guilty about taking rests or siestas, and ensure that they take as much exercise as they can physically cope with.

BPS and Comorbidities

One of the great problems and indeed mysteries of this bladder disorder is that it may be accompanied by one or multiple other disorders and/or pain syndromes which, when combined with the BPS, can lead to an extremely debilitating situation. These may include allergies or intolerances, gastrointestinal disorders (e.g. irritable bowel syndrome or inflammatory bowel disease), depression, migraine, vulvodynia, chronic non-bacterial prostatitis, thyroid disorders, systemic lupus erythematosus, Sjögren's syndrome or fibromyalgia. This makes an interactive, multidisciplinary treatment approach between the different care providers absolutely essential.

Coping and Self-Help

While having BPS is likely to involve at least some change in lifestyle, such changes may be minimal if the bladder disorder is mild, but when severe it may have a major impact on all aspects of life. BPS can therefore make patients feel that they have lost control over their life. The aim should be to help them to regain some feeling of being in control again, to adjust their lifestyle where necessary and to try to look at what they *can* do rather than what they *cannot* do, developing new interests to replace activities they are no longer able to undertake and developing coping strategies. While support from a partner and family can play a vital role here, support, understanding and encouragement on the part of the care provider can also make all the difference.

Diet Modification

Diet modification is a form of self-help that can help some patients with milder BPS to such an extent that they may not even need medication. Many patients will know from their own experience that certain foods and beverages appear to exacerbate their bladder symptoms and that avoidance of these items can help to reduce the symptoms. It should be emphasised that this is very individual and that what irritates one bladder does not necessarily irritate another. The long lists of foods and beverages to avoid that are found on some Web sites may be very alarming to patients, leading to some becoming paranoid about their diet and even anorexic.

The article on the "Effects of Comestibles on Symptoms of Interstitial Cystitis" by Shorter and colleagues in 2007 concluded that there is indeed a large number of BPS patients whose symptoms appear to be exacerbated by consumption of specific items. Their study identified the most bothersome foods as being items containing caffeine, citrus fruits and juices, tomatoes and tomato products, items containing vinegar, spicy food, alcohol and certain artificial sweeteners. Coffee was found to be the most bothersome with the authors suggesting, however, that the effect of caffeine may be related to its diuretic effect.

It is not only food and drink that can exacerbate the bladder but also various medications and food supplements, especially vitamin C.

Fluid Intake

When outside the home or when planning to go anywhere, BPS patients tend to restrict their fluid intake—or not drink at all—to reduce the need for toilets. However, this can lead to urine concentration and actually exacerbate the symptoms. To avoid dehydration, patients who cut down their fluid intake prior to going out should make up for this by drinking plenty when at home or within easy reach of toilets.

Avoid Constipation

Constipation can exacerbate BPS symptoms by causing pressure in the pelvic floor and on the bladder. In addition to drinking enough fluid and taking adequate exercise, the patient's diet should include sufficient fibre. However, high fibre will not be the ideal solution for BPS patients with concomitant irritable bowel syndrome since it will lead to bloating and abdominal cramp. Unfortunately, some of the drugs used to treat BPS can also be a cause of constipation (including many analgesics and antidepressants).

Hygiene and Clothing

BPS patients have easily irritated skin, especially in the urogenital area. They should preferably wash their clothes in washing agents and fabric softeners specially designed for sensitive skin that do not contain perfume or harsh chemicals. They should likewise avoid using perfumed products near the urogenital area and avoid feminine hygiene sprays. Women should do everything possible to avoid a bladder infection, including wiping from front to back following bowel movements, regularly changing tampons or sanitary pads and being scrupulously hygienic in sexual activity. BPS patients often feel more comfortable in looser clothing and should wear cotton rather than synthetic underwear.

Stress Avoidance

As every patient soon discovers, physical and emotional stress situations can cause flares and exacerbate symptoms. Patients consequently need to learn to pace themselves, plan activities and try to avoid physically exhausting or very stressful situations. This is of course easier said than done, particularly for mothers trying to run a family and those coping with a stressful job.

Patient Support Groups

Patient support groups play an important role in providing information and moral support. Patient-to-patient counselling is invaluable since only another patient truly understands what BPS is actually like and its impact on daily life. Any patient support group will tell you that patients will often tell patient telephone counsellors or patient chat forums all the very intimate and personal medical and sexual details that they feel they cannot raise with their doctor. However, in some cases trained counsellors are essential, for example in the case of suicidal patients.

Patient Education

Patient education can give patients a better knowledge and understanding of their symptoms, and therefore also of their treatment. They can learn more about BPS and associated disorders through hospital or clinic (online) patient information in their own language, reliable Web sites and patient support groups, while today many patients as well as patient advocates also consult scientific literature in order to stay abreast of medical developments and the latest insights.

Care Provider's Role

BPS patients need a great deal of support and empathy from their care provider. Many patients will often have worked their way through an entire series of doctors before reaching you. The doctor's role in emotional support for BPS patients is of great importance and should not be underestimated. When faced with a doctor who has neither time nor sympathy for them, the patient is likely to become depressed and desperate, even suicidal. The care provider's approach is going to play a crucial role in the patient's coping mechanism. If the patient goes home feeling that the doctor does not listen, does not understand or seems unsympathetic, that patient will be acutely depressed and will most likely go elsewhere. This is disastrous not only for the patient but also for the healthcare system.

The key message is that every BPS patient is different, requires an individual approach with customised treatment and needs time and an appreciation by the care provider of the impact on the patient's life, all packaged with a good dose of sympathy and understanding. It can make all the difference.

Recommended Reading

Chapple C. Introduction and conclusions. European Urology Supplements. 2007;6:573–5.

Marschall-Kehrel D. Update on nocturia: the best of rest is sleep. Urology. 2004;64(6 Suppl 1):21–4.

Meijlink JM. Interstitial cystitis: diagnosis & treatment. An overview. http://www.painful-bladder.org/pdf/Diagnosis&Treatment_IPBF.pdf (Updated yearly)

Nickel JC, Shoskes D, Irvine-Bird K. Clinical phenotyping of women with interstitial cystitis/painful bladder syndrome: a key to classification and potentially improved management. J Urol. 2009;182(1):155–60.

Shorter B, Lesser M, Moldwin RM, Kushner L. Effect of comestibles on symptoms of interstitial cystitis. J Urol. 2007;178(1):145–52.

Van de Merwe JP. Interstitial cystitis and autoimmune diseases. Nat Clin Pract Urol. 2007;4(9):484–91.

Chapter 29
Exploratory Research on the Social Costs and Care for Patients with Bladder Pain Syndrome

Loredana Nasta, Simone Montagnoli, and Maria Avolio

Introduction

Bladder Pain Syndrome (BPS) previously called Interstitial Cystitis (IC) [1], remains difficult to diagnose. It is often mistaken for bacterial cystitis and a broad range of unclassified disorders which are often believed to be psychogenic in nature [2]. Its symptoms are diverse and heterogeneous: they basically include chronic pelvic pain and a burning sensation originating from the bladder which then extends to the entire pelvic floor, with the involvement of other organs and functions; a frequent micturition urge can become seriously disabling, to the detriment of the patient's quality of life. Over a decade ago, a study conducted in the United States showed that the disease-induced distress could be more disabling than several forms of nephropathy with its associated time-consuming dialysis. Given its low prevalence (less than 5:10,000 inhabitants in the EC), Interstitial Cystitis/BPS was classified by the Italian Ministry of Health, through Ministerial Decree Nr. 279/2001, as a Rare Disease. Such classification implies a free access for patients to the diagnosis, monitoring, treatment, and prevention of BPS; the disease-related disability has been recognized and such condition has been included into the National Registry of Rare Diseases.

L. Nasta (✉)
Italian Interstitial Cystitis Association, Viale Glorioso 13, 00153, Rome, Italy
e-mail: l.nasta@aici-onlus.it

S. Montagnoli
Social Health Division, Dynamic and Clinical Psychology, Research Department, Institute of Social Affairs, Rome, Italy

M. Avolio
Institute of Public Health and Preventive Medicine, National Observatory in Health in the Italian Regions, Catholic University "Sacro Cuore", Rome, Italy

J. Nordling et al. (eds.), *Bladder Pain Syndrome: A Guide for Clinicians*,
DOI 10.1007/978-1-4419-6929-3_29,

Although a definition of Rare Disease is often based on inconsistent, not always shared epidemiology criteria, such a classification is aimed at depicting a social phenomenon rather than evoking some nosological reference or clinical–medical notions [3]. Exploratory studies of rare diseases and of the emerging needs of patients are virtually nonexistent: this lack of data creates even more confusion in the identification of the most typical elements emerging from such a general "container."

This is the reason why we decided to carry out a fact-finding survey. We attempted to explore BPS not only from a medical standpoint but also especially in terms of social costs and care needs of patients with BPS and their families. The same aspects were examined and compared for 11 low-prevalence disorders, in order to identify any differences or similarities.

Using the "rare disease" classification as a social categorization identifying a typical series of social issues can turn into a readily available, specific reference allowing any welfare measure to suggest and develop a decisive paradigm shift in the field of rare diseases. Rare diseases should not be simply seen as a highly diverse set of pathologies but as a series of recurrent social problems and issues. In line with this new approach, we performed a societal study. We did not simply focus on the individual patients or their disease, but rather on their family setting.

The idea to conduct our survey was promoted by several entities which have been dealing with rare diseases, their problem aspects, and possible interventions: the Institute for Social Affairs was the scientific entity which interpreted this fact-finding and exploratory survey along with "UNIAMO" Federazione Italiana Malattie Rare (Italian Federation of Rare Disease); the latter did involve a number of federated patients' groups: Associazione Italiana Cistite Interstiziale (Italian Association for Interstitial Cystitis) provided data and took part in the design phase; Orphanet Italia (European Portal of Rare Diseases and Orphan Drugs), and Farmindustria (Association of pharmaceutical companies—member of Confindustria). A collaborative effort with the above organizations and groups allowed the Institute for Social Affairs to focus on a number of development areas, as seen directly through the eyes of patients, their families, clinicians, and pharmaceutical investigators. This study exemplifies how research can be directly geared toward a very real social demand, acting as a practical tool to promote future lines of development.

We evaluated direct costs (any expense directly related with the disease management) as well as indirect costs (such as poorer occupational activities for patients and/or their families) and intangible costs (the emotional experience and quality of affect). Such costs have an impact on the resources and criticalities identified in the system of care and, more broadly, on the social context.

Aim of this survey was to investigate the needs while analyzing social costs, in order to identify and propose health programs covering these aspects as well, other than protecting the life of individuals affected from BPS.

Methodology

With this survey we investigated the social costs and healthcare needs of patients affected from a "rare disease," considering this group as a social category. Given this approach, we decided to explore several social dimensions in order to depict a complete picture of families and their social life.

In Europe, descriptive studies of the social conditions and quality of life of patients with a rare disease are virtually nonexistent: the lack of exhaustive data on this patient population affected from a rare disease and their families prevented the identification and analysis of a representative sample. In an effort to fill this information gap, we selected ten Rare Disease Associations (including AICI—Italian Association for Interstitial Cystitis) by means of a set of criteria identifying a number of fundamental features like clinical characteristics of a given pathology, presence and types of complications, early or late diagnosis, availability or lack of treatment options, characteristics of treatment and rehabilitation pathways, etc.

This is the first survey of this kind in Italy, and one of the first in Europe. Its aim was to explore the social costs and care needs of patients with a rare disease and their family members, adding up new findings to any previously performed research studies.

Our survey was conducted between May 2009 and April 2010. Different areas have been taken into account:

- Socio-demographics: Who filled out the questionnaire (patient or family member), gender, age, geographic area, education, family members, household income.
- Medical aspects (evaluation of clinical characteristics and interventions to manage the disease): Diagnosis, time spent before receiving a diagnosis, symptoms, rate of misdiagnosis, hospitalization rate, surgical procedures, availability and type of drug treatment, co-morbidities, perception of the disease severity.
- Medical care and social–healthcare services: Specializing clinics, local point of contact for the disease management, referrals to specialists to better understand and manage the disease, degree of satisfaction with how the diagnosis is communicated, satisfaction with healthcare services provided by clinics and local points of contact.
- Economic dimension (analysis of direct and indirect costs related with the disease): Costs incurred to make a diagnosis, cost of medication and care of patients, impact of the disease management on the work life of patients and their families, costs of medical examinations and travel expenses to reach the clinics/clinical centers, exemption from payment of a "ticket" (in Italy, healthcare services are paid on the basis of specific agreements and rates, with most patients having to pay at least a share of the overall cost), households' financial and economic needs related with the disease.

- Psychosocial dimension (how the disease burden impacts on the lifestyle and ability to plan one's own future): Emotions experienced before receiving a diagnosis, disease impact on family relations, need for the family to receive a form of psychological, social, and care support.

This survey was designed and realized by a collaborative group consisting of the Institute for Social Affairs, Uniamo Fimr (Italian Federation for Rare Diseases), Orphanet Italia, and Farmindustria. The Institute for Social Affairs performed the data collection and statistical analysis.

In this paper, we only address data about the Italian Association for Interstitial Cystitis (AICI).

Data were collected by means of two questionnaires: one for patients and their family members, and a second one for AICI. Questionnaires were completed by patients or their siblings either in their paper-based version or online through a dedicated platform.

The following descriptive statistics were computed and processed with the help of SPSS software, Version17.

Results

Socio-Demographics

Overall, AICI collected 65 questionnaires (16.25% of the overall sample). These latter were filled out by patients with BPS or by their siblings (59 patients and 6 siblings).

The descriptive analysis shows that most respondents are females (87.7%) while just a minority (12.3%) is males (Fig. 29.1). As to the geographic distribution of regions where respondents live, 34.4% of patients live in Northern Italy, 45.3% live in central Italy, and 20.3% live in Southern Italy (Fig. 29.2).

Our analysis shows that highly educated patients account for 15%; 51.7% have a medium level of academic education and 33.3% a low level of education.

Medical Aspects

In this sample, BPS patients seem to perceive their disease as a severe condition: over 64.5% of respondents perceive their health conditions as poor/very poor (Fig. 29.3).

Over 72% of subjects present with some co-morbidities (Fig. 29.4) [4, 5]. Thirty percent of patients have been admitted to a hospital (29.4% were hospitalized for 2 weeks to 1 month, 29.5% for more than 1 month); 55.9% of subjects underwent a surgical procedure.

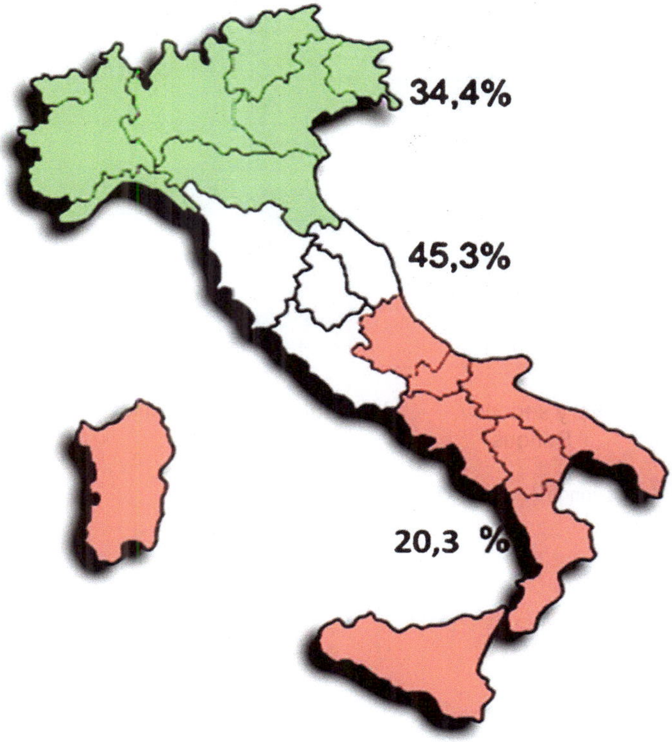

Fig. 29.1 Population Pyramids

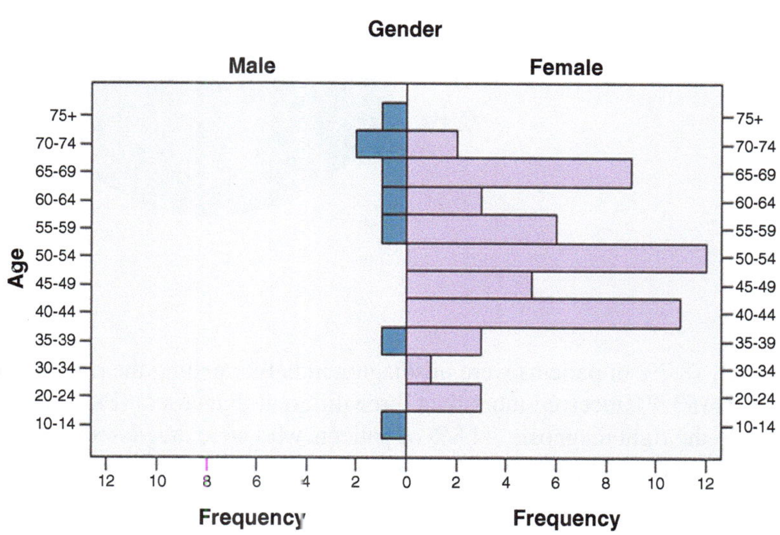

Fig. 29.2 Patient geographical distribution

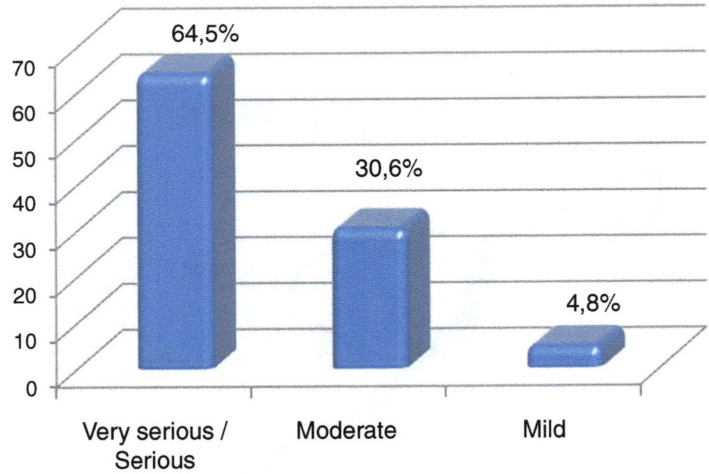

Fig. 29.3 Health conditions perceived

Fig. 29.4 Presence of co-morbidities

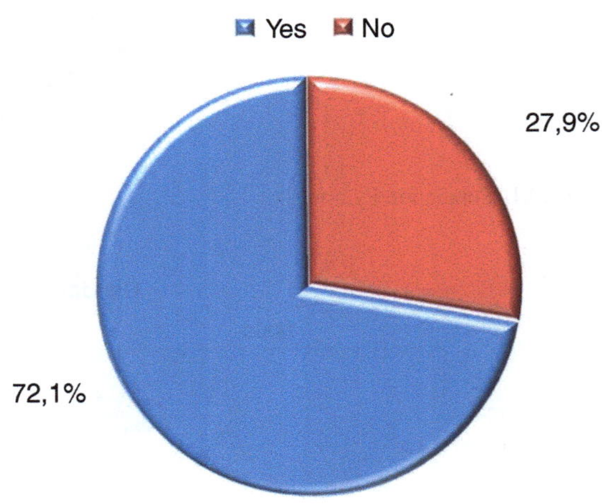

Overall, 78.7% of patients were misdiagnosed before getting the right diagnosis (Fig. 29.5) (53.9% received more than three different diagnoses) (Fig. 29.6); as to the time to the right diagnosis, 44.8% of patients who were diagnosed before 1975 eventually received the right diagnosis over 10 years later. In recent years, however, the time to get the right diagnosis seems to have remarkably reduced and improved.

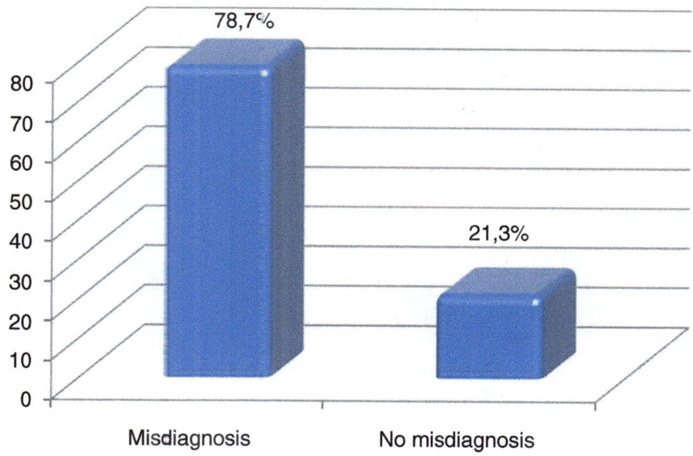

Fig. 29.5 Occurrence of misdiagnosis

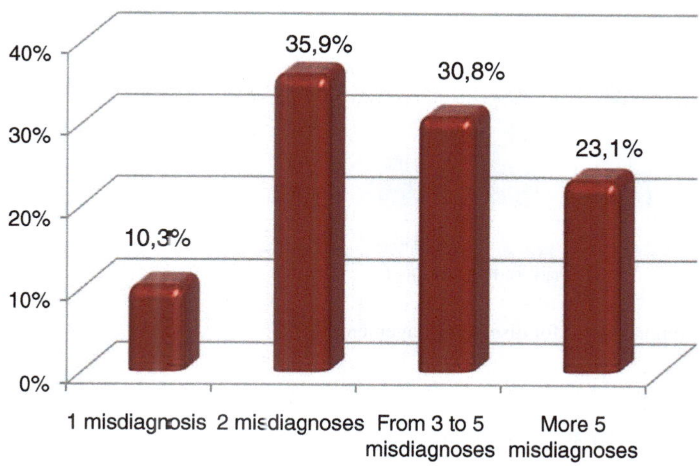

Fig. 29.6 Number of occurrence of misdiagnosis

Care and Social–Healthcare Services

Nearly all patients found a center of reference providing specialized healthcare services. However, 50.9% of such centers are located in a region different from where they live; 23% of patients do not have a local center of reference or a clinical institution in the region where they live (Fig. 29.7).

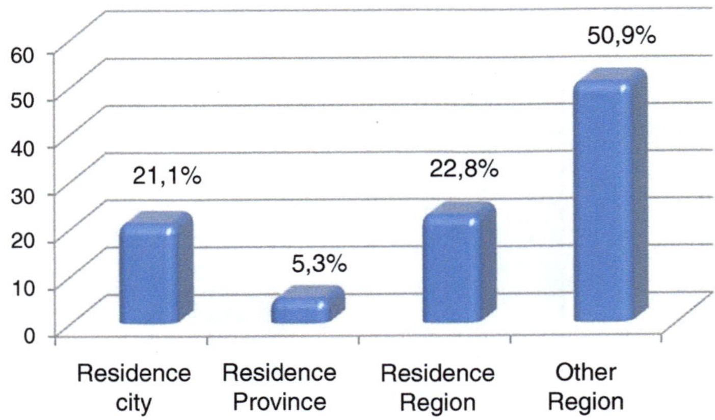

Fig. 29.7 Distance of healthcare referent centers

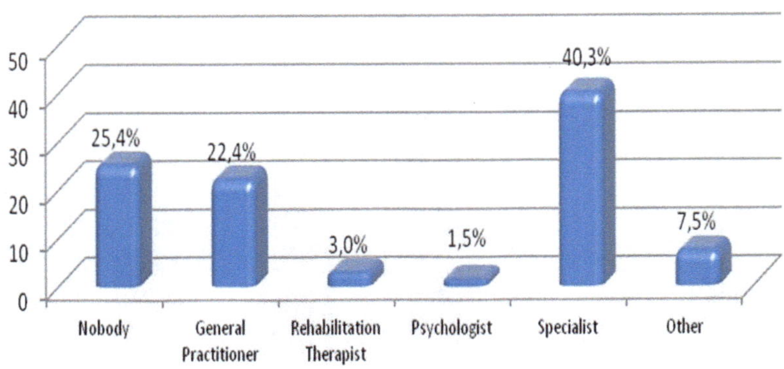

Fig. 29.8 Support people for disease management

According to 40.3% of patients, specialists have greatly helped them to acquire knowledge about the disease and its management. Several subjects (25.4%) could not find a local doctor of reference and only 22.4% of patients considered their family doctor as a local reference (Fig. 29.8).

With respect to diagnosis, 35.5% of patients are dissatisfied about the way their doctor told them the diagnosis; after receiving a diagnosis, 37.1% of patients feel the need to seek a second specialist opinion (Figs. 29.9 and 29.10).

Financial–Economic Dimension

Nearly all patients had to bear some medical expenses (clinical tests, visits, etc.) to receive a diagnosis; of these, 70% spent over 1,000€. As to treatment, 91.8% receive

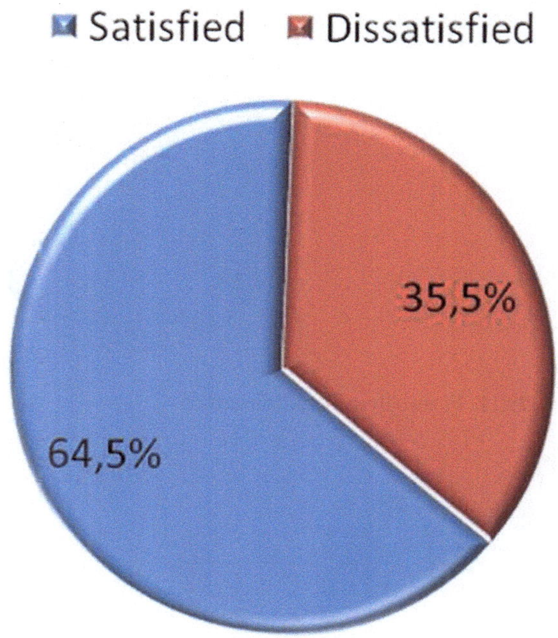

Fig. 29.9 Satisfaction level about diagnosis communication

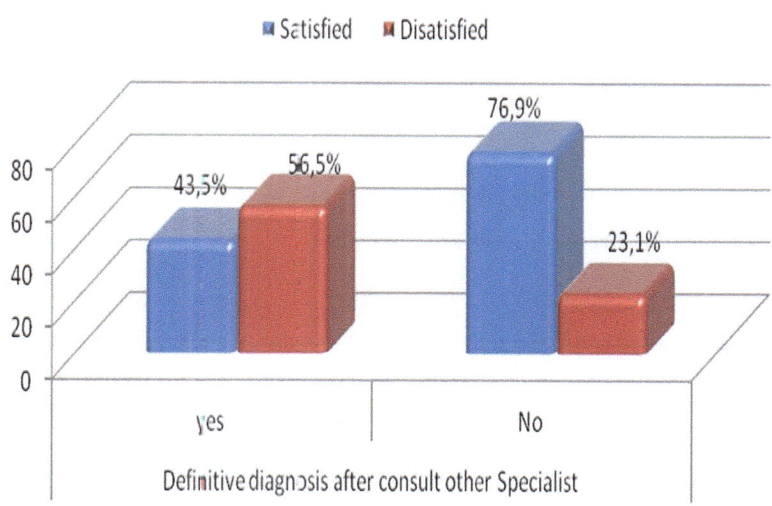

Fig. 29.10 Final diagnosis after other specialist consulting

a drug therapy and 31.5% pay the full cost of drugs; in fact, 24.2% have not received a payment exemption yet, despite their entitlement; in Italy, in fact, BPS was included in the list provided for by DM 279/2001 (exemption from payment of a "ticket" for those affected from a rare disease). In this respect, 21.5% of subjects

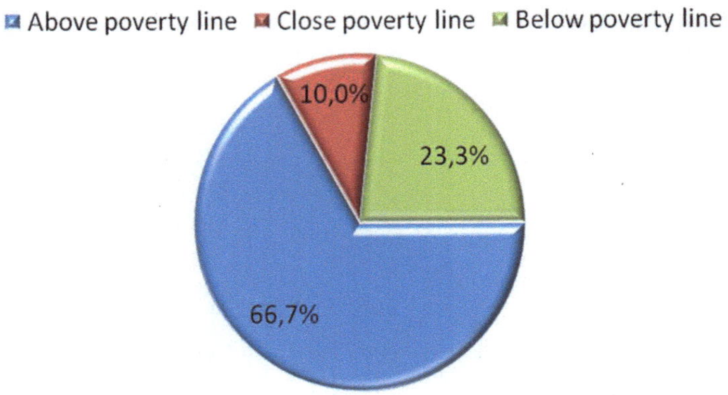

Fig. 29.11 Financial–economic dimension

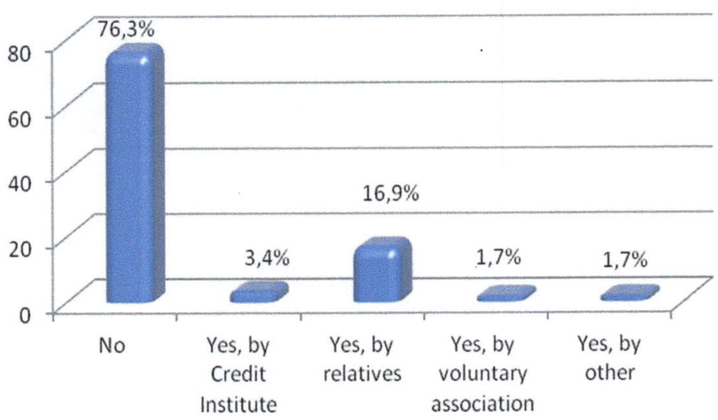

Fig. 29.12 Household income in relation to poverty line

had to request some form of financial support to manage such disease-related costs; financial support is generally provided by relatives (71.4%); finally, the disease seems to have a negative impact on the work career of both patients (73.8%) and their families; this entails a remarkable indirect cost on the household income-generating capacity; likewise, it is quite difficult to pay the indirect costs associated to the disease management: for example, travel costs to reach medical centers (76.7% of patients need to travel with an accompanying person, most commonly a sibling who, in turn, cannot go to work; in 73.3% of cases, such work leave is not paid by the employer). Moreover, in the event patients need to travel out of town for a medical visit, they are likely to spend the night in some hotel (42.9%) (Fig. 29.11).

In summary, 33.3% of our sample is below or close to the poverty line (Fig. 29.12).

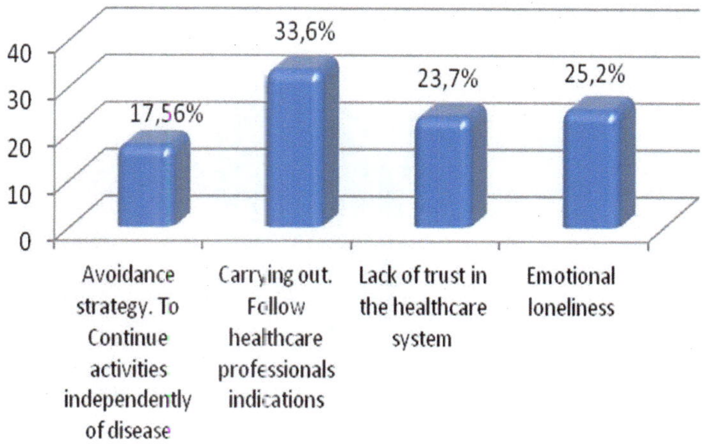

Fig. 29.13 Emotional experience of patients before definitive diagnosis

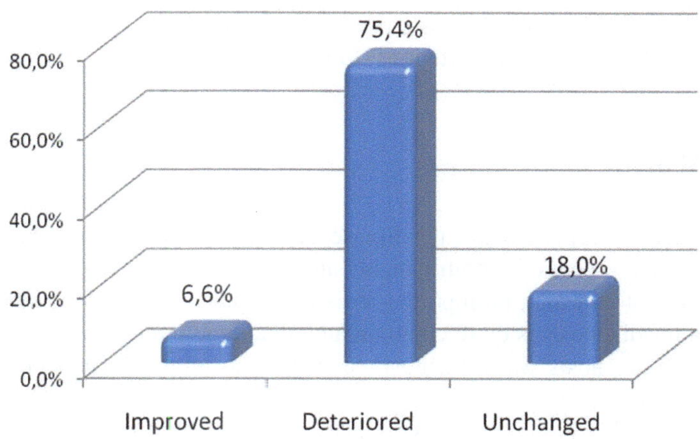

Fig. 29.14 Impact of disease on family relationships

Psychosocial Dimension

BPS patients report feelings of loneliness (25.2%) and mistrust toward the healthcare system (23.7%) (Fig. 29.13); 75.4% of subjects report a deterioration of their family relationships as a result of their disease (Fig. 29.14).

This community of patients finds no psychological, social, and healthcare support in social networks and, in particular, AICI (36%). It should be noted that the disease management is very difficult, especially when there is no local specialist

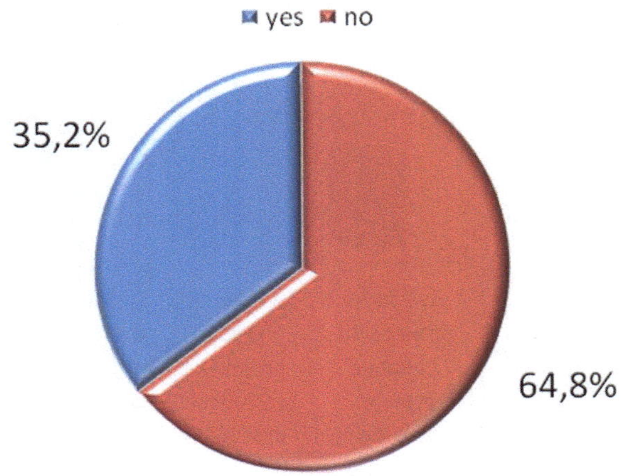

Fig. 29.15 Need of support in disease management

or specialized clinic close to where patients live. This is even more significant in the light of patients' perception of their overall health as poor/very poor. Finally, 35.2% of households report that, as a result of the disease, they needed some form of support in their daily living activities (Fig. 29.15).

Conclusions

Diagnosis is essential to manage the disease and start an appropriate treatment plan and an adaptive process for both patients and their family members. This survey helps prove that an exact, prompt diagnosis represents a crucial problem for BPS patients: a misdiagnosis is quite common and, in a large number of cases, patients receive a late diagnosis. Such diagnosis-related issues imply, for patients and their families, the activation of ineffective adaptive processes, which may lead them to feel desperate. This situation makes their distress even more serious, with ensuing feelings of solitude and mistrust vis-à-vis the healthcare system. In addition, the nature of BPS symptoms affects the sexual life of patients. To couples, this characterizes and may exacerbate any existing relationship problems. On the contrary, such couples would need to elaborate their condition and properly organize their distress. Receiving a diagnosis allows to facilitate the mental processes required for such processing.

In recent years, the time to a right diagnosis and the number of misdiagnosis seem to have remarkably improved; however, it is still necessary to do more to improve the physician's ability to promptly diagnose BPS. Moreover, the clinical benefits resulting from an early instead of late diagnosis are undisputed, given the chronic, degenerative course of BPS. Symptoms include an acute, severely disabling pelvic pain from the very beginning of the disease, and the acute phase is both unpredictable and recurrent [6, 7].

Our survey shows that when physicians report their diagnosis to patients, they tend to emphasize clinical aspects only, overlooking the significance of emotional aspects. Also, they seem to pay little or no attention to prompting some form of adaptation from patients [8]. This determines a huge dissatisfaction with respect to how the diagnosis is communicated and, in this context, the adaptive burden appears to be shifted from doctors to families.

Once the diagnosis has been confirmed, family members keep playing a significant role in the disease management and its healthcare-related aspects. Since 2001, in our country a formal network of hospital clinics specializing in the treatment of rare diseases has been established, although they are still somewhat scattered across the country: half of patients refer to a healthcare center far away from where they live, even in a different region. In order to reach a medical facility/clinic, patients must pay for travel costs (and any other additional costs). Such trips often call for a practical and emotional support which is generally provided by an accompanying person.

Reinforcing local healthcare services seems to be crucial in order to strengthen the healthcare system capacity to support these patients. This is even more important in the light of the present situation, where one in four patients have not identified a local clinic and cannot find a specializing center in the region where they live [9].

In our country, these criticalities make the support network (like the association of patients affected from rare diseases) even more important, along with help and support given by family members [10]. These latter seem to be fundamental in the patients' lives.

All the above factors create an overload of appointments and hassles for family members, with siblings hardly being able to go on with their life. The negative influence of this disease on the work career of patients and their families is as important, especially given the disease impact on the household income-generating capacity. This is why, perhaps, one-third of the sample is below or close to the poverty line.

These patients are especially vulnerable with respect to the financial burden implied in the disease management. They are often forced to seek financial support, i.e., to borrow money, from relatives.

Therefore, our findings confirm that the onset of the disease does worsen family relationships: social costs are high, with a number of implications not only for patients but for their families as well.

We strongly believe that it is necessary to keep addressing these issues: these data represent a major tool to review and set the course of any welfare policies aimed at helping patients with a rare disease, as well as at supporting their families [11].

References

1. van de Merwe JP, Nordling J, Bouchelouche P, et al. Diagnostic criteria, classification, and nomenclature for painful bladder syndrome/interstitial cystitis: an ESSIC proposal. Eur Urol. 2008;53(1):60–7. Review.

2. Bodden-Heidrich R. Psychosomatic aspects of urogynaecology: model considerations on the pathogenesis, diagnosis and therapy. Zentralbl Gynakol. 2004;126(4):237–43. Review (German).
3. Ratner V. Rediscovering a “rare” disease: a patient’s perspective on interstitial cystitis. Urology. 1987;29(4 Suppl):44–5.
4. Buffington CA. Comorbidity of interstitial cystitis with other unexplained clinical conditions. J Urol. 2004;172(4 Pt 1):1242–8. Review.
5. Mathieu N. Somatic comorbidities in irritable bowel syndrome: fibromyalgia, chronic fatigue syndrome, and interstitial cystitis. Gastroenterol Clin Biol. 2009;33 Suppl 1:S17–25. French.
6. Hanno P, Lin A, Nordling J, et al. Bladder Pain Syndrome Committee of the International Consultation on Incontinence. Neurourol Urodyn. 2010;29(1):191–8. Review.
7. Hanno P, Nordling J, Fall M. Bladder pain syndrome. Med Clin North Am. 2011;95(1):55–73. Review.
8. Carli R. Correggere il deficit o promuovere la salute? In: Molinari E, Labella A, editors. Psicologia clinica. Milano: Springer; 2006.
9. Donini G. Verso una nuova epistemologia del medico di famiglia: prendersi cura di una società inquieta. Urbino: Quattro venti; 2005.
10. Cohen C, Wills TA. Stress, social support, and the buffering hypothesis. Psychol Bull. 1985;98(2):310–57.
11. Folgheraiter F. La logica sociale dell’aiuto: fondamenti per una teoria relazionale del welfare. Trento: Erickson; 2007.

Index

J. Nordling et al. (eds.), *Bladder Pain Syndrome: A Guide for Clinicians*,
DOI 10.1007/978-1-4419-6929-3,

O

P

MIX
Papier aus verantwortungsvollen Quellen
Paper from responsible sources
FSC® C105338

If you have any concerns about our products,
you can contact us on
ProductSafety@springernature.com

In case Publisher is established outside the EU,
the EU authorized representative is:
Springer Nature Customer Service Center GmbH
Europaplatz 3, 69115 Heidelberg, Germany

Printed by Libri Plureos GmbH
in Hamburg, Germany